Health Disparities in the United States

Introduction to US Health Policy: The Organization, Financing, and Delivery of Health Care in America, fourth edition (Johns Hopkins University Press, 2016)

Introduction to Biosocial Medicine: The Social, Psychological, and Biological Determinants of Human Behavior and Well-Being (Johns Hopkins University Press, 2015)

Questioning the Premedical Paradigm: Enhancing Diversity in the Medical Profession a Century after the Flexner Report (Johns Hopkins University Press, 2010)

Health Disparities in the United States

Social Class, Race, Ethnicity, and the Social Determinants of Health

THIRD EDITION

Donald A. Barr, MD, PhD

JOHNS HOPKINS UNIVERSITY PRESS   BALTIMORE

Published in previous editions as *Health Disparities in the United States:
Social Class, Race, Ethnicity, and Health.*

Johns Hopkins University Press
2715 North Charles Street
Baltimore, Maryland 21218-4363
www.press.jhu.edu

Library of Congress Cataloging-in-Publication Data

Names: Barr, Donald A., author.
Title: Health disparities in the United States : social class, race, ethnicity,
and the social determinants of health / Donald A. Barr, MD, PhD.
Description: Third edition. | Baltimore : Johns Hopkins University Press, 2019. |
Includes bibliographical references and index.
Identifiers: LCCN 2018057306 | ISBN 9781421432571 (hardcover : alk. paper) |
ISBN 1421432579 (hardcover : alk. paper) | ISBN 9781421432588 (pbk. : alk. paper) |
ISBN 1421432587 (pbk. : alk. paper) | ISBN 9781421432595 (electronic) |
ISBN 1421432595 (electronic)
Subjects: | MESH: Health Status Disparities | Socioeconomic Factors | Healthcare
Disparities—ethnology | Ethnic Groups | Prejudice—ethnology | United States
Classification: LCC RA418.3.U6 | NLM WA 300 AA1 | DDC 362.1089—dc23
LC record available at https://lccn.loc.gov/2018057306

A catalog record for this book is available from the British Library.

*Special discounts are available for bulk purchases of this book. For more information,
please contact Special Sales at 410-516-6936 or specialsales@press.jhu.edu.*

Johns Hopkins University Press uses environmentally friendly book materials,
including recycled text paper that is composed of at least 30 percent
post-consumer waste, whenever possible.

For Adam

CONTENTS

One of the best things about being a college professor is that I have the opportunity to learn from my students. This book grew from things I learned working with one student in particular. She came to my office and asked if I would help her undertake an independent research project as part of the undergraduate honors program at Stanford University. I asked her to describe the issue she would like to research. Her response was both immediate and focused: she wanted to know if African Americans in California who develop multiple myeloma, a form of bone marrow cancer, were referred by their physicians for bone marrow transplantation less often than whites with multiple myeloma.

It was unusual for an undergraduate to have a project in mind that was so fully conceptualized. I asked how she had developed her interest in and knowledge of the treatment of multiple myeloma in African Americans. She proceeded to tell me the story of her mother.

Her mother was in her late forties. As part of the routine care for her high blood pressure, she had undergone a series of blood tests. Her only symptom had been fatigue, which she had attributed to her work as a high-ranking health official in a midwestern state. An abnormally high level of protein in the blood led to additional testing and an eventual bone scan and bone marrow biopsy, establishing a diagnosis of multiple myeloma. The cancer specialist to whom she had been referred explained to her and her husband (also a health professional) that, even though the myeloma was in an early stage, little could be done. He had advised her to resume her work and return for chemotherapy when the disease became more symptomatic.

Despite a sense of hopelessness, she persisted in learning more about her disease. She consulted the National Institutes of Health to obtain more information and sought a second opinion about treatment options from another cancer specialist. The second oncologist immediately recognized the importance of intervening before the disease became more advanced. He acted quickly to initiate chemotherapy and referred her to a regional center for consideration for a bone marrow transplant, a treatment that had been shown to have substantial benefit in early stages of the disease. She was recommended for immediate transplant, which she underwent four months after her initial diagnosis.

While she was on the transplant ward of the hospital, an African American nurse commented how pleased she was to be taking care of another black person. For the nurse, that was unusual, for, despite the higher incidence of multiple myeloma in the black population, nearly all the patients receiving transplants at the center were white.

My student explained to me that the first cancer specialist was white, while the second specialist—the one who, in the student's mind, had saved her mother's life—was black. I had the opportunity to speak with the mother several years after her transplant, and I learned that at that time she remained in remission and was feeling fine.

I helped the student link up with a cancer researcher at Stanford. The student was able to obtain the records of all persons in California diagnosed with multiple myeloma over a three-year period. Linking this cancer registry data with data about all patients discharged from the hospital in California during that same time period, she was able to determine that, even after taking into account socioeconomic status and the availability of health insurance, African Americans in California with multiple myeloma were less likely than whites to be treated with bone marrow transplantation.

The student is well on her way to becoming a leader in the medical profession, having combined her medical training with graduate training in public health focusing on the issue of health disparities. Before working with this student, I had been unaware that the incidence of multiple myeloma in African American women was 2.4 times greater than that in white women in the United States. For African American men, the rate is twice as high (data from the US National Cancer Institute 2018). As well-done research so often does, the student's project raised more questions than it answered, at least for me. Why was the rate of myeloma so much higher in blacks than in whites? There are few genetic links associated with the concept of race as conceptualized in the United States; I had difficulty attributing the higher incidence to genetics. Was it the environment? Knowing that the educational attainment and income level of African Americans is, on average, lower than that of whites, is it a matter of socioeconomic status? Yet the student's mother had a graduate degree and was a highly respected health professional.

Why, also, did cancer specialists in California provide bone marrow transplantation, a treatment proven to be effective, to African Americans less often than to whites? I had been practicing medicine in California for more than 20 years and had never seen a case of conscious racism on the part of my physician colleagues. I had recently had the disturbing experience of treating a patient with a sore knee, whom I describe in Chapter 9, so I knew that my colleagues sometimes unconsciously applied inappropriate racial stereotypes in their treatment decisions. What was going on?

Being a sociologist as well as a physician, I decided to try and find out what was going on. I immersed myself in the literature describing the nature, causes, and consequences of racial and ethnic disparities in health status and access to high-quality health care. What I found seemed crucially important to medical practice and delivery of health care in the twenty-first century. I decided to organize a course for undergraduates at Stanford, many of them, like their student colleague before them, on their way to becoming future leaders in professions such as medicine, public health, and the law. The course has been a remarkable success, typically drawing a diverse group of undergraduates. More recently, I have also been asked by the Stanford School of Medicine to broaden my focus to include issues pertaining to health disparities among children. This book is a direct outcome of the teaching I have done.

To teach effectively a topic as complex as health disparities, one must have available research literature from a wide range of academic disciplines. As the title of this book suggests, I will be looking at both the association of race and ethnicity with health status and the impacts of a range of other social determinants on health status. In the past decade especially, there has been growing attention to the social determinants of health (SDH). The World Health Organization (WHO) defines the social determinants of health as "the conditions in which people are born, grow, work, live, and age. These circumstances are shaped by the distribution of money, power . . ." The WHO then goes on to say, "The social determinants of health are mostly responsible for health inequities—the unfair and avoidable differences in health status seen within and between countries" (World Health Organization 2018). The Centers for Disease Control and Prevention of the US Department of Health and Human Services define SDH as, "the complex, integrated, and overlapping social structures and economic systems that are responsible for most health inequities" (CDC 2018).

The types of social determinants cited by the WHO and the CDC often exert their effect on health status independent of race and ethnicity. In the United States especially, race and ethnicity have played a powerful role in affecting health status. In this book I refer to a range of research addressing both race and ethnicity and SDH as drivers of health disparities. Simply presenting research data, however, is not conducive to effective learning. The data need to be threaded together into a theoretical framework. In this book, I have attempted those tasks.

Chapter 1 offers an introduction to the concept of health disparities, emphasizing how the United States has lower levels of life expectancy and higher rates of infant mortality than nearly all other developed countries, despite all the money Americans spend on health care. Rather than being a result of health care expenditures, disparities in health status appear instead to be a reflection of social and economic inequality. Additionally, we will see that the association between social inequality and health status is a continuous one, across all levels of income and education.

In Chapter 2, I consider the question, "What is health?" Before comparing health status across social, racial, or ethnic groups, we must first appreciate that the concept of health can be defined in different ways and measured with different scales, depending on the context. A consideration of six different individuals, each with a form of poor health, demonstrates that the way in which we define and measure health will largely determine how healthy or unhealthy is any particular individual.

Chapter 3 builds on the headline of a newspaper story from 1997: "They Call It 'Poor' Health for a Reason." The chapter defines the concept of socioeconomic status (SES) and traces the consistent association, over time and across places, between poverty and poor health. By looking at data gathered by the federal government, we will see evidence of this association for a wide range of conditions.

In Chapter 4, I extend the exploration of SES to look at the issue of inequality, the multiple forms inequality can take, and the association between inequality and poor health across the SES spectrum. I introduce the concept of allostatic load— the physiologic response to the stress of being in a position of social disadvantage, which over a period of years can result in physiologic injury and illness.

Because much of the inequality I explore is inequality among racial or ethnic groups, Chapter 5 attempts to explicate the concepts of race and ethnicity as they have been used in the United States. As early as the mid-1700s, the principal racial categories used today by the US Census Bureau were described by scientists as biological in nature, representing fundamental divisions of the human species. I investigate the research looking at racial categorization as biologically derived versus that suggesting it is socially constructed. Additionally, I look within racial groups to see how ethnically heterogeneous they are. For example, various ethnic groups within the race defined as "black" actually have strikingly different health status and health outcomes.

Chapter 6 summarizes the data showing consistently that those in minority racial or ethnic groups are likely to be in a position of low SES. If the health status of those minorities is consistently lower than that of a comparable population of whites, is it because those with poor health tend to be minority, or tend to have lower SES, or both? The chapter presents consistent evidence that being in a minority racial or ethnic group can be a form of social disadvantage in and of itself, even after taking into account SES.

Many of the same questions are asked in Chapter 7, while focusing on health disparities among children. With children of Hispanic and other immigrant parents comprising a rapidly increasing share of the US population, the demographics of the United States is changing. In parallel with this demographic change has been our growing understanding of and appreciation for the powerful effects social inequality can have on early child development, both psychological and biological. The inequality of poverty and residential racial segregation experienced by many children, in particular black children in low-income families, has been shown to contribute to observed disparities in conditions such as asthma and obesity. Identifying and implementing policies for early intervention in the sources of children's health disparities will be a crucial step toward reducing future disparities when today's children are adults with children of their own.

Chapter 8 moves from disparities in health status to examining a second type of disparity: disparity in access to health care. A principal determinant of access to health care in the United States is the availability of health insurance. As is the case with health status, those from lower SES groups in the United States also have worse access to health care, based on this economic fact of life. However, a growing body of research has shown that, even when people have the same level of health insurance and are treated for the same disease by the same physicians and hospitals, those from minority racial or ethnic groups often get worse care—either not receiving care when appropriate or receiving care that is lower in quality.

In Chapter 9, I present research on racial or ethnic bias on the part of physicians, distinguishing unconscious bias from the conscious racism that plagued the United States for much of the twentieth century. For a variety of medical conditions, a consistent stream of research has shown that, based largely on unconscious processes, physicians in a number of settings provide a different level of care to blacks or other minorities than they do to whites.

Chapter 10 discusses when, if ever, a physician or other health practitioner is justified in using racial or ethnic categorization in deciding the course of a patient's treatment. The chapter looks at recent trends toward and potential problems with race-based pharmaceuticals—using one drug for white patients, and a different drug for black patients with the same condition.

Chapter 11 starts with the caveat that not all disparities need to be eliminated as a matter of public policy. Irrespective of race or ethnicity, women live longer on average than do men. However, racial and ethnic health disparities are of a different type from many gender disparities. In this book I have chosen not to include an extended discussion of gender disparities, nor of other disparities such as those based on age, sexual orientation, or disability. In narrowing my focus, I do not mean to suggest that these other types of disparities are unimportant. Rather, they exist in a different context and stem from different causes, and they deserve their own examination and policy analysis.

I end this book by suggesting a framework with which we can identify those disparities stemming from SES, race, or ethnicity that need to be reduced or eliminated as a matter of public policy.

Before proceeding into the chapters themselves, I would like to explain the nomenclature I use in this book. How to name racial or ethnic groups has been an evolving topic with both social and political overtones. As part of the 2010 census, the US Census Bureau identified the five historic racial categories, using the following nomenclature:

1. White
2. Black or African American
3. American Indian and Alaska Native
4. Asian
5. Native Hawaiian and Other Pacific Islander

The US Census Bureau then identifies a second division, independent of race and based on ethnicity, with two possible categories:

1. Hispanic Origin
2. Not of Hispanic Origin

To simplify the text, I have taken the first word or words from each of these categories to describe the categories. I speak of whites, blacks, Asians, American Indians, and Native Hawaiians, meaning by these terms the full description provided by the Census Bureau. In addition, when I use the term "Hispanic," I will mean "Hispanic of any race"; when I use the terms "white" and "black," I mean "white and not of Hispanic origin" and "black and not of Hispanic origin."

At many places throughout this book I reference data provided by the Centers for Disease Control and Prevention of the US Department of Health and Human Services. In these citations, I simply refer to the CDC, the common acronym for this essential federal agency. In the list of references at the end of this book, I will include these citations under the heading "US Department of Health and Human Services, Centers for Disease Control and Prevention" and then list them by date and by topic.

In the late 1980s, the Council on Ethical and Judicial Affairs of the American Medical Association undertook a study of racial disparities in health status and health care that persisted more than 20 years after the enactment of landmark civil rights legislation. Their conclusion was not encouraging: "Persistent, and sometimes substantial, differences continue to exist in the quality of health among Americans. Blacks have higher infant mortality rates and shorter life expectancies than whites. Underlying the disparities in quality of health among Americans are differences in both need and access" (1990, p. 2344).

Fifteen years later, Dr. Nicole Lurie, a former federal health official then at the RAND Corporation, looked over the previous 15 years of research and dialogue, and concluded "Less Talk, More Action."

> For most of the areas studied, disparities between white patients and black patients have not substantially improved during the past decade or so. Rather than simply dismissing these findings as more documentation, how might we use them to enhance our knowledge and inform strategies to eliminate disparities?
>
> More widespread redesign of systems—particularly, outside of the traditional health care system—will be required to address the complex interplay of social determinants of health and health care outcomes, and this change will probably be longer in coming. (2005, pp. 727–29)

In 2009 the Commission on Social Determinants of Health issued a report titled "Action on Health Disparities in the United States." Looking at the continuing pattern of disparities in the United States and our continued low ranking relative to other developed countries, the Commission recommended increased national attention to the need to "improve the circumstances in which people are born, grow, live, work, and age," and to "tackle the inequitable distribution of power, money, and resources—the structural drivers of conditions of daily life" (p. 1170).

The national effort to reduce health disparities is a continuing one. I hope this book, by contributing to the education of future—and current—health professionals from all fields, will provide a meaningful contribution to that process.

Health Disparities in the United States

CHAPTER ONE

Introduction to the Social Roots of Health Disparities

Why are some people healthy and others not? This is a question that has gained increasing attention in the United States over the last several years. It is also the title of a book published in 1994. The contributors to that book come to two basic conclusions.

First, in trying to improve health in developed societies, we have traditionally focused most of our attention on improving the quality and availability of health care.

> Modern societies devote a very large proportion of their economic resources to the production of *health care*. . . . Such massive efforts reflect a widespread belief that the availability and use of health care is central to the health of both individuals and populations. (Evans and Stoddart 1994, p. 27)

Second, most of the variability in health status we find in the United States and other developed countries has little to do with health care and everything to do with one's position in the social hierarchy.

> Some of the best-kept secrets of longevity and good health are to be found in one's social, economic, and cultural circumstances. . . . The largest gap lies between the richest and the poorest. But the middle classes are also affected. The lower one is situated on the social hierarchy . . . the lower one's probability of staying in good health and the lower one's life expectancy. (Renaud 1994, p. 322)

Nowhere has the emphasis on improving health through advancing the technology of health care been more evident than in the United States. As shown in Figure 1.1, the proportion of the US economy that goes for providing health care rose from just under 11 percent in 1988 to 17.9 percent in 2016.

Some of the most recent increases in health care costs are a result of the expansion in access to health insurance under the Affordable Care Act (ACA). Most of the cost increases are due to our heavy investment in new medications, new facilities, and the new technology of advanced procedures, reflecting the faith of the

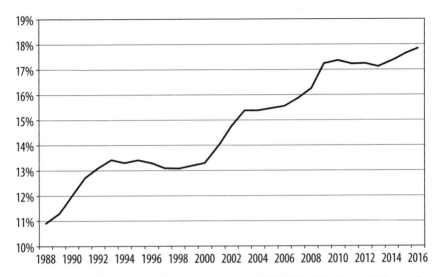

Figure 1.1. National health expenditures as percentage of GDP, 1988–2016. *Source*: US Centers for Medicare and Medicaid Services, National Health Expenditures.

American public in the power of health care to improve health status. Yet, in comparing ourselves to other developed countries that have made different policy decisions about investing national resources in health care, we find a striking inconsistency. We spend much more of our national economy on health care than any other developed country in the world (Table 1.1). However, using two common measures of population health, our population has worse health status than the population in any of these other countries.

Life expectancy estimates how many years, on average, a baby born today can expect to live. (Given consistent difference between males and females, this figure is typically broken down by gender.) Babies born in the United States in 2015 can expect to live between two and six years less than babies born in other developed countries.

Infant mortality estimates the following statistic: of a thousand babies born alive, how many will die before their first birthday? We see that the United States has the highest infant mortality rate of any of the countries listed. In fact, in 2015 the United States had a higher infant mortality rate than 31 of the 35 countries in the Organisation for Economic Co-operation and Development, an association of the most developed countries in the world. The US infant mortality rate was only better than the rates found in Chile, Turkey, and Mexico.

Table 1.1. Health Indexes, Selected OECD Countries, 2016–17

Country	% GDP Spent on Health Care (2017)	Infant Mortality Rate (2016)	Male Life Expectancy at Birth (2017)	Female Life Expectancy at Birth (2017)
Japan	10.7	2.0	81.0	87.1
Sweden	10.9	2.5	80.6	84.1
France	11.5	3.7	79.2	85.5
Germany	11.3	3.4	78.6	83.5
Switzerland	12.3	3.6	81.7	85.6
Greece	8.4	4.2	78.9	84.0
Canada	10.4	4.7	79.8	83.9
United Kingdom	9.7	3.8	79.4	83.0
United States	17.1	5.9	76.1	81.1

Source: Data from OECD, http://www.oecd.org/statistics/, accessed 7/2/18. Infant mortality data for Canada are from the World Bank, https://data.worldbank.org/.

A New Challenge: Falling Life Expectancy in the United States

In December 2017, the National Center for Health Statistics, the principal government data source that tracks population health statistics, reported some startling news. After rising consistently every year since 1950, life expectancy in the United States fell for two consecutive years (Kochanek et al. 2016). There had been some warning earlier that the rate of decline in death due to cardiovascular disease was decreasing (Sidney et al. 2016). While death rates due to heart disease and cancer—the top two causes of death—continue to decrease, albeit at a somewhat slower rate, the death rate for unintentional injuries, the third leading cause of death, increased 17 percent between 2014 and 2016. Unintentional injuries include accidents and poisonings. The principal increase in this category has been due to what the US Department of Health and Human Services (2018) has described as the "Opioid Epidemic," involving deaths from prescription opioids as well as illicit opioids. Often death from an overdose of opioids is intentional rather than accidental, suggesting a substantial overlap between accidental opioid deaths and suicide by opioid overdose. Oquendo and Volkow (2018) describe suicide as "A Silent Contributor to Opioid-Overdose Deaths." They conclude that "The significant increases in both opioid-overdose deaths and suicide rates in our country have contributed to reduced life expectancy for Americans" (p. 1569). Case and Deaton (2017) refer to these deaths as "deaths of despair." Stein and colleagues (2017) have analyzed the patterns of these deaths over time and conclude that they occurred principally among non-Hispanic whites living outside large urban areas, and "were primarily caused by self-destructive health behaviors likely related to underlying social and economic factors in these communities" (p. 1541).

I discuss these issues in greater depth in Chapter 4. There is extensive data confirming the impression that deaths of despair and the opioid epidemic are strongly associated with social, racial and ethnic, economic, as well as geographic differences among population groups.

Where Does Health Come From?

How is it that we, as a country, invest so much of our economy in providing *health care*, but we get so little in return in the form of *health*—at least health as measured by these common statistics? Perhaps our basic assumption—that more health care will lead, necessarily, to better health—is flawed. Perhaps something other than health care drives the health of a community or a society.

Economist Victor Fuchs addressed this issue in 1983 in his seminal book *Who Shall Live?* Fuchs tells us "A Tale of Two States" (pp. 52–54), comparing demographic characteristics and health status in two adjacent states in the United States—Nevada and Utah. Using data from the 1960s and 1970s, he found that the two states had similar populations using measures such as income, education, age distribution, and access to health care. However, the health of those who live in Nevada was substantially worse than that of those who live in Utah. Infant mortality was 40 percent higher in Nevada than in Utah. Death rates were consistently higher in Nevada for all age groups—about 40 percent higher for young adults, 50 to 70 percent higher for those ages 40 to 49. When one looks at two specific illnesses with known causes, the differences in death rates are even more striking. The combined death rate in Nevada from lung cancer (associated with cigarette smoking) and cirrhosis of the liver (associated with alcohol abuse) ranged from 100 percent higher to nearly 600 percent higher than the comparable rate in Utah, depending on the age range and the gender studied.

You will no doubt recognize why Nevada and Utah had such strikingly different health statistics, despite having populations that were generally similar in demographic characteristics and their access to health care. The influence of the Mormon Church in Utah has led to much lower rates of smoking and alcohol abuse in that state. In addition, those in Utah experienced lower rates of divorce and migration. Nevada, on the other hand, has an economy and a culture that includes higher rates of smoking and alcohol consumption, higher divorce rates, and higher rates of geographic migration. Life in Nevada is fundamentally different from life in Utah. Those lifestyle factors, and not the availability of health care, drove the differences between the two states in terms of health status. As described by Victor Fuchs, "The basic finding is the following: when the state of medical science and

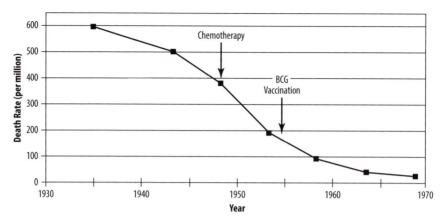

Figure 1.2. Mean annual death rates (standardized to 1901 population) from respiratory tuberculosis, England and Wales, 1935–70. *Sources*: Evans et al. (1994); McKeown 1979.

other health-determining variables are held constant, the marginal contribution of medical care to health is very small in modern nations. . . . For most of man's history, [per capita] income has been the primary determinant of health and life expectancy—the major explanation for differences in health among nations and among groups within a nation" (1986, pp. 274–76).

To illustrate the relationship between the availability of health care, the standard of living, and mortality rates, let us look at death rates from tuberculosis (TB) in England and Wales. There was a decline in the death rate from TB following the discovery in the late 1940s of the first drugs that were effective against TB and the development in the 1950s of the first vaccine used to prevent TB (Figure 1.2).

It appears that the advent of antituberculosis drugs and a tuberculosis vaccine—two key additions to the health care regimen available to treat TB—were effective in reducing the death rate. However, when one takes a longer time frame, the picture that emerges is quite different. Figure 1.3 shows the decline in the death rate from TB in England and Wales from 1840 to 1970.

From the longer-range perspective, it appears that the health care developments of the mid-twentieth century had relatively little effect on the overall death rate from TB. In fact, half of the decline in the rate of death from TB took place before the tubercle bacillus responsible for TB was discovered. While the number of deaths declined by 51 percent between 1948 and 1971 following the introduction of medications and a vaccine, most of the overall decline had taken place before any effective medical treatment was available (McKeown 1979).

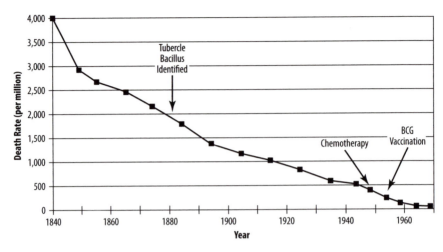

Figure 1.3. Mean annual death rates (standardized to 1901 population) from respiratory tuberculosis, England and Wales, 1840–1970. *Sources:* Evans et al. (1994); McKeown 1979.

If health care was not responsible for the decline in death rates from TB, then what was? Consistent with Fuchs's comments above, the rising standard of living seen in England and Wales in the nineteenth and twentieth centuries can explain the falling death rates. Better nutrition, better sanitation, better housing, and less crowding, combined with public health measures to prevent the spread of TB, accounted for most of the decline in death rates over the last 200 years.

To illustrate this point, and to underscore the role income and standard of living play in reducing the chance of death from TB, let us consider two fictional persons, one from the world of music and one from the field of literature. The opera *La Bohéme*, first performed in 1896, tells the story of Mimi, a poor seamstress struggling to survive in the Latin quarter of Paris. She meets and falls in love with Rodolfo, an equally poor poet who has to burn the pages of a play he was writing to stay warm. The opera tells us of the love between Rodolfo and Mimi and of Rodolfo's hesitance when he learns Mimi has TB. The lovers struggle to stay together (and to stay warm), only to have Mimi die tragically, succumbing to her disease.

Thomas Mann first began writing his novel *Magic Mountain* in 1912. It tells the story of Hans Castorp, the son of a well-to-do German family who goes to visit his cousin in a TB sanatorium high in the Swiss Alps. What was originally intended as a stay of only a few weeks extends to seven years of intensive therapy, as it turns out that Hans himself has developed TB. Seven years of sumptuous meals, fresh air, exercise, and companionship help Hans to fight off his disease, only to be drafted into the German army at the beginning of World War I (a conflict in which he is likely to be killed).

What if their roles had been reversed? If Mimi had been from a wealthy French family and Hans from a poor German family, which one would have survived TB? For more than a century, where you are on the social hierarchy has been a strong predictor of whether you live or die from a disease such as TB.

The standard of living available to those lower on the social hierarchy has been a powerful predictor of how many of them would die from the many infectious diseases that ravaged Europe and North America during much of the twentieth century. From 1900 through 1970, the United States experienced a steady decline in the overall death rate. As was the case in England and Wales, the rising standard of living seen in the United States during this period was associated with a steady fall in the rate of death from infectious diseases such as measles, tuberculosis, pneumonia, diphtheria, typhoid, and polio. It was also the case that the antibiotics and vaccines to treat these diseases were among the important medical discoveries of the twentieth century. However, as with the case of tuberculosis in England and Wales, most of the decline in the death rate for each of nine most feared infectious diseases occurred before the medical treatment for that disease was discovered (McKinlay and McKinlay 1997). Better health, in this case measured by reduced death rates from infectious diseases, was associated principally with rising levels of income and improvements in the standard of living. Advances in medical care played a smaller role in reducing the death rate from these illnesses.

By the end of the twentieth century, deaths from infectious diseases had declined substantially and were largely replaced by deaths from three major chronic diseases: heart disease, cancer, and stroke. With the tremendous advances in medical care seen during the last part of the twentieth century, we might expect to see death rates from these and other chronic diseases falling substantially. Yet, when we look at the actual death rates in the United States from the six leading causes of death, adjusted for changes in the age distribution of the population over this time, we see a mixed record of success (Jemal et al. 2005). The death rate from heart disease and accidents showed a sharp decline from 1970 through 2002, while the death rate from stroke declined at a slower rate. The death rate from cancer and diabetes changed relatively little during this time, and the death rate from chronic lung disease actually rose. By 2011 heart disease, cancer, chronic lung disease, and stroke accounted for 59 percent of all deaths in the United States (National Center for Health Statistics, 2013).

If measles, tuberculosis, and pneumonia have now been replaced by heart disease, cancer, and stroke as principal causes of death, will Fuchs's point—that differences in income are the principal determinant of differences in health status—still hold? An answer to this question has been provided by the Whitehall study, conducted over a period of several decades in England. The study has been following employees in the British Civil Service, recording many aspects of their health status over time. It compares the health of four principal groups of employees:

1. the administrators who work at the highest ranks of the Civil Service
2. the professional and executive employees who carry out much of the work of the Civil Service, under the supervision of the administrators
3. the clerical workers who provide the staff support for their professional and executive supervisors
4. the other workers, not in any of these employment categories, who clean the floors, take out the trash, and serve the food in the cafeteria

As one might expect, the level of education and training required to work in each of these categories is quite different. The administrators tend to have more education than the executive employees, who in turn have more education than the clerical workers, and so on down the line. Also not surprisingly, the income of each category tends to be higher than the income of the category immediately below it.

Each category of worker is fully employed, and each tends to work in similar physical surroundings. Each has access to the full level of health care provided by the British National Health Service. Will we see the same hierarchical difference in death rates in British Civil Service workers that we saw between Mimi and Hans when faced with tuberculosis? Figure 1.4 provides an answer to this question.

Figure 1.4 graphs the cumulative death rate from all causes over 10 years of observation for each of the four categories of employee described above. It seems clear that administrative employees have a substantially lower rate of death than the janitors, cafeteria workers, and "others" in this category. If Hans had been an administrator in the British Civil Service and Mimi a maid who cleans the bathrooms for the Civil Service, she would be more likely to die during this time period than he.

However, the comparison between the highest class of worker and the lowest is only part of the story. Each category of worker has a lower death rate than the category immediately below it. With each step down the employment hierarchy, health deteriorates and the chance of death goes up. Repeating Renaud's comment from the beginning of this chapter, "the lower one is situated on the social hierarchy . . . the lower one's probability of staying in good health and the lower one's life expectancy" (Renaud 1994, p. 322).

The Whitehall study is not a study of how poverty is related to the chance of death or illness. It is a study of people who are employed and who have regular ac-

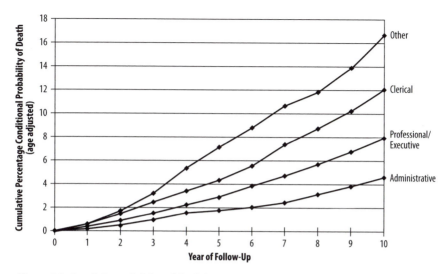

Figure 1.4. Cumulative probability of death based on occupational category within the British Civil Service—the Whitehall study. *Source*: Marmot et al. 1984, used by permission of Elsevier Limited.

cess to health care. It is important to appreciate that the relationship between income and health is not dichotomous, with only those who fall below some threshold of poverty suffering the health consequences of being at the bottom of the social hierarchy. Even though the majority of research published between 1975 and 2000 on the relationship between social class and health focused on the effects of poverty, it is clear from the Whitehall study and numerous others that the relationship between social class and health—between one's position on the social hierarchy and one's likelihood of either illness or death—is a continuous relationship that spans all levels of the social hierarchy, from the very lowest to the very highest (Adler and Ostrove 1999).

Figure 1.5 illustrates the two conceptual models of the relationship between income and health. The horizontal axis measures income—typically family income. The vertical axis represents the likelihood that an individual at a given income level will enjoy good health, whether measured by the rate of illness or the chance of death. In the threshold model, those who live in poverty have lower health status than those who live above the poverty line (the poverty line measured by the federal government and used to qualify those who fall below it for a variety of benefits). Once a family receives a level of income sufficient to meet its basic needs for food, clothing, and housing, there is no further health benefit to a rising standard of living.

By contrast, the continuous model in Figure 1.5 suggests that there is, indeed, a health benefit to escaping poverty. However, the farther a family gets from

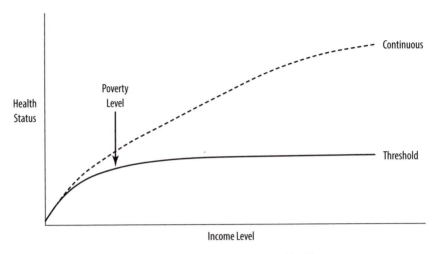

Figure 1.5. Two models of the association between income level and health status.

poverty—the higher its income and associated standard of living—the better its health becomes. Even though neither lives in poverty, an executive employee brings in more income than a clerical employee and accordingly enjoys better health. That better health status extends to the members of the executive's family as well. An administrative employee, in turn, enjoys a higher standard of living and better health than the executive employee who works under their direction. This is the message of the Whitehall study.

Health psychologist Nancy Adler and colleagues have looked thoroughly at the association between socioeconomic status (SES) and health status. (SES measures status within the social hierarchy according to a number of measures in addition to income. Chapter 3 details how income and SES are associated.) In a series of publications (Adler et al. 1994; Adler and Ostrove 1999), they summarized the research in this area that firmly supports the continuous model of this association. They analyzed the results of eight separate studies, each measuring the association between SES and the mortality rate—either the overall adult mortality rate for those at a given level of SES or the infant mortality rate. In each of these studies, with every step down the SES hierarchy, the chance of death, either adult death or infant death, goes up.

Adler and colleagues also summarized studies investigating the association between SES and health measured as the rate of certain chronic illness within a given SES group. Again, the relationship is clearly a continuous one. With every step down the SES hierarchy, the chances go up of having arthritis, high blood pressure, and other chronic diseases that reduce one's quality of life. Of course, this does not mean that every person in a lower SES category will have a higher rate of illness and earlier death than every person in a higher SES category. The mortality rates and illness rates are statistical averages that accurately state the likelihood that an individual within the indicated category will have the outcome that is being measured. In 1900 a poor seamstress was more likely to die from tuberculosis than was the son of an affluent family. In 2015 a poor seamstress was more likely to contract high blood pressure and arthritis, to have her infant die before its first birthday, and herself to die earlier than the son of an affluent family. While the circumstances in which Mimi and Hans Castorp lived have changed dramatically over the decades following their fictional lives, with countless medical advances, their health status relative to each other has changed little.

This association between social status and health status holds both for the United Kingdom and for the United States. In the United Kingdom, all residents are provided health care through the British National Health Service. The United States has taken a more fragmented and incremental approach to providing health care to its residents. Rather than a right of citizenship, health care in the United States has historically been treated largely as a market commodity, available to those who are willing (and able) to pay for it. As described in 1986 by health economist Uwe Reinhardt: "Americans have . . . decided to treat health care as essentially a private consumer good of which the poor might be guaranteed a basic package, but which is otherwise to be distributed more and more on the basis of ability to pay" (Reinhardt and Relman 1986, p. 23).

Since the 1960s the federal and state governments have provided coverage for certain of the most vulnerable segments of our society, including the elderly and the very poor. However, in 2012, two years after the Affordable Care Act (ACA) was signed into law, 48 million people, most of them in low- to moderate-income working families, had no health insurance and as a result had little access to health care (US Census Bureau 2013). Beginning in 2014, the changes enacted as part of ACA reduced the number of uninsured Americans by nearly 18 million people, while still leaving 27 million people without health insurance (American Community Survey 2016).

In understanding the association between social position and health in the United States, we cannot ignore the very real economic barriers to health care that still exist. It seems clear that income and other measures of social position affect health directly, as well as affecting it indirectly through impaired access to health care. This relationship is illustrated in Figure 1.6, in which the width of the arrows indicates the strength of the relationship.

Before we can understand these relationships and the causal factors behind them more fully, we first need to look at the SES concept in more depth. What are the

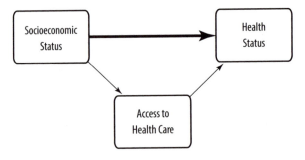

Figure 1.6. The association between social position, access to health care, and health status.

measures of SES other than income? Does it matter how long one is in a position of disadvantaged SES? Chapter 3 explores these and other aspects of the relationship between SES and health in more depth.

Before looking at the relationship between SES and health, we must first understand what we mean by "health." Is there more than one way to measure health? Which is more important, health as perceived by the individual or health as measured by objective scales or the impressions of health professionals? These are the subjects of Chapter 2.

CHAPTER TWO

What Is "Health"?

How Should We Define It? How Should We Measure It?

In Chapter 1 we saw that the United States fares relatively poorly when compared to other developed countries using measures of a population's health status such as life expectancy and infant mortality. In order to compare the health of individuals rather than of countries, however, we need different types of measures. How "healthy" one person appears, or feels, relative to another person will depend to a large extent on how health is defined and measured in this context.

Consider, for example, the following descriptions of six different people. Each is drawn from an actual person I have known in my years as a practicing physician and professor. As you read the descriptions, ask yourself the following two questions:

1. Who is the healthiest?
2. Who is the least healthy?

Six People: Healthy or Unhealthy?

1. The CEO of a large company who has between 6 and 10 alcoholic drinks every 24 hours
2. A student at Stanford University in the middle of studying for final exams
3. A teenager born weighing two pounds who exhibits problems with coordination and cognition
4. A paraplegic person (that is, someone with a spinal cord injury who is paralyzed from the waist down) who bikes to work each morning as an engineer at a major high-tech company (using a hand-crank bike)
5. A teenager who is 25 pounds overweight and is sad and discouraged because she has few friends
6. A 94-year-old who has lived in the same house for 20 years and who has the beginnings of kidney failure and is in the early stages of Alzheimer disease

When I present this list to my students at Stanford, there typically is little consensus on the answer to either question. The CEO is obviously successful and probably has a substantial income. He would be at the top of most social hierarchies. However, he is an alcoholic, exhibiting the characteristics of chronic alcohol abuse identified by the National Institute on Alcohol Abuse and Alcoholism. There are few outward signs that this person is unhealthy—no heart disease, with blood pressure within reasonable limits. Yet a physician who has accurate information about his alcohol consumption would have to view him as unhealthy.

Most Stanford students enjoy excellent physical health. Yet each year a few students develop potentially serious emotional problems when under the stress of final exams. Fortunately, the exams last only a few days, and with proper support and counseling the students who experience the emotional cost of the stress triggered by exams recover completely and are ready to resume classes after a short period of rest.

There has been careful research on the health outcomes of babies born prematurely at extremely low birth weight (usually defined as weighing less than 1,000 grams at birth). A two-pound baby weighs less than 1,000 grams. Twenty or 30 years ago such an infant faced a substantial risk of experiencing fairly high levels of permanent disability as a result of prematurity. Some of these former preemies have significant problems with muscular coordination and mental ability. How should we view a teenager in this situation?

Rather than developing physical disabilities as a result of prematurity, many otherwise healthy individuals, at some time during their childhood or early adulthood, are involved in an accident that damages their spinal cord, leading to permanent paralysis from the waist down, known medically as paraplegia. How are we to view a person with this level of disability? Does it matter that this person graduated from a top university and has a successful career as a computer professional, or has superb cardiovascular health based on an excellent diet and regular, vigorous exercise?

A teenager who is 25 pounds overweight is probably obese (that is, the ratio of a person's height to weight exceeds the guidelines established by the National Institutes of Health). There are few abnormal signs or symptoms due to the obesity for this teenager. The health effects of obesity more typically show up in adulthood. However, this person, in addition to being obese, is consistently sad and discouraged and has few friends. (In Chapter 4 we will see that having few friends and social contacts is associated with worse health outcomes independent of other factors.) I would be concerned about this person's health—her emotional health now and the long-term health consequences of obesity and social isolation later.

Finally, we have the 94-year-old. Clearly, she has chronic medical problems that will affect her daily life and may eventually lead to her death. Can we consider a person such as this to be healthy? When students pose this question, I respond: what would this woman say herself? Few 94-year-olds have the luxury of being able to stay in their own home until the end of their life. This particular 94-year-old had a regular circle of friends who visited her every day, took her to church every week, and helped her with shopping and going to the doctor. As 94-year-olds go, this one was fairly healthy—at least, she thought so.

It should by now be clear that there is a principle we must acknowledge in measuring health:

- How healthy or unhealthy a person is will depend on which definition of health we use.

There is an associated principle that we must also consider:

- How you define health will depend on the level at which you analyze health, with different measures used:
  — at the level of an individual
  — at the level of a community or neighborhood
  — at the level of a country or society

Defining Health at the Level of an Individual

The World Health Organization (WHO) attempted to define what "health" means for an individual anywhere in the world. The constitution of the WHO was first adopted at the International Health Conference held in New York in 1946. The preamble to that constitution states: "Health is a state of complete physical, mental and social well-being and not merely the absence of disease or infirmity."

The intent of the global community adopting this definition was to make it clear that the health of any individual is measured not simply by the presence or absence of disease. Health involves health of the body, health of the mind and the emotions, and health of the social context in which one lives. While this definition has clear value in broadening our understanding of health, it has limited value from a policy context. It defines a level of health that few can ever hope to achieve. I certainly have relatively few moments when I am in such a complete state of well-being. My arm is often bothered by tendonitis; sometimes I have a hard time sleeping because of stressful issues at work. I often wish I could find more time to spend with friends. In addition, it is a rare student in my class who can state that they are in a state of complete health. The potential danger in setting what for many may be an unrealistic goal is that it puts us in the position of always falling short, no matter how hard we try.

Beyond setting an expectation that few can hope to attain, this definition gives us little guidance on how to measure health. It seems to create a dichotomy: either we are healthy, or we are not. We have no way of stating, for example, that we are "79 percent healthy." Based on this definition alone, we have no way of following our health over time to determine whether it is improving or declining. Similarly, we have few mechanisms to compare one individual with another.

This is not to say that the WHO definition is without merit. On the contrary, by creating an awareness of the many aspects of health, it gives us an opportunity to explore the three axes of health the definition includes: physical health, mental health, and social well-being. I explore each of these aspects of individual health in sequence, and then ask whether there might be a way to combine them into a composite measure of health that can be used in a policy context.

Physical Health: The Medical Model

Sociologist Andrew Twaddle provided a definition of health that the US medical profession relied on for much of the twentieth century. He stated that "health must be understood first as a biophysical state" and that "illness is any state that has been diagnosed as such by a competent professional" (1979, pp. 145–46). Twaddle identified two fundamental dimensions of health according to the medical model:

1. an absence of symptoms—sensations noticed by the patient and interpreted as abnormal
2. an absence of signs—objective characteristics noted by a health professional, of which a patient may often be unaware

This approach to defining health tells us what the concept of health *is not*. A person with abnormal signs or symptoms is not healthy. It does not tell us what health *is*. In the practice of medicine, this might be referred to as a "rule-out" definition. One looks for the presence of abnormal signs or symptoms, and when one determines that there are none, it is possible to rule out ill health. If one does not have ill health, then one is by definition healthy, at least from the medical perspective.

There are potential problems, though, with using this approach in isolation. What if the patient and the doctor disagree? Whose definition of "health" then takes precedence? Say, for example, a person is bothered by a headache (an abnormal symptom) and goes to a doctor for advice. Knowing that headaches can be either benign, with no specific treatment indicated, or serious, with aggressive therapy indicated, the doctor will look for abnormal signs on tests such as a physical examination or a CAT scan. Having looked and found no abnormal signs of illness, the doctor might reassure the person that they are healthy (that is, the doctor has "ruled out" ill health). However, the patient may still feel the headache and may both feel unhealthy and expect to be treated as unhealthy.

What are we to make of a condition that has no abnormal symptoms? An important example of this is high blood pressure, also referred to as hypertension; persons with hypertension develop symptoms only after a number of years. Should we consider a person with somewhat elevated blood pressure to be unhealthy, based on our knowledge that their blood pressure will *eventually* lead to further problems? What might be the consequences of labeling such a person as "unhealthy," even if they feel fine?

Another potential problem with the medical approach to health are the problems that have been identified in the reliability of what would otherwise seem to be objective evidence of abnormal signs of illness. On tests such as EKGs, CAT scans, and certain laboratory tests, different individuals reviewing the tests might interpret the same test as either normal or abnormal. There have even been studies in which the same reviewer has been given the same set of tests to interpret on two occasions, separated by a period of time, with some of the interpretations differing— even though it was the same test. This phenomenon is thought to contribute to the marked variation in the rates at which certain procedures, such as prostate or heart surgery, are done on similar populations of patients. Wennberg and colleagues documented these "area variations" in a number of contexts, variations that seem to involve doctors in different parts of the country interpreting differently what should be considered a "normal finding" and what constitutes an "abnormal finding" (Wennberg et al. 1982; Wennberg 1993).

Health as Functioning at a Normal Level: The Sociocultural Model

Sociologist Talcott Parsons looked at health as reflecting the extent to which an individual is able to maintain a normal level of functioning within their social context. He noted that "health may be defined as the state of optimum *capacity* of an individual for the performance of roles and tasks for which he has been socialized" (1979, p. 122). Parsons does state that "*all* processes of behavior on whatever level are mediated through physiologic mechanisms." However, his approach to health focuses more on what a person is able to do with their body than on the physiological state of that person's body. Also, rather than comparing a person's level of functioning to some lofty ideal state, as the WHO definition does, it looks at the person in the context of their own social circumstances. From this perspective, a person with a medical condition that consistently has abnormal signs or symptoms who is nonetheless able to perform customary roles and tasks should be considered healthy. Thus, from this perspective, health is not the absence of something (signs and symptoms), but rather the presence of something—the ability to function normally.

While there are some attractive aspects of adopting this perspective on health, it too has some potential drawbacks when used in isolation to define health. The same level of physical functioning for two individuals may imply different states of health, depending on the social roles and tasks they face. Thus, a concert violinist with arthritis in their fingers may be seen as unhealthy and deserving of intervention because of the extent to which the arthritis impairs their ability to perform. A house cleaner with the same degree of arthritis in their fingers may warrant little attention, as it is possible to go on cleaning houses despite the discomfort of the arthritis. Given the degree to which inequalities continue to exist in educational opportunities, with inequalities in educational attainment leading to strikingly different socially defined roles and tasks, adopting the sociocultural model of health in isolation may perpetuate inequalities according to race, ethnicity, or gender.

As we will see when we take another look at the health of the 94-year-old described above as patient 6, the ability to perform common tasks is especially important in evaluating the health of elderly people and of those with physical disabilities. There are five common tasks that most of us take for granted; being unable to perform them directly affects the quality of a person's daily life. These tasks are commonly referred to as activities of daily living (ADLs). They are:

1. feeding one's self
2. bathing one's self
3. dressing one's self
4. being able to use the toilet without assistance
5. being able to transfer one's self without assistance (for example, from a bed into a chair)

It should be apparent that a person who is unable to perform any of the ADLs without assistance is in a state of relatively poor health from this perspective. A simple summation of the number of ADLs a person requires assistance with is commonly used as a measure of health and disability. Often this measure is used to determine a person's eligibility for extra benefits, such as home health care.

Health as a General Feeling of Well-Being: The Psychological Model

The first two models of health rely on an assessment of an individual's health by an independent evaluator. The perceptions and attitudes of the individual in question affect the health assessment, but do not determine it. A third model of health relies on the individuals themselves to provide an assessment of their own health. For example, it is possible to ask an individual a question such as, On a scale of 1 to 10, how would you rate your overall feeling of well-being today?

A number of scales have been developed to measure a person's health based on that person's own perceptions. These measures are often time specific; a person may give one answer in the face of an immediate stressor and another answer a short time later after that stressor has been removed. Think, for example, of patient 2 above, the Stanford student during final exams. While this student may report a rather low sense of well-being in the midst of final exams, the same student may report a substantially improved well-being after finals are over and they have had a chance to spend time with family and friends at home.

Since 1996 the US Agency for Healthcare Research and Quality (AHRQ) has conducted an ongoing survey of the health status of the US population, referred to as the Medical Expenditure Panel Survey (MEPS). One of the questions they ask of individual respondents is how they would rate their overall health status, based on the following five categories: Excellent, Very Good, Good, Fair, or Poor. Davis and colleagues (2017) have analyzed the pattern of responses to this question for older adults in the US, defined as age 65 or greater. They categorized those who responded either Excellent or Very Good as "healthy" adults, and then followed the trends in the number of healthy adults in the US between 2000 and 2014. Overall, the number of healthy older adults increased from 14.0 million (42.4 percent) to 22.4 million (48.2 percent). The authors also found that, after controlling for age and gender, both African American and Hispanic respondents reported lower rates of health, as did those from lower incomes and those with lower levels of education. The authors report that, "our new finding regarding widening gaps by race/ethnicity and socioeconomic status is concerning. This finding supports the notion of '2 different Americas' having formed" (p. 1684).

Another Look at Our Six Patients

Having considered three ways to define health (medical, sociocultural, psychological), we can now take another look at our hypothetical six patients to reconsider who is the healthiest and who is the least healthy.

The CEO of a large company who has between six and 10 alcoholic drinks every 24 hours. From the medical perspective, a perceptive physician would determine that this person is quite unhealthy. While the individual may have few symptoms to complain of at this time, the physician knows that chronic alcoholism will, in all likelihood, lead to serious diseases and has the potential to impair significantly social role functioning. This is why many physicians ask probing questions about alcohol consumption as part of routine health screening, and many validated screening instruments have been developed to look for signs of possible alcohol abuse.

From a sociocultural perspective, this person is doing quite well. So long as he can effectively maintain his role as CEO, the alcohol abuse may not impair his health. Once again, however, this person is at high risk of a substantial decline in health if the alcohol abuse begins to impair his functioning at work. In addition, we know little about this person's personal or family situation. If the alcohol abuse were associated with impaired social relations outside of work, then we would have to consider this person to have serious health impairment.

It is difficult to evaluate this person from a psychological perspective. It may well be that the drinking is masking an underlying psychological problem that the person may initially fail to acknowledge. Were the person to stop drinking, that psychological impairment may become more apparent. It is difficult to predict how this person would rate his own health from this perspective.

In summary, the health of the alcoholic CEO is currently impaired in terms of the medical model, and either impaired or significantly threatened from the standpoint of the other models. We should regard this person as generally unhealthy.

A student at Stanford University in the middle of studying for final exams. This person may report a very high level of stress from the psychological perspective. Stanford students often are short on sleep and experience high levels of anxiety during finals. However, finals only last a week, after which students get at least a week of rest with the opportunity for travel and relaxing with family and friends. For most students, the stress is short-term. From a sociocultural perspective this person is doing quite well. Simply being at Stanford suggests that the student is highly functional in a social context. Most Stanford students will have friends and social networks as well that add to their level of overall social functioning. Similarly, most young adults have little in the way of medical abnormalities that show up as abnormal symptoms or signs. So, even though this person might report experiencing high stress and anxiety right now, we have little to worry about regarding the student's overall health.

A teenager born weighing two pounds who exhibits problems with coordination and cognition. We have little to go on to evaluate the health of this person. Certainly from a strictly medical perspective this person has signs of potentially significant health impairment. The physical and cognitive difficulties many former premature infants face as teenagers often require extra help and support. They may be less able to participate fully in academic, athletic, and social activities. One might expect such a child to feel discouraged or depressed about the life they face. Later in this chapter I return to this issue by looking at research that has actually followed former premature infants into adolescence, and has asked these types of questions of the children, their teachers, and their parents.

A paraplegic person who bikes to work each morning as an engineer at a major high-tech company. This person has evidence of a health impairment on only one level—the use of his legs. He appears to have compensated for this impairment quite effectively through the use of a mechanical assist device—the hand-crank bike. I would expect him to have excellent upper-body strength (from all that cranking) and superb cardiovascular fitness (from biking to work every day rather than driving a car). From a sociocultural perspective this person seems to be doing superbly. Engineers at high-tech companies are generally highly educated, tend to face interesting and challenging work, and enjoy generous incomes. There is no reason to think that this person's family life has been impaired by paralysis. Unless he finds the paralysis itself so discouraging that it affects his own perceptions of his quality of life, one would expect this person to report fairly high perceptions of his own health. An isolated physical impairment does not necessarily make someone unhealthy, and in the face of other signs of positive health takes on less significance in this regard.

A teenager who is 25 pounds overweight and is sad and discouraged because she has few friends. Here is someone we should worry about. This person is showing significant health impairment on all fronts. The obesity itself will very likely be associated with other serious medical problems, either now or in the near future (diabetes and high blood pressure, for example). With few friends this person is showing evidence of poor social role functioning. The sadness and discouragement reported by this teenager is a clear statement of her own perception of poor emotional health. Any health professional who encounters this person would be quite concerned, and would want to evaluate possible interventions on a number of levels.

A 94-year-old who has lived in the same house for 20 years and who has the beginnings of kidney failure and is in the early stages of Alzheimer disease. At first, most of my students place this person squarely in the "unhealthy" category, many at the bottom of the list. In response, I ask the students to consider if their own grandparent were in this situation, how that grandparent would respond to the question, "How are you doing?" This person represents an actual patient I took care of until she eventually died of her worsening kidney failure. There was treatment that would have kept her alive longer, but she refused it. She said she was happy being who she was, and she wanted to die happy. And she did. For her, the impaired memory and physical weakness from her kidneys was of little importance. What *was* important was that at 94 she still lived in the house she had lived in for decades and that she needed no help with her ADLs. She cooked for herself, she dressed herself, and she bathed herself. Her many neighbors and friends helped her with shopping, visited her regularly, and took her to church every week. From this person's own perspective, life didn't get any better. I knew she had signs of poor memory and an abnormal kidney test, but I believe I enjoyed our visits together almost as much as she did.

So who is the healthiest? For me, the 94-year-old and the bike-to-work engineer are at the top of the list. Who is the least healthy? From my perspective, it has to be either the CEO or the overweight and depressed teenager. For the Stanford student I'll need to wait until after finals to be sure. The former preemie who now has substantial impairments may yet surprise us.

Health as a Multidimensional Concept

It seems apparent that each model of health we have considered tells us something about a person's state of health, but tells us little about a person's *overall* state of health. Rather than being one-dimensional, health has multiple dimensions, three of which we have considered so far. Wolinsky (1988) suggests that we think of health as a three-dimensional concept. As represented in Figure 2.1, each of the three axes represents one of the three ways of approaching health we have discussed: health as the absence of disease, health as social role functioning, and psychological health.

Wolinsky suggests that we dichotomize each dimension into "well" and "ill." Overall health is measured by the ratio of "well" dimensions to "ill" dimensions. Someone who is well on the psychological and social dimensions but ill on the medical dimension should be seen as more healthy than someone who is well along the medical dimension but ill along the social and psychological dimensions. The approach suggested by Wolinsky gives equal weight to each of the three dimensions, and does not allow for gradations along the three axes.

What if each dimension is continuous, as represented in Figure 2.1, rather than dichotomous, as suggested by Wolinsky? (That is, what if the measurement on each

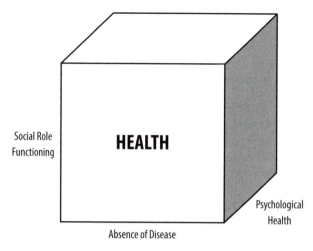

Figure 2.1. Health as a three-dimensional concept. *Source*: Based on Wolinsky 1988.

of the three dimensions can assume any of a wide range of values, rather than simply "well" or "ill"?) From this perspective overall health could be any of a large number of points within the three-dimensional space represented by the diagram. If it were possible to measure health reliably at any point along the medical, social, and psychological dimensions, and then combine these measurements into a measurement of overall health, such a tool would be very useful both as a policy tool and in following the health of an individual over time.

John Ware and colleagues developed such an instrument: the 36-Item Short-Form Health Survey, often referred to simply as the SF-36 (Ware and Sherbourne 1992). Developed for use in the Medical Outcomes Study, Ware used the SF-36 to compare the health outcomes over time of patients enrolled in alternative health care delivery systems. The SF-36 uses an approach similar to that proposed by Wolinsky, but treats each dimension of health as continuous rather than dichotomous. As shown in Table 2.1, it uses 36 individual questions, each asking about a specific aspect of health such as the ability to climb stairs, walk several blocks, or engage in vigorous activities. It also asks about limits on activities as the result of emotional problems.

Using statistical modeling, the SF-36 uses various combinations of these 36 questions to create eight separate scales, each measuring a different dimension of health. It then combines four of these dimensional measures to create an overall measure of physical health, and the other four to create an overall measure of mental health.

Table 2.1. The SF-36 Health Status Survey Instrument

1. In general, would you say your health is:				
Excellent	Very good	Good	Fair	Poor

2. Compared to one year ago, how would you rate your health in general now?				
Much better now than one year ago	Somewhat better now than one year ago	About the same	Somewhat worse now than one year ago	Much worse now than one year ago

The following questions are about activities you might do during a typical day. Does your health now limit you in these activities? If so, how much?

Yes, limited a lot	Yes, limited a little	No, not limited at all
3. Vigorous activities, such as running, lifting heavy objects, participating in strenuous sports		
4. Moderate activities, such as moving a table, pushing a vacuum cleaner, bowling, or playing golf		
5. Lifting or carrying groceries		
6. Climbing several flights of stairs		
7. Climbing one flight of stairs		
8. Bending, kneeling, or stooping		
9. Walking more than a mile		
10. Walking several blocks		
11. Walking one block		
12. Bathing or dressing yourself		

During the past 4 weeks, have you had any of the following problems with your work or other regular daily activities as a result of your physical health?

Yes	No
13. Cut down on the amount of time you spent on work or other activities	
14. Accomplished less than you would like	
15. Were limited in the kind of work or other activities	
16. Had difficulty performing the work or other activities (for example, it took extra effort)	

During the past 4 weeks, have you had any of the following problems with your work or other regular daily activities as a result of any emotional problems (such as feeling depressed or anxious)?

Yes	No
17. Cut down on the amount of time you spent on work or other activities	
18. Accomplished less than you would like	
19. Didn't do work or other activities as carefully as usual	

20. During the past 4 weeks, to what extent has your physical health or emotional problems interfered with your normal social activities with family, friends, neighbors, or groups?				
Not at all	Slightly	Moderately	Quite a bit	Extremely

21. How much bodily pain have you had during the past 4 weeks?					
None	Very mild	Mild	Moderate	Severe	Very severe

Table 2.1. (*continued*)

22. During the past 4 weeks, how much did pain interfere with your normal work (including both work outside the home and housework)?				
Not at all	*A little bit*	*Moderately*	*Quite a bit*	*Extremely*
These questions are about how you feel and how things have been with you during the past 4 weeks. For each question, please give the one answer that comes closest to the way you have been feeling. How much of the time during the past 4 weeks				

All of the time	*Most of the time*	*A good bit of the time*	*Some of the time*	*A little of the time*	*None of the time*
23. Did you feel full of pep?					
24. Have you been a very nervous person?					
25. Have you felt so down in the dumps that nothing could cheer you up?					
26. Have you felt calm and peaceful?					
27. Did you have a lot of energy?					
28. Have you felt downhearted and blue?					
29. Did you feel worn out?					
30. Have you been a happy person?					
31. Did you feel tired?					
32. During the past 4 weeks, how much of the time has your physical health or emotional problems interfered with your social activities (like visiting friends, relatives, etc.)?					

All of the time	*Most of the time*	*Some of the time*	*A little of the time*	*None of the time*
How TRUE or FALSE is each of the following statements for you?				

Definitely true	*Mostly true*	*Don't know*	*Mostly false*	*Definitely false*
33. I seem to get sick a little easier than other people				
34. I am as healthy as anybody I know				
35. I expect my health to get worse				
36. My health is excellent				

Source: 36-Item Short Form Survey (SF-36). Developed at RAND as part of the Medical Outcomes Study. Used with permission.

The four subscales used to measure overall physical health include:

1. Physical Functioning
2. Role Limitations Due to Physical Problems
3. Bodily Pain
4. General Health Perceptions

The four subscales used to measure overall mental health include:

1. Vitality
2. Social Functioning
3. Role Limitations Due to Emotional Problems
4. General Mental Health

Researchers have translated the SF-36 into other languages and found it to be equally reliable. Changes in an individual's SF-36 score over time have been found to be associated with the cost of providing health care services, with those patients with worse health as measured by the SF-36 requiring more health care.

An excellent example of how the SF-36 can be used in research on health status is a study published by Sjogren and Thulin (2004). The authors wanted to know more about the ways in which heart surgery affected the health status of individuals who were 80 years old or older, concerned that surgery of this magnitude might worsen overall health status rather than improve it. It compared findings on the eight different health status scales incorporated into the SF-36 for patients who underwent surgery, comparing them to age-matched patients without heart disease. They found that those patients who had surgery reported lower physical functioning but less bodily pain than the comparison group. Otherwise the two groups were not significantly different on any of the other six scales.

Using instruments such as the SF-36 allows us to assess health along medical, social, and psychological dimensions. Wilson and Cleary (1995) offer us a way of understanding how these different aspects of health are associated with each other. They suggest that the three dimensions of health are linked causally, with changes in physical health triggering subsequent changes in role functioning and ultimately in emotional health, and that each dimension is influenced by characteristics unique to the individual patient as well as characteristics of the environment in which that person lives. In addition, they suggest that the three aspects of health are not the final outcomes we should focus our attention on, but rather are each intermediate factors that affect in various ways the ultimate thing we should be measuring: quality of life. I have illustrated Wilson and Cleary's model of health in Figure 2.2.

In their model, biological and physical abnormalities are the fundamental causes of poor health. These abnormalities in turn lead to symptoms that are characteristic of disease. The person's perception of poor physical health leads to a reduction in functional status. Under this model it is the reduction of functional status in response to perceived illness that leads to a feeling of poor general health. It is the person's perception of a reduction in general health status that then reduces the quality of life they enjoy.

For each of these causal links, characteristics unique to the individual and characteristics of the environment in which the individual lives and works can have either buffering or enhancing effects on the chain of causality—from biologic abnormalities to a reduced quality of life. For example, someone with strong social and psychological supports may respond to a given set of symptoms with a smaller

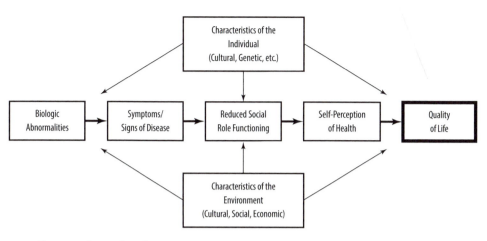

Figure 2.2. Factors that affect health status. *Source:* Based on Wilson and Cleary 1995.

reduction in functional status than another person with similar symptoms but a weaker support system. Conversely, someone who tends to amplify the symptoms they perceive, or who has little motivation to be healthy, may experience a substantially reduced functional status in response to those symptoms. Similarly, individual motivation and preferences coupled with the nature of one's social and emotional support system will directly affect the quality of life one experiences.

This perspective brings up the important questions of the extent to which gender will affect perceptions of overall health status, and whether gender should be included as a variable in studies of factors affecting perceived quality of life. Stefanick (2017) has described a pattern of research on a range of human health issues that exclude gender as a variable. Stefanick points out the distinction between the concepts of sex and gender, with sex as a biologic quality based on chromosomes and sex hormones, while gender refers to a person's self-perception and self-representation in a broader social and cultural context. For a range of diseases, from cardiac disease to mental illness, gender has been shown to play an important role. It would therefore be important to include self-identified gender in analyses and discussions of health as a general feeling of well-being. Braveman (2017) argues that the issue of health equity is becoming increasingly central in national discussions. Gender will also be a central element of analyses of health equity.

Thus, quality of life is powerfully affected by symptoms of illness, functional limitations, and perceptions of well-being. However, the presence of these problems does not necessarily mean that a person will experience a reduced quality of life. A case in point is that of premature infants weighing less than 1,000 grams (referred to as extremely low birth weight [ELBW]).

In the 1970s and 1980s, medical science was in the transition from being nearly helpless to being very successful in the treatment of ELBW infants. ELBW babies born in that time frame often survived, but often with substantial levels of physical and cognitive disability. Saigal and colleagues (1996) reported on a study of 141 ELBW babies born between 1977 and 1982 who had survived and were then teenagers, comparing them on a number of scales to a comparison group of teenagers, matched on age, sex, and social class, who were born at full term weighing at least 2,500 grams (normal birth weight [NBW]).

The authors first compared the two groups of teenagers on six scales of disability: cognition, sensation, mobility, self-care, emotion, and pain. For each of the six scales, the ELBW teenagers reported a higher frequency of problems than the NBW group. All these differences were statistically significant ($p \leq .05$) except for emotion and pain. Using objective measures of disability, the ELBW teenagers had both lower physiological health (cognition and sensation) and lower functional health (mobility and self-care) than the NBW group. From the model proposed by Wilson and Cleary, can we assume that the ELBW teenagers will also report a lower quality of life? Saigal and colleagues addressed this question by assessing each subject's perception of their own quality of life, using a standardized assessment tool that measured quality of life on a scale from 0 to 1. What they found was essentially no difference in the distribution of the quality of life score between the two groups.

There is a danger in assuming that an individual who has objective evidence of physiologic abnormalities that are associated with measurable physical impairment will necessarily experience a lower quality of life than someone without those impairments. Nor can we assume that these physiologic and functional impairments will necessarily constrain other important activities of those affected with them. Saigal and colleagues (2006) followed these same teenagers into early adulthood, comparing the ELBW and NBW subjects on educational attainment, employment or educational status, independent living, getting married, and having children. They found few differences, concluding that "a significant majority of former ELBW infants have overcome their earlier difficulties to become functional young adults" (p. 667).

Imagine if, instead of comparing ELBW infants with NBW infants, we were instead comparing 94-year-olds living in their own home with 44-year-olds. On objective scales of dimensions such as cognition, sensation, mobility, self-care, emotion, and pain, the 94-year-olds would likely register worse health than the 44-year-olds, much the same as the comparisons of the ELBW and NBW children above. If we asked the same subjects to rate their quality of life—based on my ex-

with the 94-year-old woman used as an example at the beginning of this

ight expect something similar to the quality-of-life comparisons of the

ELBW and NBW children. Despite their physical frailty and cognitive impairme.. when asked about how they feel they are doing, these 94-year-olds may well suggest, "I'm doing just fine, thanks."

The Danger of Approaching Health as a Moral Imperative

I have described health as a multidimensional concept that is directly affected by individual and environmental circumstances. Should we expect everyone to be healthy? Should we expect those with behavior patterns that are unhealthy to overcome them and to attain the level of health characterized by the absence of abnormal signs and symptoms? There is a hidden danger if we do—especially if we do so in the role of health professionals.

Faith Fitzgerald published a seminal essay in 1994, warning us to avoid what she called the "tyranny of health in which those who are unwell are assumed to have misbehaved" (p. 197). It is easy for a physician or other health professional to look at a person and recognize right away that their own behavior (e.g., smoking, lack of exercise, obesity) is impairing their attainment of full health. Should we then blame the person for that behavior and for the resulting ill health? Fitzgerald suggests that as health professionals, or even as friends or family members, it can be problematic, and perhaps harmful to an individual, to approach behaviors associated with poor health as an issue of individual moral worth.

> What harm can this do? Much harm. If health (physical, mental, and social) is normal and the failure to be healthy is someone's fault, then when a person becomes ill he or she may have done something wrong. If we root out that wrongness, or better yet, prevent it, we can restore that person to normal health and can benefit society. In effect, we have said that people owe it to society to stop misbehaving, and we use illness as evidence of misbehavior. (Fitzgerald 1994, p. 197)

It is easy to think of behaviors that fall into this category. They include:

- obesity
- smoking
- lack of exercise
- high cholesterol
- poor diet
- alcohol abuse
- drug abuse

ɔe associated over time with adverse health outcomes. Each is a
ιch an individual seemingly has control. However, as we will see
, each is also a behavior that differs markedly in terms of the social
ι one belongs. Those who have higher levels of educational attain-
age, will consistently smoke less than those with lower educational
attainmeι.. Ɔften these behaviors will have additional cultural associations, with those from differing racial or ethnic groups yet similar levels of educational attainment having consistently differing patterns of health-related behaviors. Is it the individual that determines behavior based on individual will and choice, or is it a characteristic of human behavior to follow patterns established by the social group? These are issues we will commonly confront, as health professionals, as co-workers, and as friends or family.

We separate the issues of blame versus responsibility, with regard to health-related behaviors. A person who develops lung cancer after several decades of smoking certainly bears responsibility for the behavior that contributed to the development of the cancer. Yet it is possible to approach that responsibility in a context devoid of moral judgment; that is, without assigning blame. Blame implies weakness; responsibility acknowledges the causal relationships involved. It is often difficult to look at someone we care for, or someone we are caring for as health professionals, who is engaging in what appears to us to be self-destructive behavior, without attributing some form of moral weakness to that person. Again in the words of Fitzgerald, "We must beware of developing a zealotry about health, in which we take ourselves too seriously and believe that we know enough to dictate human behavior, penalize people for disagreeing with us, and even deny people charity, empathy, and understanding because they act in a way of which we disapprove" (1994, p. 197).

Measuring the Health of a Community or a Society

Until now I have been discussing how to understand the health of an individual. The available measurements we have identified—symptoms, signs, SF-36 score, and the like—all pertain to a specific individual. What if we want to compare the health of different communities or of different societies? We will need measures that apply to groups of people rather than to individuals. Two general categories of health indicator are commonly used to define and compare health at this level: rates of illness and rates of death. Table 2.2 compares the rates of several illnesses and selected rates of death for four states from four different regions of the United States: California, Iowa, Mississippi, and New York.

Table 2.2. Comparative Health Indexes for Four States

Condition	California	Iowa	Mississippi	New York
Asthma (2015)	7.7%	7.6%	7.8%	9.9%
Diabetes (2015)	9.6%	7.7%	13.6%	8.9%
Hypertension (2015)	25.8%	30.6%	42.4%	29.3%
Obesity (2016)	25.0%	32.0%	37.3%	25.5%
Breast cancer deaths (2015)	19.6	18.5	21.8	19.2
Heart disease deaths (2014–16)	279	312	453	348
Infant mortality (2016)	4.2	6.1	8.6	4.5
Median family income (2015)	$64,500	$54,736	$40,593	$60,850

Sources: Data from the US Centers for Disease Control and Prevention.
Asthma: 2015 Adult Asthma Data: Most Recent Asthma State or Territory Data, https://www.cdc.gov/asthma/most_recent
_data_states.htm.
Diabetes: Age-Adjusted Percentage, Adults with Diabetes—Total, 2015, by State, https://gis.cdc.gov/grasp/diabetes
/DiabetesAtlas.html.
Hypertension: Data Trends & Maps—Hypertension, https://www.cdc.gov/dhdsp/maps/dtm/index.html.
Obesity: Adult Obesity Prevalence Maps, https://www.cdc.gov/obesity/data/prevalence-maps.html.
Breast cancer deaths: Age-Adjusted Death Rate—Female Breast, per 100,000 persons in 2015, https://gis.cdc.gov/Cancer/USCS
/DataViz.html.
Heart Disease Death Rate per 100,000, 35+, All Races/Ethnicities, Both Genders, 2014–16, https://nccd.cdc.gov/DHDSPAtlas
/Reports.aspx.
Infant mortality: Infant mortality rates, by state: United States, 2016, https://www.cdc.gov/nchs/pressroom/sosmap/infant
_mortality_rates/infant_mortality.htm.
Data for median family income from the US Census Bureau, 2015, https://www2.census.gov/programs-surveys/demo/tables
/income-poverty/glassman-acs.xls.

Rates of Illness

Table 2.2 compares the prevalence rates of four common illnesses for the four states. The rates reflect the percentage of adults within the state who were found to have the specified condition. Using these four illnesses, it is fairly straightforward to identify the state with the lowest level of health. Mississippi has substantially higher rates of hypertension (high blood pressure), diabetes, and obesity than any of the other states. However, Mississippi has a relatively low rate of asthma, a condition often made worse by the air pollution that is common to large, metropolitan areas. While having the highest rate of asthma, New York has the second lowest rate of obesity and the second lowest rate of diabetes—a condition often associated with obesity. California and Iowa do well with hypertension, while Iowa does especially well with diabetes.

From these data it should be clear that rates of illness can provide a very interesting look at certain states. The disease or diseases one selects as the measure of comparative health will have a great deal to do with how a state will fare. Certain diseases will reflect the degree of urbanization within a state. Other diseases, such as obesity, diabetes, and hypertension, will tend to clump together.

Rather than looking at specific disease rates, Montez and colleagues (2017) suggest that the rates of disability among older adults (aged 45 years and older) may also vary across states due to concurrent differences in rates of educational attainment within a state and the social and economic circumstances within the state. Analyzing rates of disability based on limitations in ADLs, they found the highest rates of disability in most states to be concentrated in the population of older adults with low levels of education, defined as not having completed high school. The states with the highest levels of disability among this population group were Mississippi, Kentucky, and West Virginia. They suggest that this association may be largely due to the "personal and contextual socioeconomic circumstances of low-educated adults" within a state, with these factors varying substantially among lower-income states and higher-income states (p. 1106).

Rates of Death

The federal government reported that a baby born in the United States in 2016 could expect to live, on average, 78.6 years (Kochanek et al. 2017). This life expectancy varies by sex at birth, with an expectancy of 76.1 years for male babies and 81.1 years for female babies. This difference is due to a combination of sex and gender, as these categories are described above.

Life expectancy at birth differs substantially by where the family into which a baby is born lives. Dwyer-Lindgren and colleagues (2017) have analyzed changes in life expectancy over the period 1980–2014 at the level of the county. They found that, in 2014, combined life expectancy for males and females varied by as much as 20 years between counties with the lowest and those with the highest levels. Based on their analysis that includes a range of individual and demographic variables, the authors were able to conclude that "inequalities in life expectancy among counties are large and growing, and much of the variation in life expectancy can be explained by differences in socioeconomic and race/ethnicity factors, behavioral and metabolic risk factors, and health care factors" (p. 1004).

Table 2.2 provides data on several of the conditions associated with reduced life expectancy in four individual states: California, Iowa, Mississippi, and New York. A principal contributor to reduced life expectancy is the rate of infant mortality within a state. In 2016 Mississippi had the second-highest rate of infant mortality of all 50 states, while California had the fifth-lowest rate. (Alabama had the highest rate and Vermont had the lowest rate.)

Rates of diabetes, hypertension, and obesity vary among these states in a consistent pattern, while New York has the highest rate of asthma. When we look at the rate of death from heart disease, we find Mississippi to have the highest rate of all 50 states. Iowa at 312 deaths and California at 279 deaths were in the midrange of the distribution among the states. (The lowest rate was Minnesota, with 225 deaths per 100,000 population over age 35.) As with disease rates, rates of death give a fairly consistent picture of the health of a state relative to other states. However, the relative health ranking may change depending on the specific measure one uses.

One should also note the final statistic given in Table 2.2: the median income in that state for a family of four. Mississippi has by far the lowest level of family income of any of the four states studied. In 2015 the median income for a family of four in Mississippi was the lowest of all 50 states. As we explore the association between health status and income in more depth, we will see that there is a strong association between economic well-being and health status.

In Chapter 4 we will look at not only the level of income in differing states and differing countries but also at the level of economic inequality—the distance between the best-off residents and the worst-off—among differing states and countries. In addition to being toward the bottom of the distribution in family income, Mississippi has one of the higher levels of economic inequality among its residents. We will see that both the absolute income and income relative to others are associated with health status.

Comparing Health Status Globally

When comparing health among countries globally, we can use a series of standard indicators gathered and reported by agencies such as the World Health Organization (WHO). Principal among these are

- Male life expectancy at birth—the number of years, on average, a male baby born in the year for which the data are reported can expect to live
- Female life expectancy at birth—the number of years, on average, a female baby born in the year for which the data are reported can expect to live
- Infant mortality rate—of a thousand babies born alive, the number who will die before their first birthday
- Maternal mortality rate—of one hundred thousand women giving birth, the number who will die as the result of complications during the birthing process

It is more difficult to use rates of illness to compare the health of differing countries. While this can be done, different illnesses are unique to certain geographic or climatic areas. In addition, the types of illness found in countries of varying

Table 2.3. Health Indexes for Fifteen Countries, 2015–16

Country	Male Life Expectancy at Birth (years)	Female Life Expectancy at Birth (years)	Infant Mortality Rate[1]	Maternal Mortality Rate[2]	Per Capita Income ($US)
Argentina	74	80	10	52	20,270
Bangladesh	71	74	28	176	4,040
Brazil	71	79	14	44	15,160
Canada	81	85	4	7	45,750
Colombia	71	78	13	64	14,170
Democratic Republic of the Congo	59	62	72	693	870
Greece	79	84	3	3	27,820
Haiti	61	66	51	359	1,830
India	67	70	35	174	7,060
Mexico	74	79	13	38	17,740
Nigeria	55	56	67	814	5,680
Norway	81	84	2	5	63,530
Russian Federation	66	77	7	25	24,893
Singapore	81	85	2	10	90,570
United States	76	81	6	14	60,200

Sources: World Health Organization 2018, http://www.who.int/gho/publications/world_health_statistics/2018/en/. Levels & Trends in Child Mortality (Infant Mortality), http://www.childmortality.org/files_v21/download/IGME%20report%202017%20 child%20mortality%20final.pdf. World Development Indicators 2017 (Per capita income), http://wdi.worldbank.org/tables.
[1] Infant mortality—deaths per 1,000 live births (2016)
[2] Maternal mortality—deaths per 100,000 live births (2015)

levels of economic development are often quite different. Accordingly, it is more common to use the types of mortality statistics cited above to compare countries.

Using data from the WHO, Table 2.3 shows these indexes for 15 countries from around the globe, drawn from each of the 5 largest continents. In addition, it presents the per capita share of the gross national income for the countries listed.

There are wide disparities in each of the indicators listed. Infant mortality ranges from 2 per 1,000 births in Singapore and Norway to 72 per 1,000 in the Democratic Republic of the Congo. Life expectancy goes from a low of 56 years for women and 55 years for men in Nigeria to 85 years for women (in Canada and Singapore) and 81 years for men (in Canada, Norway, and Singapore).

Health status and socioeconomic status are inextricably linked. As we saw in Chapter 1, as socioeconomic status rises over time, health status improves. Using both illness rates and mortality rates, the same is true in comparing health among different states in the United States. To examine this relationship in a global context, I have taken the data from Table 2.3, which lists the countries alphabetically, and instead sorted the countries by per capita income. Table 2.4 shows the 15 countries by income from lowest to highest.

Not surprisingly, of the 15 countries listed, the Democratic Republic of the Congo has the lowest per capita income ($870), while Singapore has the highest

Table 2.4. Health Indexes for Fifteen Countries, by per Capita Income

Country	Male Life Expectancy at Birth (years)	Female Life Expectancy at Birth (years)	Infant Mortality Rate[1]	Maternal Mortality Rate[2]	Per Capita Income ($US)
Democratic Republic of the Congo	59	62	72	693	870
Haiti	61	66	51	359	1,830
Bangladesh	71	74	28	176	4,040
Nigeria	55	56	67	814	5,680
India	67	70	35	174	7,060
Colombia	71	78	13	64	14,170
Brazil	71	79	14	44	15,160
Mexico	74	79	13	38	17,740
Argentina	74	80	10	52	20,270
Russian Federation	66	77	7	25	24,893
Greece	79	84	3	3	27,820
Canada	81	85	4	7	45,750
United States	76	81	6	14	60,200
Norway	81	84	2	5	63,530
Singapore	81	85	2	10	90,570

Sources: World Health Organization 2018, http://www.who.int/gho/publications/world_health_statistics/2018/en/. Levels & Trends in Child Mortality (Infant Mortality), http://www.childmortality.org/files_v21/download/IGME%20report%202017%20child%20mortality%20final.pdf. World Development Indicators 2017 (Per capita income), http://wdi.worldbank.org/tables.
[1]Infant mortality—deaths per 1,000 live births (2016)
[2]Maternal mortality—deaths per 100,000 live births (2015)

($90,570). As we follow the columns showing mortality rates, we see that as we go up the income ladder, infant and maternal mortality declines and life expectancy increases nearly in lockstep. With a few exceptions, as the average income within a country goes up, the health of the country improves. We note that despite relatively low rates of infant and maternal mortality, the Russian Federation has relatively low life expectancy for both men and women when compared to countries with similar levels of per capita income. These discrepancies suggest the need for more focused research on the reasons these countries deviate from the general pattern linking per capita income with these health indexes.

Finally, we see that, despite having one of the highest per capita income of all those listed, the United States ranks fifth of the five higher-income countries listed for each health indicator. In the following chapters I explore in more depth why the United States consistently ranks so low among developed countries in these core health indicators.

In comparing health statistics among countries with strikingly different levels of development, there is one caveat. These comparative statistics are valid only to the extent that they are gathered in the same way, using standardized methods of measurement. Countries may differ in either their ability or their willingness to gather accurate statistics. For example, Liu and colleagues (1992) looked at the way different countries gather and report infant mortality data. In order for the death of an infant to be seen as contributing to the infant mortality rate, the infant must be born alive. In Western countries this means with a spontaneous heartbeat and other signs of vital organ functioning. However, in a country that has no resources to provide intensive medical care to premature infants, the infant has to survive the first 24 hours of life before being counted as a "live birth." In some countries it has become a matter of policy to count as "live births" only those infants who do survive 24 hours following birth. Similarly, if an infant dies close to their first birthday, in some countries the health care system may not be aware of the death, and as a result the death may not be counted as an infant death. For these and other similar reasons, comparisons of mortality data among countries globally may have some inherent inaccuracies.

Kontis and colleagues (2017) have published an insightful analysis of future trends in life expectancy across 35 industrialized countries through the year 2030. The basic conclusion of this analysis is "that life expectancy will increase in all of these 35 countries with a probability of at least 65% for women and 85% for men, although the increase will vary across countries" (p. 1325). They caution, however, that "projected life expectancy is lower in countries with higher levels of young adult mortality and major chronic disease risk factors, and possibly less effective health systems. These countries also tend to have higher social inequalities, which might lower national life expectancy by affecting the entire population or through the poor health of the worst-off social groups and communities, which in turn affects the national average" (p. 1334). They also predict that by 2030, life expectancy in the United States will fall even further behind other industrialized countries.

Another measurement instrument that is commonly used in assessing health in a global context is the disability-adjusted life year (DALY). DALY provides a means of estimating the magnitude of the burden created by a disease or condition. DALY is based on the concept of potential years of life lost due to certain causes, while also incorporating an estimation of the level of disability attributed to the disease for those who develop the disease but do not die from it. Using a methodology described by the World Health Organization (2018), living one year with a disease that reduces one's level of functioning by 50 percent would mean the loss of 0.50 DALY. Thus, dying five years prematurely would create the loss of the same number of DALYs as living with a disease for 10 years with the loss of 50 percent of one's functional ability. Living 10 years with a 50 percent disability and then dying five years prematurely would mean the loss of 10 DALYs (five DALYs for the effect of the disability when alive, and an additional five DALYs for the premature death).

Table 2.5. Global Impact of Four Major Diseases, by Gender and Age Group, 2001 (Impact measured in thousands of DALYs)

Disease	Age (in years)						Total
	0–4	5–14	15–29	30–44	45–59	60–69	
Diarrhea							
Male	27,878	705	548	587	482	280	30,480
Female	25,682	667	443	420	396	292	27,900
Worm Infection							
Male	229	914	12	8	10	6	1,179
Female	244	890	10	5	7	5	1,161
Tuberculosis							
Male	731	616	4,401	6,990	5,969	2,799	21,506
Female	655	663	3,393	3,760	2,606	1,318	12,395
Ischemic Heart Disease							
Male	104	219	1,070	4,207	14,072	13,452	33,124
Female	75	170	1,022	2,014	6,735	10,077	20,093

Source: World Bank—Global Burden of Disease and Risk Factors (2006), https://openknowledge.worldbank.org/handle/10986/7039.

Table 2.5 provides an example of the manner in which DALYs have been used in a policy context to assess what is referred to as The Global Burden of Disease (GBD), a metric intended to provide "a comprehensive picture of what disables and kills people across countries, time, age, and sex" (Global Burden of Disease 2018). Using data from 2001 gathered by an international group of researchers, it shows the global burden (measured in thousands of DALYs) of four major diseases: diarrhea, worm infection, tuberculosis, and ischemic heart disease. From the table it can be seen that, among children, diarrheal illness inflicts by far the largest health burden globally, affecting primarily young children. While ischemic heart disease places a substantial burden on those over 60 years old, its global impact is comparable to half that of diarrheal illness.

The Global Burden of Disease international research group (GBD 2015 Obesity Collaborators 2017) has also examined a different question pertaining to which risk factors play the largest role in affecting early death rather than the specific causes of death. They note that, "Since 1980, the prevalence of obesity has doubled in more than 70 countries and has continuously increased in most other countries" (p. 13). More than two-thirds of deaths globally that were associated with a high body mass index (BMI) were due to cardiovascular disease. In an editorial that accompanied the GBD article, Gregg and Shaw (2017) voice their concerns over the data showing that "the global obesity epidemic is worsening in most parts of the world and that its implications regarding both physical health and economic health remain ominous" (p. 80). It is interesting to note that among the 20 largest countries globally, the highest rate of death associated with increased BMI was found in Russia. Fortunately, the United States has experienced a flattening in the rate of obesity and associated diabetes over time, presumably as a result of the growing national emphasis on reducing caloric intake (especially in sugared beverages) and increasing levels of physical activity.

Taksler and Rothberg (2017) suggest that it might be valuable from a public health perspective to focus years of life lost from specific illnesses in the United States as well as death rates. They give the example of heart disease as causing the most deaths in the country in 2015, while cancer caused 23 percent more years of life lost than heart disease. They do not incorporate level of disability in their analysis.

The group of researchers from the United States that help to gather and evaluate data for the GBD reports has reported DALYs lost in the United States for the period 1990–2016 (US Burden of Disease Collaborators 2018). In 2016 the three leading causes of loss of DALYs in the United States were ischemic heart disease, lung cancer, and chronic obstructive pulmonary disease. Six individual risk factors account for most of this loss: smoking, high body mass index (BMI), poor diet, alcohol and drug use, high fasting plasma glucose (that is, diabetes), and high blood pressure.

It is interesting to note that the authors were also able to identify a substantial change in risk factors over this time period. "Opioid use disorders moved from the 11th leading cause of DALYs in 1990 to the 7th leading cause in 2016, representing a 74.5% change" (p. 1444). I will address the rising impact of opioid use disorders in the United States in more depth in Chapter 4.

One should not confuse the DALY with another measure, the QALY (quality-adjusted life year). The QALY is commonly used in developed countries as part of cost-effectiveness analysis. Rather than estimating premature death and disability, the QALY is typically used to evaluate the effectiveness of a specific treatment in prolonging the lives of those with specific diseases. It first estimates the number of years a person's life is extended by the treatment, then estimates the health-related quality of life (HRQL) experienced by that person during those additional years. Living an additional year with a 50 percent HRQL constitutes 0.50 QALY; living an additional year with no impairment in HRQL constitutes 1.0 QALY (Miller et al. 2006).

The Relationship between Socioeconomic Status and Health, or, "They Call It 'Poor Health' for a Reason"

In 1997 the *New York Times* published an article by Richard Shweder reporting on his research into the health of the US public. The subtitle for this chapter is taken from the title of that article. Shweder looked at a variety of diseases and conditions, and concluded that "lower-middle-class Americans are more mortal, morbid, symptomatic, and disabled than upper-middle-class Americans. With each little step down on the educational, occupational, and income ladders comes an increased risk of headaches, varicose veins, hypertension, sleepless nights, emotional distress, heart disease, schizophrenia, and an early visit to the grave."

Cardiovascular disease (CVD), which includes both heart disease and stroke, has for many years been the leading cause of death in the United States. In 2018 a group of leading cardiologists nationally published a report on the association between socioeconomic status (SES) and the outcomes of CVD (Schultz et al. 2018). They summarized the known risk factors for developing CVD, which include hypertension, high cholesterol, diabetes, and smoking. As important as each of these factors is, the authors were able to conclude that "Low SES has been linked to the development of CVD and may confer a cardiovascular risk that is equivalent to traditional risk factors. The increased burden of CVD in people with low SES is attributable to a constellation of biological, behavioral, and psychosocial risk factors that are more prevalent in disadvantaged individuals" (p. 2167).

In Chapter 1 we considered the fictional lives of Mimi, the poor seamstress in *La Boheme,* and Hans Castorp, the son of a well-to-do family in *Magic Mountain.* Each had tuberculosis; Mimi died, Hans survived. This pattern has been the same throughout history. When the plague swept through Europe in the Middle Ages, commoners were more likely to die from it than aristocrats. When world wars ravaged the twentieth century, sergeants were more likely than generals to die on the battlefield from wounds and to die in the barracks from a heart attack.

From the Whitehall study discussed in Chapter 1, we saw that blue-collar workers in the British Civil Service are more likely than white-collar workers to die from a variety of causes. The Black Report—a government-financed study that examined the health status of a full range of social classes in England and Wales, using occupation as a marker for social class (London Department of Health and Social Security 1980)—also found consistent differences in health status that were associated with one's position on the hierarchy of occupational status. Both the Black Report and the Whitehall study were in a country that had health care available to all under the British National Health Service. The consistent differences in health status could not be attributed to differences in access to health care.

On October 29, 2012, Hurricane Sandy struck coastal areas of New York, New Jersey, and surrounding areas. The Red Cross reported that 117 people died from the storm. Of those who died, half were over the age of 55, with drowning as the most common cause of death (US Department of Health and Human Services 2013).

We saw similar patterns in 2005, when Hurricane Katrina, characterized by the US Centers for Disease Control and Prevention as "one of the strongest hurricanes to strike the United States during the past 100 years and was likely the nation's costliest natural disaster to date" (US Department of Health and Human Services 2006, p. 240), destroyed much of the city of New Orleans and surrounding areas. Thousands of people were treated for illnesses and injuries caused by the storm, and nearly 1,000 people died (CDC 2006).

Might we expect illnesses and deaths due to natural disasters such as hurricanes to follow the same pattern as tuberculosis in the nineteenth century and the plague throughout history?

Greenough and colleagues (2008) surveyed a random sample of evacuees from Katrina who were staying in Red Cross shelters. They found that, prior to the storm, those being housed at shelters were disproportionately unemployed or underemployed, low-income, unmarried, with chronic medical problems, yet lacking health insurance. Brunkard and colleagues (2008) examined the death records of those who died from the storm in Louisiana, finding half of them to be older than 75, with drowning once again the most common cause of death. While the racial distribution of those who died and those being housed at shelters largely matched the racial distribution of the local population, for those coming from Orleans Parish, the hardest hit section of New Orleans, the death rate of blacks over the age of 18 was consistently higher than for whites, with the black/white ratio for different age groups ranging from 1.7:1 to 4:1.

Heat waves are another form of natural disaster. In July 1995 Chicago and the surrounding areas experienced a severe, intense heat wave. The temperature climbed above 100 degrees and stayed there for several days. The rise in temperature was soon followed by a sharp rise in the number of deaths due either to the heat alone or due to cardiovascular disease made worse by the heat. More than 700 people in Chicago died from heat-related causes.

Semenza and colleagues (1996) reported on a detailed analysis of the nature of the deaths in Chicago that were a result of the heat wave and of the social and demographic characteristics of those who died. They were able to identify a series of factors that were associated with an increased likelihood of dying during the heat wave:

- people with known medical problems who were confined to bed
- people who did not leave home each day
- people who lived alone
- people who lived on the top floor of a building
- people with few regular social contacts
- people with no working air conditioner
- people with no access to transportation
- people who had nailed their windows shut for safety

As we might expect, people with known medical problems who were confined to bed were more likely to die from the heat. We might expect frail elderly people to be more susceptible to the heat. But the pattern does not stop there. Two general categories of risk factor emerge from the analysis.

1. *Those with few social contacts.* Those who lived alone and did not leave home at least daily were more likely to die, as were those with few social contacts with friends and family. (In Chapter 4 we will see evidence that weak social networks are associated with a variety of health risks.)

2. *Those with evidence of low income.* In many neighborhoods in Chicago, in which the buildings are not air-conditioned and many do not have elevators, the rent for apartments on the top floor will be less than for those on lower floors. Those who rent these apartments are also less likely to be able to afford the cost of having their own air conditioner or to have access to their own means of transportation. It should also be clear that those who find it necessary to nail their windows shut for safety will be living in lower-income neighborhoods than those who leave their windows operable (and thus available to create a cooling cross-draft).

In a heat wave, people are more likely to die if they are sick, are poor, and have few social contacts. In a hurricane, similar patterns emerge. As with the infectious diseases from centuries past, those today with lower income or other forms of socioeconomic disadvantage are more likely to die from natural disasters such as heat waves or hurricanes.

Terminology: Socioeconomic Status or Socioeconomic Position?

As reflected in the title of this chapter, I refer to a person's place on the hierarchy of social and economic attainment as their "socioeconomic status." This is a term that has been used commonly by social scientists for quite some time. Nancy Krieger and colleagues have suggested that a more appropriate term to describe this hierarchy might be "socioeconomic position," which they define as "an aggregate measure that includes both resource-based and prestige-based measures . . . [that] refer to individual's rank or status in a social hierarchy" (1997, p. 345). They go on to suggest that "'socioeconomic status' blurs the distinction between two different aspects of socioeconomic position: (a) actual resources, and (b) status, meaning prestige- or rank-related characteristics" (p. 346).

In the literature on health disparities, one commonly encounters both phrases. To explore the differences in the intended meaning of these two terms, I consulted the *Oxford English Dictionary*. The OED defines the word "status" as "social or professional rank, position, or standing; a person's relative importance." It defines "position" as "a person's circumstances, condition, or situation, esp. as affecting his or her influence, role, or power to act."

Both terms seem to reflect common perceptions of a rank-ordered hierarchy. For example, when I was a Boy Scout, I was fully aware that an Eagle Scout was in a position of higher status, that is, higher respect and influence, than was a mere First Class Scout. Does "status" also subsume the level of one's resources, whether economic or otherwise? To me it does. Accordingly, I use the term "socioeconomic status" to refer both to one's access to resources as well as to one's place in a hierarchy of influence and prestige.

What Is Socioeconomic Status? How Should We Measure It?

So far I have been talking principally about the association between income and health status. Those with lower levels of income tend to have lower health status than those who have higher levels of income. I have been using income as a measure of SES. Sometimes I use the income earned by an individual; sometimes, the total income earned by all the people in the household of which the individual is a member.

However, we also saw from the Whitehall study and the Black Report from the United Kingdom that the relative status of one's occupation is also strongly associated with health status over time. For these studies, occupational status was used as a measure of SES. We would certainly expect those with higher-status occupations also to enjoy higher incomes. In fact, the median or average income associated with a certain type of occupation often serves as the metric for assigning the place of an occupation on the scale of occupational status.

Beyond income and occupational status, the level of education one has completed is a third way in which SES is often measured and reported. Those with higher levels of education will typically enjoy better health. By means of example, Montez and Zajacova (2013) looked at the change in mortality rates among white women in the United States between the ages of 45 and 84, comparing women of differing levels of education. They found that mortality rates decreased for college educated women, remained fairly constant for high school graduates without a bachelor's degree, and increased for women who did not graduate from high school. The end result was widening disparities in mortality rates based on education.

While the level of education attained is strongly associated with death rates and other aspects of health inequality, perhaps not surprisingly, those with higher levels of education will also tend to have higher levels of income, and they will tend to occupy occupations with higher levels of occupational status. This association is illustrated in Figure 3.1.

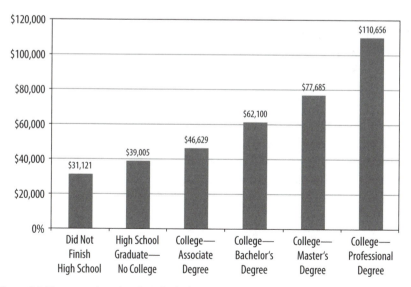

Figure 3.1. Mean annual earnings for individuals in 2017, by highest level of education. *Source*: US Census Bureau, Current Population Survey, 2018.

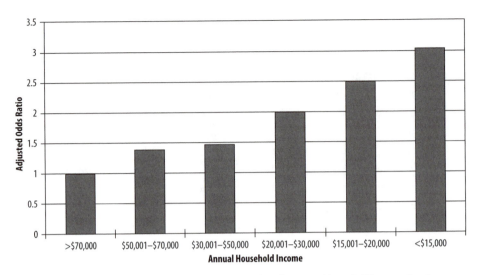

Figure 3.2. Adjusted odds ratio for all-cause mortality, based on annual household income. Data from 1972–89; income is indexed to 1993 dollars. >$70,000 = 1.00. *Source*: Based on McDonough et al. 1997.

Using data for 2017 gathered by the US Census Bureau, we are able to see the median yearly income in the United States for adults aged 25–64 who worked full time, sorted by level of education. With each step up the educational ladder, income goes up. The incremental increase is largest for those with a college degree and various levels of graduate or professional education after college. Thus, we should view income and education as two sides of the same SES coin. Both income and education will in turn be closely associated with occupational status.

McDonough and colleagues (1997) published an earlier analysis of the association between household income and the odds of dying from any cause. Using data from the period 1972–89, they identified a strong stepwise association (Figure 3.2). Using as a point of reference the death rates of those households with an income greater than $70,000 (measured in 1993 dollars), it should be apparent that, for every step down the income ladder, the odds of dying go up.

Rather than looking at the odds of dying, Grol-Prokopczyk (2017) looked at the level of pain experienced by people in the United States in association with SES. The author followed a cohort of people older than 50 for a period of 12 years and found significant stepwise differences in the level of pain experienced, "with pain scores monotonically lower with each categorical increase in education or wealth" (p. 315). The author did not find significant differences in the level of pain experienced among different racial and ethnic groups.

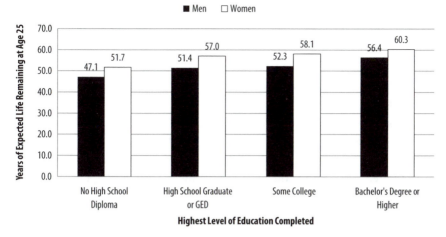

Figure 3.3. Additional life expectancy at age 25, United States 2006, by sex and education level. *Source*: National Center for Health Statistics, Health, United States, 2011.

Using data from 2006, the relationship between education as a measure of SES and the life expectancy at age 25 is illustrated in Figure 3.3. The chart shows how many more years, on average, a 25-year-old man or woman in 2006 could expect to live, based on the highest level of education completed. For those aged 25, each step up the educational ladder brings with it the expectation of additional years of life.

Confirming the association between education, income, and health status, the US Congressional Budget Office (2008) looked at changes in life expectancy in the United States and concluded that overall life expectancy had steadily increased between 1950 and 2004. "Accompanying the recent increases, however, is a growing disparity in life expectancy between individuals with high and low income and between those with more or less education. The difference in life expectancy across socioeconomic groups is significantly larger now than in 1980 or 1990" (p. 1).

Isaacs and Schroeder (2004) published a discussion of these associations in a paper entitled "Class: The Ignored Determinant of the Nation's Health." They note the tremendous advances medicine made over the course of the twentieth century, citing an Institute of Medicine report and stating that "Americans today, as compared with those in 1900, 'are healthier, live longer, and enjoy lives that are less likely to be marked by injuries, ill health, or premature death.'" However, the authors go on to acknowledge that "any celebration of these victories must be tempered by the realization that these gains are not shared fairly by all members of our society. People in upper classes—those who have a good education, hold high-paying jobs, and live in comfortable neighborhoods—live longer and healthier lives than do people in lower classes, many of whom are black or members of ethnic minorities. And the gap is widening" (p. 1137).

In a study of changes in life expectancy and death rates in the United States over the period 1980–2015, Bor et al. (2017) confirmed that the gap between the upper classes and the lower classes has continued to grow. In addition to widening health inequality, the authors also identified widening income inequality over this time period, "driven largely by soaring top incomes . . ." In the face of this growing income inequality, they also found that "the widening of survival inequalities has occurred lower in the distribution—i.e., between the poor and the upper middle class" (p. 1475).

Vega and Sribney (2017) reported similar findings. They reported that 30 years ago, the gap between life expectancy at the lowest quintile of income and the highest was five years. That gap had widened to a current difference of 12 years for men and 14 years for women. In their report, the authors make a very important point about the nature of these inequalities: "It is not income status per se that predisposes to disease; rather, income inequality creates a propensity to disease pathways over the course of human development through environmental exposures and learned behavior in specific social contexts" (p. 1606). A review by Cunningham and colleagues (2018) confirmed that, compared to higher income individuals, lower income individuals, especially those with chronic medical problems, had higher rates of behavioral health problems such as smoking, obesity, and serious psychological stress.

Rather than focusing on income at the level of the individual, Egen and colleagues (2017) assessed the links among poverty, social conditions, and health outcomes at the level of the county. They grouped the 3,141 counties in the United States into groups based on median household income within the county, with each group comprising 2 percent of counties (63 counties per group). They then rank-ordered the 50 groups of counties by income, and compared these groups on several health indices. They found gaps in life expectancy between the best off and the worst off group of 7.1 years for women and 9.5 years for men. They also found differences in several key health indicators between the best off and the worst off groups of counties, with lower high school graduation rates and greater rates of smoking and obesity in the lowest group.

Singh and colleagues (2017) adopted a geographical perspective, comparing changes in health outcomes over the period 1990–2013. They compared outcomes in Appalachia, defined as covering 428 counties in 13 states, based on the definition adopted by the Appalachian Regional Commission, a federal–state partnership. They reported that infant mortality, while not differing substantially between Appalachia and the rest of the United States in 1990–92, was 16 percent higher in Appalachia in 2009–13. Combined life expectancy for men and women increased in both areas, while the gap between them widened. Life expectancy was 0.6 years shorter in Appalachia than in the United States in 1990–92, and widened to a difference of 2.4 years by 2009–13. Perhaps not surprisingly, "smoking-related diseases accounted for more than half of the life-expectancy gap between Appalachia and the rest of the country" (p. 1427). The states of Kentucky and West Virginia had the highest rates of smoking and secondhand smoke exposure in the country.

The association between SES as measured by educational attainment and death rates has been found consistently in studies of other developed countries. Marmot and colleagues (1995) summarized the results of studies done in Hungary, Finland, Denmark, Sweden, and Norway in addition to England and Wales. For all these studies, the age-standardized death rate falls continuously with increasing years of education. Similarly, Semyonov and colleagues (2013) examined the association between wealth (as opposed to income) and health in the United States and in 15 European countries. They found that in all these countries, "rich persons tend to be healthier than poor persons," and that "the positive association between wealth and health holds even after controlling for socio-demographic attributes and household income" (p. 10).

Martinson (2012) made a direct comparison between the United States and England, comparing the income gradient in health across a range of conditions such as diabetes, hypertension, heart disease, and stroke. Despite the fact that the English population exhibits better overall health and has universal health insurance through the British National Health Service, "inequality in health by income was quite similar" in both countries (p. 2054).

Makaroun and colleagues (2017) also compared health in the United States and England. Using wealth rather than income as a measure of SES, they found a consistent pattern in both countries of higher rates of death and disability in the lower quintiles of wealth. This disparity became apparent among individuals 54 years of age and older. The authors "found a more than 100-fold difference in wealth across quintiles," with "the largest difference in mortality . . . found between Q1 and Q2, with minimal difference between Q4 and Q5" (p. 1747). Similar to the findings of the earlier study by Martinson, these authors found no substantial difference in the two countries in the relationship between wealth and either mortality or disability.

They suggested that "One potential explanation for our findings is that poor health outcomes may stem from cumulative long-term stressors throughout life resulting from low wealth, such as unstable housing, exposure to trauma, and susceptibility to drug and alcohol addiction. Our study suggests that the ability of health care to ameliorate these stressors and improve health later in life is modest" (p. 1751).

A study published by Cadar and colleagues (2018) looked at factors associated with increased rates of dementia among elderly individuals in England. They analyzed data from a nationally representative sample of aged 65 or greater who had no signs of dementia at the beginning of the study. The study followed these individuals for up to 12 years, measuring the rate at which signs of dementia began to appear. They found that the risk of developing dementia was 1.68 times greater for those in the lowest quintile of wealth than for individuals in the highest quintile. This association was independent of other factors such as educational attainment, level of deprivation, and other health indicators. In England, as in the United States, wealth appears to be an important aspect of SES with consistent association with health status.

Is Race a Measure of SES Independent of Education, Income, and Occupation?

As we will see in Chapter 6, there is a complex relationship among race, SES, and health. Using data for 2015, Table 3.1 shows age-adjusted death rates in the United States broken down by race and gender. For both men and women, black Americans have death rates that are substantially higher than those of white Americans. The death rate of black men is 21 percent higher than that of white men. For black women the death rate is 13 percent higher than that of white women.

One possible explanation for these disparities in age-adjusted death rates is the level of educational attainment for black and white Americans. Using data gathered between 2003 and 2007, Kaplan and colleagues (2015) report on a study that followed more than 30,000 black and white adults over the age of 45 for six years. They

Table 3.1. US Age-Adjusted Death Rate, by Race and Gender, 2015

	Male	Female
Black	1,040	711
White	862	627

Source: Murphy, S. L., Xu, J., Kochanek, K. D., et al. Deaths: Final Data for 2015. *National Vital Statistics Reports.* November 27, 2017: 66(6), https://www.cdc.gov/nchs/data/nvsr/nvsr66_06.pdf.

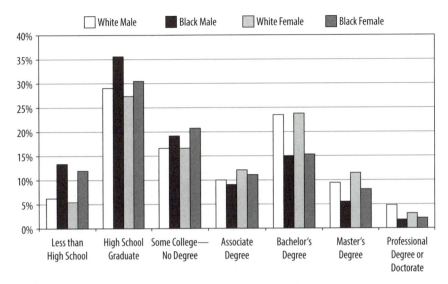

Figure 3.4. Educational attainment of adults 25 years and over, by race and gender, 2017. *Source:* US Census Bureau.

identified "a consistent pattern in the relationship between educational attainment and all-cause mortality in which less educational attainment was associated with higher risk of mortality" (p. 326). After controlling for individual demographic and risk factors, this association between educational attainment and risk of mortality applied equally to black subjects and white subjects with the same level of education.

Figure 3.4 compares the educational attainment of whites and blacks in the United States in 2017, sorted by gender.

From Figure 3.4, we see that blacks in the United States are more likely than whites

- never to graduate from high school
- to graduate from high school but not go on to college

At the other end of the educational spectrum, substantially more whites

- finish college
- obtain a master's degree
- obtain a doctorate or professional degree

With education as a principal measure of SES as well as mortality risk, and lower average educational attainment among blacks as compared to whites, we would expect higher death rates among the black community.

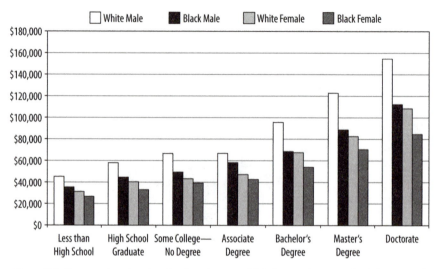

Figure 3.5. Mean earnings by educational attainment of full-time workers age 25–64, by race and gender, 2017. *Source:* US Census Bureau, Current Population Survey.

When we compare the average level of earnings for blacks and whites broken down by educational attainment and by gender, we find that at all levels of educational attainment, black men and women earn lower incomes than white men and women with the same level of education. These data are shown in Figure 3.5.

Even for those who stop with a high school education and for those who never finish high school, white men earn more than black men. In this case we find that educational attainment does indeed predict income, but it does so differently for blacks and whites. This might lead us to ask whether we will also see differences in health status of blacks and whites at the same level of SES.

Using data gathered between 1979 and 1989, Isaacs and Schroeder (2004) identified persistent racial differences in health even when we compare those with similar levels of income (Table 3.2). Using income reported in 1980 dollars, we see a dual relationship:

- Those with lower incomes had higher death rates than those with higher incomes, with the ratio in the death rate of lowest income to highest income ranging from 2.4 to 2.9.
- At a given level of income, blacks died at a higher rate than whites, with the ratio ranging from 1.04 for higher-income men to 1.65–1.67 in lower- and middle-income women.

Table 3.2. Average Annual Age-Adjusted Rates of Death from Heart Disease among Persons 25 to 64 Years Old, 1979–89

	Men			Women		
Annual Income	White	Black	Ratio of Black Men to White Men	White	Black	Ratio of Black Women to White Women
	No. of deaths / 100,000 person-years					
<$10,000	324.1	390.8	1.21	112.2	184.7	1.65
$10,000–$14,999	255.4	292.8	1.15	71.3	119.2	1.67
$15,000–$24,999	136.9	142.2	1.04	43.7	64.8	1.48
Ratio of lowest to highest income	2.4	2.7	—	2.6	2.9	—

Source: S. L. Isaacs and S. A. Schroeder, "Class: The Ignored Determinant of the Nation's Health," *New England Journal of Medicine* 351(11): 1137–42. Copyright © 2004 Massachusetts Medical Society. All rights reserved. Reprinted with permission.
Note: Data on income ranges (in 1980 dollars) and ratios of black men to white men and black women to white women are from Williams 2001, p. 69.

(Note: To compare 1980 dollars with more current data: in 1980 the median household income in the United States was $17,710; in 2017 it was $61,372.)

Developing a Model of the Various Measures of SES

It may be useful at this point to summarize our understanding of the association between SES and health. So far we have determined:

- The association between SES and health is not due to a threshold effect, with all those above the threshold enjoying equal levels of health. Rather, the association between SES and health appears to be continuous, with health status increasing with each increment in SES.
- The association between SES and health has to do with more than simply a person's position in the hierarchy of income distribution. That association reflects multiple forms of the social hierarchy, including the hierarchies of education and occupation, and possibly an additional hierarchy of race.

Lynch and von Hippel (2016) have reviewed these issues, asking, "Does higher education improve health (causation)? Do the healthy become highly educated (selection)? Or do good health and high educational attainment both result from advantages established early in the life course (confounding)?" (p. 18).

It is important to keep in mind a fundamental principle of statistical analysis. For any two variables (let us call them *a* and *b*), stating that "*a* is associated with *b*" does not in itself prove that "*a* is the cause of *b*." There are three possible explanations for this association:

- *a* is the cause of *b* (often illustrated as *a* → *b*)
- *b* is the cause of *a* (often illustrated as *b* → *a*)
- Some missing third factor is the cause of both *a* and *b*, often illustrated as:

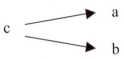

It is possible to consider various possibilities for the missing third factor *c* in this model. These include time preference, self-efficiency, and social anomie and a loss of trust in society.

Time Preference

It is possible that one's position in the hierarchy of a social system leads to an individual's having a sense of time preference that differs from the time preference of others in a different position. To be successful in obtaining an education, especially an education that includes a college or graduate degree, one must be willing to postpone the payoff for one's investment of time and effort. Similarly, to take seriously the warnings of the dangerous health outcomes caused by smoking cigarettes, one must have a clear perception that it is worthwhile to forgo the immediate satisfaction gained by smoking to avoid the health consequences that will likely not appear for years, if not decades. Those who find it difficult to forgo satisfaction in the present in order to obtain even greater satisfaction in the future may also find it difficult to stop smoking or to persist in their education.

Mischel and colleagues (1988) and Shoda and colleagues (1990) demonstrated the effects of differences in time preference and the ability to delay gratification in a study of four- and five-year-olds from a reasonably affluent university community. These children were shown two possible reward objects—for example, a plate with one marshmallow and a second plate with two marshmallows—and were asked which they preferred. Not surprisingly, most children preferred two marshmallows to one. The children were then told that they could have the preferred reward, so long as they would wait while the researcher stepped outside of the room for a while, with the promise of returning soon. However, the children were also given the option of ringing a bell, which would bring the researcher back into the room right away. The reward system was fairly straightforward. If the children waited for the researcher to return without ringing the bell, they would get the two marshmallows. If they rang the bell to bring the researcher back sooner, the children would get one marshmallow.

Some children were able to wait for the researcher to return, thus gaining the increased reward by delaying that reward. Others found that too difficult, and chose instead to accept the smaller reward without the required wait. Some were able to delay gratification in return for a greater reward; others had difficulty delaying gratification.

The fascinating part of this study came several years later, when the researchers tracked these study subjects into adolescence. They compared the two groups of children—the delayed gratifiers with the immediate gratifiers—on a number of scales that might predict future SES. They found consistent differences, in that the delayed gratifiers as adolescents demonstrated better academic and cognitive abilities, better verbal fluency, better ability to plan and attend to detail, and a better ability to deal with frustration and stress. As described in a *New York Times* op-ed about these studies,

> The children who waited longer went on to get higher SAT scores. They got into better colleges and had, on average, better adult outcomes. The children who rang the bell quickest were more likely to become bullies. They received worse teacher and parental evaluations 10 years on and were more likely to have drug problems at age 32. . . . The Mischel experiments, along with everyday experience, tell us that self-control is essential. Young people who can delay gratification can sit through sometimes boring classes to get a degree. They can perform rote tasks in order to, say, master a language. They can avoid drugs and alcohol. (Brooks 2006)

Psychologists have delved more deeply into the issue of time perspective. Zimbardo and Boyd (1999) were able to assess a person's time perspective based on their answers to a series of questions. They identified forms an individual's time perspective might take, including:

- Future—"characterized by planning for and achievement of future goals . . . with consideration of future consequences, conscientiousness, preference for consistency, and reward dependence, along with low levels of novelty and sensation seeking"
- Present—Fatalistic—"reveals a belief that the future is predestined and uninfluenced by individual actions, whereas the present must be borne with resignation because humans are at the whimsical mercy of 'fate'"

- Present—Hedonistic—"orientation toward present enjoyment, pleasure, and excitement, without sacrifices today for rewards tomorrow . . . a lack of consideration of future consequences . . . low ego or impulse control"

Zimbardo and Boyd used these scales in a study of more than 500 college students in California, and were able to determine a series of significant correlations between their scales of time perspective and an individual's personal characteristics and academic performance. Students who demonstrated a "Future" perspective had higher grades in college and spent more hours per week studying. They were also less likely to exhibit aggressive tendencies or to lack impulse control. By contrast, those students who demonstrated a "Present—Fatalistic" perspective showed more aggression and more impulsive behavior, and had lower grades.

These results are strikingly similar to the results of the Mischel study, when they followed their subjects into high school. Might it be that, at the age of four, children have already adopted their own perspective on time, and that this time perspective stays with them as they enter and subsequently move through school?

Will the time perspective adopted in childhood persist into the adult years? In 2009, Guthrie and colleagues used the Zimbardo scales of "Time Perspective" in a study of more than 500 adults recruited from hair salons and barber shops in a suburb of Washington, DC. They found that those adults who exhibited a "Future" perspective tended to be more highly educated, and as a consequence more likely to be in a professional occupation. By contrast, those with a "Present—Fatalistic" perspective had the reverse—tending to be less educated and less likely to be in a professional occupation. They did not find an association between the "Present—Hedonistic" perspective on either education or occupation.

Time perspective, whether measured as a child, as a college student, or as an adult, seems to be an important predictor of educational and occupational attainment. We know also that these outcomes are strongly associated with one's health status as an adult.

Self-Efficiency

Based on differences in childhood experience and family dynamics, some individuals may grow into adulthood with strikingly different perceptions of their own ability to direct their own life and influence their own existence. If a person has a sense that they are free to choose from alternative actions and is principally responsible for their own successes and failures, it may be much easier to pursue long-term goals such as higher education. By contrast, a person who has developed the sense that their life will be directed by forces outside their control may be more likely to approach choices as if they were up to luck or fate, and correspondingly may be less likely to invest in longer-term outcomes such as education or the positive health consequences of avoiding harmful behavior such as smoking. Recall from Chapter 2 that I distinguished between attaching responsibility to an individual for his unhealthy behaviors and attaching blame. Blame carries with it the connotation of personal weakness and failure. If a person has never developed the sense that they are actually in charge of their own life, it would not be appropriate to assign to them the negative connotations of blame for unhealthy behaviors that they may view as out of their own control.

Social Anomie and a Loss of Trust in Society

Sociologist Emile Durkheim (1897) spoke of the deleterious effects that develop when an individual loses faith that the norms of the society in which they live will treat them fairly and equally with others. When society appears to hold out one normative message, yet reacts with another, an individual may come to distrust society and its system of norms. In the face of a loss of normative faith, one tends to become isolated and alienated from the norms of society. In the face of such "social anomie," it may be extremely difficult for a person born into a position of disadvantage (whether it be economic, social, or racial) to adhere to the behaviors identified by the norms of that society as leading to healthy outcomes.

Taking a step back from the individual associations of income, education, occupation, and race with health status, it is possible to envision a relationship in which all of these markers of SES are in turn caused by being born into and/or growing up in a position of general social disadvantage. It is being a member of this disadvantaged "class" that makes one substantially more likely to experience the sense of isolation, powerlessness, alienation, and foreshortened time preference that leads directly to lower levels of education, with resultant lower occupational status and lower income. Graham (2004) refers to this causal cascade as the "social determinants of health" (Figure 3.6).

Understanding the Nature of a Social Hierarchy

In the preceding section I considered the possibility that a missing factor caused individuals to have both low SES and poor health. I then considered certain psychological and behavioral characteristics that may devolve over time as a result of a person being born into or growing up in a position of relatively low social position.

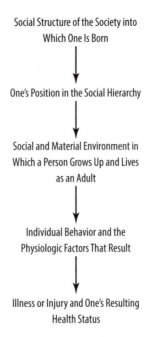

Social Structure of the Society into
Which One Is Born

One's Position in the Social Hierarchy

Social and Material Environment in
Which a Person Grows Up and Lives
as an Adult

Individual Behavior and the
Physiologic Factors That Result

Illness or Injury and One's Resulting
Health Status

Figure 3.6. The causal cascade of the social determinants of health. *Source*: Based on Graham 2004.

It is the long-term effects of occupying a low position in the overall social hierarchy that eventually leads both to low SES and to poor health outcomes. In addition, this association between social position and social outcomes is a continuous one that spans all levels of social status. Marmot and colleagues (1995) described research that illustrates these points. They looked at the mortality rate of men in England and Wales for the period 1976–81. Recognizing the differing rates of death within different age groups, they separated the men into three age groups: 15–64, 65–74, and 75 or older. They then considered the following characteristics of the men under study:

- Did they own a car?
- Did they own their dwelling or rent it?
- Did their principal occupation involve nonmanual labor or manual labor?

Within each age group they broke their subjects down sequentially by these three dichotomies. They first divided the subjects by car ownership: owning a car or not owning a car. They then broke each of these groups down by type of housing: owner-occupied or rental. These groups were further broken down by type of occupation: nonmanual or manual. The authors then graphed the mortality rate for these men according to which of the eight possible groups they fell into. They found a consistent pattern:

- Those who owned a car had lower rates of mortality than those who did not own a car.
- Within both categories of car ownership, those who owned their home had lower mortality than those who rented their home.
- Within both categories of car ownership, and further within both categories of home ownership, those with nonmanual occupations had lower mortality than those with manual occupations.

Mortality rates generally increased in stepwise fashion from those who owned a car, owned their home, and worked in a nonmanual occupation (with the lowest mortality) to those who did not own a car, rented their home, and worked in a manual occupation (with the highest mortality).

Each of the three dichotomies in this study describes a position of social advantage/disadvantage. The study illustrates the following principle: the more forms of social advantage a person has, the lower the chances of death over time.

If having several markers of low status is associated with poor health, does it matter how long one experiences the resulting social disadvantage? Will those who are able to move out of a position of disadvantage over time have better health than those who remain disadvantaged over time? This was the question addressed by a long-term study conducted not in England and Wales, but in Alameda County, situated in California across the bay from San Francisco. Alameda County has some sections that are quite well-to-do and other sections that have high concentrations of poverty and inadequate housing.

The Alameda County study is one of the longest running health studies that has followed a single cohort of subjects over time. It initially gathered data on nearly 7,000 adults who were representative of the overall population of the county. There have been numerous publications from the study describing a wide range of psychological and behavioral factors and measuring health outcomes in terms of both death rates and a range of other measures of illness and disability.

Lynch and colleagues (1997) looked at the health histories of nearly 1,100 adults who had been followed from 1965 through 1994. In 1994 the median age of these subjects was 65 years. The authors recorded the subjects' reported income at three times—1965, 1974, and 1983—determining whether that income fell below or above a figure that represented twice the federal poverty line.

The federal government publishes annually the amount of money a family of a given size requires each year to pay for the basic necessities such as food, clothing,

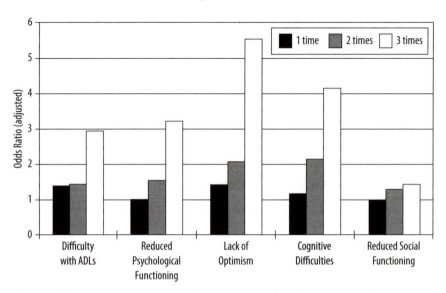

Figure 3.7. Effect of sustained poverty on odds of reporting health problems. Shows odds ratio based on the number of times subjects reported being in poverty. *Source*: Based on Lynch et al. 1997.

and shelter. Those who fall below this poverty line are officially deemed to be living in poverty. Those with incomes marginally above this poverty level are not impoverished, but are in a position of relatively low income. Thus, those with up to twice the poverty line in the study group include working individuals and families as well as poor individuals and families. However, all are in a position of relative economic disadvantage described by the authors as "economic hardship." The authors measured how many times over the study period subjects reported experiencing this economic hardship. The maximum number of times was three. They then compared a variety of health measures for those reporting economic hardship one, two, or three times to those never reporting economic hardship. The results are shown in Figure 3.7.

Those reporting economic hardship only once during the 18-year study period had health outcomes that were nearly identical to those never experiencing economic hardship (shown as an odds ratio of 1 in the vertical axis). For those reporting two episodes of hardship, the odds of experiencing poor health outcomes were up to two times greater than those of people with no experience of hardship. For those reporting three episodes of economic hardship, suggesting that they had experienced continuous hardship for 18 years, the odds of experiencing a poor health outcome were typically three to five times greater than for those with no hardship. Not only does economic hardship expose one to the risk of poor health outcomes, but also the longer one is in a disadvantaged economic state, the greater one's chances of having a poor health outcome.

Frank and colleagues (2003) reported on a fourth follow-up episode for the Alameda County study. They examined data from subjects responding in all four surveys between 1965 and 1994, focusing on the presence of the following conditions:

- high blood pressure
- perceived health
- depression
- heart trouble
- trouble breathing
- trouble feeding
- sick days

The authors found substantial consistency in the pattern of the data. They sorted subjects according to which percentile of family income they fell into in 1965. Using this rank ordering of individual subjects by income, they then compared subjects on the percentage reporting one of the above problems. To rule out gender effects, they examined this relationship between baseline income percentile and health outcomes separately for men and women.

There is a consistent downward gradient for the relationship between income percentile and the percentage reporting poor or fair health. For women this association is nearly linear, while for men it is somewhat curvilinear. The same general pattern is true for all of the outcomes studied. In Alameda County, California, the lower the income you start with and the longer you face the social disadvantage coincident with economic hardship, the worse your health will be on a variety of different measures that capture all three general aspects of health as discussed in Chapter 2.

One can look at any of the major causes of death in the United States and find similar social gradients in mortality rates, including:

- lung cancer
- other cancers
- coronary heart disease
- strokes
- other cardiovascular disease
- chronic bronchitis and other respiratory disease
- gastrointestinal disease
- genitourinary disease
- accidents and violence

Galea and colleagues (2011) reviewed nearly 30 years of published research addressing how various forms of social inequality are associated with increased rates of illness and mortality. Using a mathematical model they developed based on this research, they estimated the number of deaths that take place each year in the United States that are attributable to social factors such as these. Of the approximately 2.3 million deaths that occurred in 2000 in the United States, they reported that approximately 873,000 (38%) were due to the effects of various forms of social inequality, principally low levels of education, residential racial segregation, poverty, and low levels of social support.

As summarized by Frank and colleagues, "Among health researchers, there is widespread consensus that 'something' about SES, as indicated by readily available markers such as income or education, is a fundamental determinant of human health. But there is no agreement on what that something is. However, the shape of SES-health gradients may hold clues as to the key mechanisms by which gradients are created and maintained over the life-course" (p. 2306). They go on to suggest two broad categories of factors, each of which is a core aspect of overall social structure that may be this "something." These are:

1. material deprivation
2. the perception of relatively less privilege, which then may lead to "psycho-neuro-endocrinological/immunological cascades" that have clinical health effects

In Chapter 4, I examine both possible factors and the mechanisms through which they may work in affecting health.

The Association of Transition among SES Categories and Health Outcomes

Until now I have been speaking of SES as if it were fixed, with little opportunity for an individual or a family to transition up or down the SES spectrum over time. This, of course, is not an accurate reflection of American society. One of the core historical values of American culture has been the opportunity, often through education, for someone from a lower stratum of SES to be able to move into a higher stratum.

Similarly, it is possible for one to move down the SES ladder. Often illness or disability will impair one's ability to function at a high level, and over time one's SES may decline. Given the opportunity to move up in SES, or to move down, how would we expect such transitions to affect health status? If they do indeed affect health status, will the effect of a transition up be similar in magnitude to a transition down?

Pensola and Martikainen (2003) addressed this question in a study of more than 110,000 men born in Finland between 1956 and 1960. They followed these men, recording how many of them died as young adults during the period 1991–98. They placed each subject in the study in one of two SES categories at the time of their birth and again at the time of their death. The SES at birth was determined by whether the head of the child's household at the time of birth was engaged in a manual labor occupation (lower SES) or a nonmanual labor occupation (higher SES). The SES in the 1991–98 study period was determined by the occupation of the subject himself, using the same SES dichotomy. Occupational data were obtained from the Finnish census.

Thus, these subjects could fall into one of three categories:

1. The subject was low SES at both birth and as an adult.
2. The subject was high SES at both birth and as an adult.
3. The subject had changed SES categories between birth and adulthood.

This third category could be further subdivided into

3a. Those who were low SES at birth and high SES as an adult.
3b. Those who were high SES at birth and low SES as an adult.

The researchers found that the mortality rate is nearly three times as high for the men born into lower SES and remaining in lower SES, when compared to men who were born into and remained in higher SES. By contrast, the mortality rate for those men who transitioned from one SES category to another between childhood and adulthood had a mortality rate that was midway between the rates for the constant SES categories.

These findings mirror those from the Alameda County study, described above. The longer one stays in a lower SES position, the more that person's health declines. This study is able to address a question the Alameda County study did not. Are the health effects different if you transition over time from low SES to high SES, as compared to transitioning from high SES to low SES? Among those subjects experiencing a transition between SES groups, substantially more subjects experienced an upward transition between childhood and adulthood than experienced a downward transition. Those who made the upward transition had a mortality rate as young adults that was nearly as low as the rate for those who were both born into and remained in the high SES category. By contrast, those who were born into high SES but ended in low SES as adults had a mortality rate that was indistinguishable from that experienced by those who both were born into and remained in low SES. Thus, these data suggest the following:

- Those who remain in a low SES category between birth and adulthood will have substantially worse health as adults than those who are born into and remain in a high SES category.
- For those who transition between SES categories, the SES into which they were born and spent their childhood has less predictive power for their health as an adult than does their SES category as an adult.

The Social Roots of Health Inequality: "The Status Syndrome"

In this chapter we have seen that SES is associated with health across the full spectrum of SES—from the least well-off to the most well-off. SES can be approached in a variety of ways, but the association with health status seems fairly constant. A person can improve their chances of enjoying better health by moving up the SES ladder through education, but the longer one remains in a position of disadvantaged SES, the worse one's health tends to be. In addition, there seems to be a lingering effect on health of the SES circumstances into which one is born and spends one's childhood.

We can appreciate how growing up under impoverished circumstances will lead to a deterioration of health over time. Crowding, inadequate sanitation, and nutritional shortages all weaken the body and contribute to illness. How, though, are we to explain why a fully employed administrative worker tends to have better health than a fully employed professional worker? Or, in the words of Michael Marmot, "Why should someone with a master's degree have a longer life expectancy than someone with a bachelor's?" He offers the following explanation: "Socioeconomic differences in health are not confined to poor health for those at the bottom and good health for everyone else. Rather, there is a social gradient in health in individuals who are not poor: the higher the social position, the better the health. I have labeled this 'the status syndrome'" (Marmot 2006, p. 1304).

Marmot has written further about this syndrome: "For people above a threshold of material well-being, another kind of well-being is central. Autonomy—how much control you have over your life—and the opportunities you have for full social engagement and participation are crucial for health, well-being, and longevity. It is inequality in these that plays a big part in producing the social gradients in health. Degrees of control and participation underlie the status syndrome" (Marmot 2004, p. 2).

How does social status in its many forms impact health across the life course and across the spectrum of status? Developing an understanding of the possible mechanisms that explain this relationship is key to understanding the social roots of health disparities. We have identified as an important contributor the material benefits that go along with increasing social status, such as sanitation and nutrition. However, it is difficult to see how better material benefits might explain health differences for those at the upper ends of the SES distribution who have more than adequate material comforts. Alternative explanations include individual behaviors. Differences in time preferences and the ability to delay gratification may explain such things as the striking gradients we see in the rate of cigarette smoking across social strata. We might also expect differences in the physical environment that follow the social status hierarchy also to contribute to health disparities. Those who live in more crowded conditions may also be exposed to more environmental pollutants over time, with resultant health effects.

What, though, about Marmot's suggestion that there may be important psychological differences that track social status? Might there be psychological effects of living in a higher- (or lower-) status condition, such as perceptions of autonomy and control, which will also affect health over time? These are the questions I address in the following chapter, in which I attempt to build a theoretical model of the many ways that being in a disadvantaged social position, whether it be socioeconomic, socioenvironmental, or sociopsychological, can affect health over one's lifetime.

CHAPTER FOUR

Understanding How Low Social Status Leads to Poor Health

As we have seen, there is substantial evidence that one's position in the social hierarchy is strongly associated with one's health over time. Those lower in the hierarchy experience on average more illness, more disability, and a shorter life span. This phenomenon of a social hierarchy of health exists across the entire spectrum of SES, from the least well-off to the most well-off.

Were the data to suggest that the association between SES and health were a threshold phenomenon (see Chapter 1 for a description of the threshold model of health status), we might look to material disadvantages associated with poverty that lead to poor health. However, SES and health do not follow the threshold model. Whatever leads to the association between social status and health exists across all levels of social and socioeconomic status.

There has been substantial research in recent years that suggests a possible source for the poor health that is associated with a position of social disadvantage. This factor is what Goode (2002b) described as "the heavy cost of chronic stress." Goode describes the effects on the human body of facing chronic levels of stress: "Prolonged or severe stress has been shown to weaken the immune system, strain the heart, damage memory cells in the brain and deposit fat at the waist rather than the hips and buttocks (a risk factor for heart disease, cancer and other illnesses) . . . stress may be a thread tying together many illnesses that were previously thought to be unrelated."

The human body has evolved a complex yet effective system for responding to stress. This system works best when stress comes in well-defined increments. Getting ready for a meeting or studying for a final exam (or, for that matter, writing a book manuscript) can each be a very stressful experience. Our bodies are able to mobilize energy reserves to help us complete the task more quickly and more effectively. Once the task has been completed and the stress level is reduced, our bodies return to their resting state and recharge their physiological reserves.

For some people, though, the stress they face is ongoing. Stress becomes a part of their everyday existence. The bodies of these people are able—at least initially—to mobilize their physiological reserves in response to stress. But for these people, the stress level never fully goes away, and as a result their bodies never get a chance to recharge. Eventually, their stress response system becomes weakened, with two effects:

1. They are less effective at responding to stress when it comes.
2. They are less able to respond to the stress of illness or injury, due to weakened immune systems.

Goode (2002b) describes the origins of this chronic stress effect in the following terms: "perhaps the best indicator of how people are likely to be affected by stress is their position in the social hierarchy."

The Physiological Response to Stress: The Hypothalamic-Pituitary-Adrenal Axis

To understand how stress exerts its effects on humans, we must first grasp the basic principles of the body's stress control mechanism. (It is not necessary to have taken a course in biology to understand this mechanism.) There are two basic parts to it:

1. the brain as the body's monitoring and control mechanism
2. the adrenal gland as the source of stress response hormones

The Brain: Sensing Stress and Turning on the Stress Response System

We often think of the human brain as the center of conscious thought and reasoning. The brain has functions that are equally important but that operate on an unconscious level. It is no accident that our body's temperature is maintained at approximately 37 degrees Centigrade (98.6 degrees Fahrenheit). In much the same way that a building's heating system uses a thermostat to turn the heater or air conditioner on and off so as to maintain a constant temperature, the body has a thermostat in the unconscious portion of the brain that monitors and maintains a constant body temperature (thermostasis). The part of the brain that performs this thermostatic function is the hypothalamus.

The hypothalamus has important functions in addition to thermostasis. One of the most important of these is monitoring and responding to stress, or allostasis (McEwen and Seeman 1999). The brain is able to detect stress in ways that are both conscious and unconscious. If a person becomes consciously aware of an immediate threat or danger, that conscious message is carried to the hypothalamus. In addition, there are the effects of psychological stress in all its many forms that trigger a stress response in the hypothalamus, which may not always lead to a conscious awareness of stress.

Once the hypothalamus senses stress, it sends a message over nerve pathways in the brain to the brain's relay center—the pituitary gland. The pituitary, situated at the base of the brain, accepts incoming messages from the brain and converts them to hormones, which it secretes into the bloodstream. Each of these hormones targets a specific part of the body, instructing it to "turn on" or "turn off." In the case of stress response hormones, the part of the body that is targeted is the adrenal gland.

The Adrenal Gland: Responding to Stress by Releasing Hormones

The adrenal gland is situated adjacent to the kidney on each side of the body. When it receives a message from the pituitary gland to "turn on" it immediately pumps into the bloodstream hormones it has stored up for just such an occasion. Two of these are epinephrine and norepinephrine (often referred to by their common names, adrenalin and noradrenalin). We all are familiar with the "adrenalin rush" we experience when we are startled or otherwise suddenly aroused. Our heart starts beating faster and harder, and we breathe more deeply. As often described in science classes, our muscles become ready for "fight or flight."

The adrenal gland produces another hormone that is equally important—cortisol (commonly referred to as cortisone). Cortisol is slower to kick in, but also slower to turn off. After the immediate assist of epinephrine and norepinephrine, cortisol helps our body to function more efficiently over the longer term. (Cortisol is also an important part of our body's circadian rhythm, or internal time clock.) After the stressful experience has been resolved, the increased levels of cortisol will once again revert to the prestress level.

This combined control mechanism involving sensing stress in the hypothalamus, sending control hormones from the pituitary that result in the release of epinephrine, norepinephrine, and cortisol from the adrenal gland, is often referred to as the hypothalamic-pituitary-adrenal axis (HPA). The level at which this allostatic control mechanism is functioning is referred to as the allostatic load. The higher the level of stress response hormones circulating in the blood, the higher the allostatic load. This mechanism is illustrated in Figure 4.1.

As described above, the normal stress response involves the body's allostatic load being maintained at a baseline state of readiness. Soon after the hypothalamus perceives stress, the allostatic load begins to rise. There tends to be a maximum level

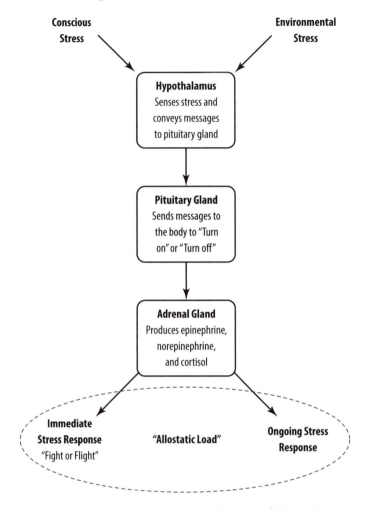

Figure 4.1. The hypothalamic-pituitary-adrenal axis and the control of allostatic load.

of allostatic load a body can attain. When a body has attained this maximum load response, the allostatic load plateaus for a while. Once the stressful event is over, the allostatic load returns to normal. This resolution phase takes somewhat more time than the rapid response phase. After resolution, the body "recharges" the adrenal gland, storing up sufficient quantities of stress response hormones for the next stress experience.

Imagine, though, that before the allostatic load has a chance to return to its baseline level, another stressor is sensed by the hypothalamus. The allostatic load will once again increase to the plateau level. Should the perception of stressors be

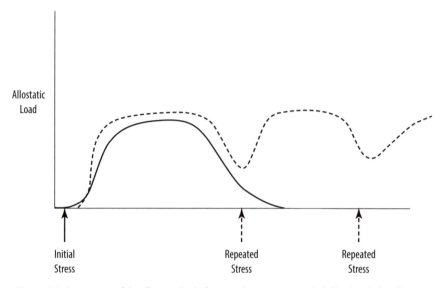

Figure 4.2. Comparison of the allostatic load of a normal stress response (solid line) with the allostatic load of a repeated stress response (dashed line).

ongoing, the allostatic load will not have the chance ever to fully recharge, and the adrenal gland will be producing an ongoing stream of stress response hormones. The body will experience chronic elevation in its allostatic load. This phenomenon is illustrated in Figure 4.2. A person experiencing repeated stressors, without the opportunity for intervals that are relatively stress-free, will experience a chronically elevated allostatic load, with higher than normal levels of circulating stress response hormones.

The Physiological Effects of Chronically Elevated Allostatic Load

Chronic elevation of cortisol and the other hormones of the allostatic stress response have been shown to trigger inflammation in cells through the release of chemicals called inflammatory cytokines (Miller et al. 2009; Cohen et al. 2012). Chronic inflammation within a cell in turn leads to the release of certain biochemical markers of cellular injury. Perhaps the most important of the types of cells adversely affected in this way are the cells that line the inside of the arteries and smaller arterioles that distribute blood throughout the body. This inflammation can cause injury to these vascular cells, which can then lead to scarring within the cell and the formation of calcium deposits. Once the scarring and calcium deposits have

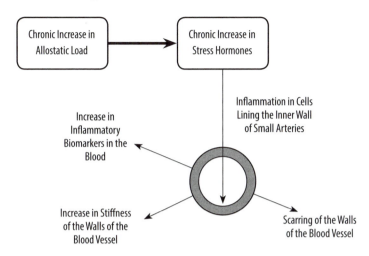

Figure 4.3. The physiologic injury caused by chronically elevated allostatic load.

occurred, the lining of the vessel itself can become thickened and stiffened, leading to narrowing of the internal lumen of the vessel. This process is illustrated in Figure 4.3.

There are several important biochemical compounds, often referred to as biomarkers that have been shown to provide a measure of the cellular injury associated with this chronic inflammation. A major biomarker is referred to as C-Reactive Protein (CRP). A broad coalition of researchers based at Cambridge University in England has summarized the role of CRP in cardiovascular disease (Emerging Risk Factors Collaboration 2012). Reviewing data from 52 separate studies, they found that elevated CRP levels were highly predictive of future cardiovascular disease such as heart attacks and stroke. Elevated levels of CRP were also associated with concurrent elevation in a second biomarker, fibrinogen, a protein that is part of the process by which blood clots and scar tissue form. Increased levels of fibrinogen in the cells lining the arterial circulation can lead to both thickening and stiffening of the interior layers of the arteries (often referred to as intima-media thickness, or IMT).

The Framingham Heart Study has been following patterns of heart disease in community-based cohorts in Massachusetts since 1948. Researchers looked at the offspring (average age 61) of the original study cohort to determine if there was a relationship between the socioeconomic position (SEP) experienced by these individuals throughout their lives and the level of these biomarkers in their blood (Loucks et al. 2010). They found "evidence that cumulative life course SEP is inversely associated with many inflammatory markers including CRP . . . and fibrinogen" (p. 191). They also noted a strong association between these biomarkers and risky health behaviors such as smoking, body mass index, high blood pressure, and high cholesterol. Perhaps not surprisingly, they also found that lower cumulative SEP was associated with a higher risk of developing coronary heart disease such as a heart attack or heart failure (Loucks et al. 2009).

The Women's Health Study has been following a nationally representative sample of female health professionals in the United States, all of whom were aged 38 or older and free of heart disease and cancer when the study was initiated between 1993 and 1996. Using blood samples from the women enrolled in the study, researchers looked at the state-level variations in biomarkers such as CRP and fibrinogen and death from cardiovascular disease. They found a consistent association between the average levels of these biomarkers within a state and the cardiovascular death rate within that state (Clark et al. 2011).

A third biomarker that contributes to this process is a biochemical substance called interleukin-6 (IL-6). IL-6 is one of a group of molecules referred to as inflammatory cytokines that increase cellular inflammation throughout the body, in particular in the cells lining blood vessels. By triggering inflammation in the cells lining arteries, IL-6 leads to the deposition of fibrinogen, with associated scarring and thickening of the IMT. Yudkin and colleagues (2000) were able to identify an association between IL-6 and CRP, suggesting that chronically elevated levels of psychological stress could trigger the release of both markers.

Johnson and colleagues (2017) conducted a systematic review of articles that studied biomarkers associated with chronic elevation in allostatic load. Among the 26 articles they identified that studied these associations, they found that the three biomarkers most often used were CRP, fibrinogen, and IL-6. For each of these three markers, they found a negative association between socioeconomic position and allostatic load in all but three of the articles.

Chronic elevation in CRP and fibrinogen, especially in the arteries supplying the heart, has been associated with a fourth biomarker, coronary artery calcium (CAC). The scarring of the lining of blood vessels associated with elevated CRP and fibrinogen will often lead to the deposition of calcium in these cells. Using computed tomographic (CT) scans of the heart, it is possible to measure the amount of calcium that has been deposited in the coronary arteries—the arteries providing blood supply to the heart muscle itself. A study of a population-based sample of nearly 7,000 men and women between the ages of 45 and 84, all of whom were initially free of heart disease, administered a CT scan to all subjects when the study was initiated between the years 2000 and 2002 (Detrano et al. 2008). They then compared the amount of CAC identified on these initial scans, and the frequency with which subjects experienced cardiovascular disease in the three- to five-year follow-up period. They found the initial CAC score to be "a strong predictor of incident coronary heart disease" (p. 1336). A subsequent analysis of the same study population concluded that adding the CAC score to the traditional model of risk factors for heart disease significantly improved that model (Polonsky et al. 2010). Although routine screening for elevated CAC is not recommended as part of preventive care, elevated levels should be seen as an indicator of elevated risk that warrants lifestyle modification and close attention to other risk factors such as blood pressure, cholesterol, and smoking (Grayburn 2012).

Yan and colleagues (2006) used repeated CT scans to measure CAC in the arteries of nearly 3,000 patients over a period of 15 years. The researchers compared the subjects according to the level of education they had completed, performing separate analyses for black and white subjects, and for men and women. They found the familiar pattern of stepwise reduction in damage to the heart, based on the education one has completed, from "less than High School" through "more than College." Each educational category showed fewer calcium deposits in the heart than the category below it, with the lowest educational category having the highest buildup of calcium over the 15-year period of the study. Cumulative damage to the tissue of the heart followed educational attainment very closely.

Stress in the Workplace, Hypertension, and the Whitehall Study

Elevated blood pressure (hypertension) is strongly associated with increased rates of heart attacks, stroke, kidney disease, and other illnesses. Maintaining a normal blood pressure during one's adult years is essential to maintaining one's long-term health. Rehkopf and colleagues (2017) reported on the efforts of a major US corporation to determine the extent to which stress experienced in the workplace environment contributes to rates of hypertension. They were able to analyze data from 6,535 individual workers from 24 different manufacturing plants. In addition to measuring a worker's blood pressure while at work, they also gathered data on the demographics and early life experiences of the workers. They then evaluated workers' reports of the level of physical, psychological, and social stress experienced while at work, and the extent to which this stress was associated with elevated blood pressure.

The authors found the strongest predictors of hypertension to be amongst individuals having lived during childhood and adolescence in a situation of high levels of income inequality, and in communities with fewer individuals who had completed a high school education. After controlling for these factors, they were able to identify significant associations between the perceived levels of psychological and social stress and rate of hypertension, with social stress demonstrating the larger effect. Interestingly, they found no significant associations with the physical demands of the job and rates of hypertension.

Recall from the Whitehall study, discussed in Chapter 1, that higher-status workers in the British Civil Service had lower rates of death than workers who were lower in status. Might differences in allostatic load explain the status-dependent association? Would these differences be work-related or independent of the work environment? Researchers from the Whitehall study have provided data to address these questions.

Blood pressure is recorded using two pressure readings:

- the systolic pressure, which measures how hard the heart is beating
- the diastolic pressure, which measures the stiffness of the blood vessels (less stiff is better)

Of these two numbers, chronic elevation of the diastolic pressure is often associated with more severe disease than comparable elevations in the systolic pressure. Historically physicians defined "normal" blood pressure as anything below 140 (systolic) and 90 (diastolic), although many have suggested that optimal blood pressure is actually lower than this.

Researchers in the Whitehall study (Marmot and Theorell 1988) went into the workplace and measured the blood pressure of a group of high-status workers and a comparable group of lower-status workers. The workers went home at the end of the day, where they again had their blood pressure measured. The researchers compared the workers' blood pressure at work and at home. The results are shown in Figure 4.4.

At work, the blood pressure of the two categories of workers was approximately the same—about 135 (systolic) and 88 (diastolic) (written as 135/88 mmHg, and spoken as "one thirty-five over eighty-eight"). At home, the blood pressure of both categories of worker had come down. However, the blood pressure of the higher-status workers had come down substantially more than that of the lower-status workers: about 3 points lower on the systolic pressure and about 8 points lower on the diastolic pressure. Something was keeping the blood pressure of the lower-status workers at a higher level than that of the higher-status workers.

With blood pressure that remains at higher levels throughout the day, never coming down to as low a "resting" state, we would expect the lower-status workers to have a higher likelihood of developing the complications associated with chronically

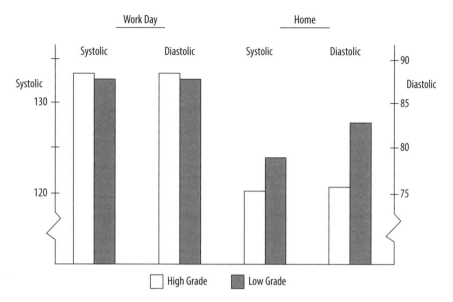

Figure 4.4. Blood pressure of high-grade and low-grade workers—at work and at home. *Sources:* Michael Marmot and Tores Theorell, "Social Class and Cardiovascular Disease: The Contribution of Work"; *International Journal of Health Services* 18, no. 4 (1988), used by permission of the Baywood Publishing Co., Inc.

elevated blood pressure. This is especially true of the diastolic pressure, as increased diastolic pressure often reflects scarring and stiffness of the lining of the blood vessels. One way to test for this association is to look for the biomarkers indicative of tissue damage that may contribute to the higher blood pressure of workers of lower occupational status.

Brunner and colleagues (1997) found a consistent association between the current occupational status and levels of fibrinogen in the blood of British Civil Service workers, with lower-status workers having higher fibrinogen levels. They also looked at the childhood experiences of these workers, and were able to determine that factors such as the socioeconomic circumstances in which the worker grew up (measured by father's social class) was also associated with fibrinogen levels as an adult (Brunner et al. 1996). Elevated levels of fibrinogen will be associated with scarring of the lining of arterioles and resulting stiffness of the arteriolar wall. This stiffness is reflected by an increased diastolic blood pressure, as described above for lower-status workers in Whitehall.

The increased allostatic load that is associated with chronically elevated levels of stress, and the biochemical markers of illness that often accompany that increase, appear to follow the same social hierarchy as other forms of illness. We can now identify a specific process by which the stress of being in a position of social disadvantage can lead to increased rates of illness.

McEwen and Seeman summarized our current understanding of allostatic load in the context of differences in social status: "Allostatic load appears to be a useful construct for conceptualizing how 'wear and tear' and increased morbidity and mortality are caused over long time intervals, not only by the more dramatic stressful life events but also by the many events of daily life that elevate activities of physiological systems. . . . All of these factors influence the temporal patterning and efficiency of turning on and turning off the hormonal mediators of stress" (1999, p. 43).

Economic Inequality as a Magnifier of Differences in Social Status

All societies have a hierarchy of social status, with an associated hierarchy of health status. However, different societies (and different communities within a society) will have differing levels of economic inequality within its social hierarchy. The gap between those at the top of the hierarchy and those at the bottom of the hierarchy may be narrow in some societies and wide in others. A growing body of research suggests that the health of an individual will be affected both by their place in the social hierarchy of their own society as well as by the level of economic inequality that exists between the best-off and the worst-off within that society. The very nature of relations among members of a society will change as the perceived level of inequality changes. As summarized by Wilkinson, "The evidence strongly suggests that as social status differences in a society increase, the quality of social relations deteriorates . . . health and the quality of social relations in a society vary inversely with how hierarchical the social hierarchy is" (1999, pp. 50–51).

To illustrate this point, let us consider what happens when children encounter candy under conditions of inequality (Rinsky 2001). Let us imagine a situation in which two young children are playing together in a room. A researcher is observing the children and their reaction to changing circumstances. The first thing the researcher does is to offer each child a bowl containing six M&M candies. Each child appreciates the added material well-being associated with the candy. Each is quite happy. The children continue to play together well.

Now the researcher introduces inequality into the equation. He removes the bowls, adds six M&Ms to one and three M&Ms to the other, and returns the bowls to the children. Each is materially better off than before. Now a new dynamic has entered the room. The child with fewer M&Ms, perceiving that the other child for no apparent reason now has more M&Ms, becomes angry and tearful: "That's not

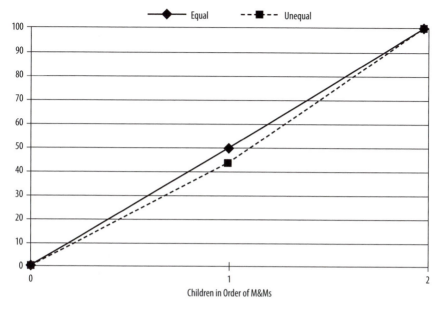

Figure 4.5. Comparison of the distribution of M&Ms under conditions of equality and inequality.

fair!" Despite being better off materially, the child has focused on the inexplicable inequality that has emerged. The play is no longer friendly or easy. For reasons that will become apparent soon, I have chosen to represent the conditions of M&M equality and inequality on a graph (Figure 4.5).

In Figure 4.5, the x-axis represents the children in rank order of the number of M&Ms in their bowls. The y-axis represents the cumulative percentage of all M&Ms in the room accounted for by the indicated child. The solid line represents the condition of complete equality: each child has 50 percent of the M&Ms, so in this case the rank ordering is arbitrary; the first child accounts for 50 percent of the total, and the first and second children combined account for 100 percent. The dashed line represents the inequality introduced into the play room: the first child, now with 9 M&Ms, accounts for only 43 percent of the M&Ms, while the second child with 12 accounts for 57 percent; the cumulative total for the second child is still 100 percent. Notice how the line for the condition of inequality lies slightly lower on the graph than the line for equality.

Imagine now that a third child has entered the room. Each of the previous children maintains their bowl of M&Ms: 9 in one, 12 in the other. The new child gets a bowl with 6 M&Ms. The child with 9 now has mixed feelings of inferiority (compared to the child with 12) and superiority (compared to the child with 6). The new child perceives glaring inequality: "How come they have more than me?" The child with 12 may be feeling a bit smug now. Interestingly, over time, this child may begin to come up with explanations as to why they have the most, and to defend their right to them. Unfortunately, the atmosphere in the room has now become somewhat chaotic. The very nature of the interaction among the children—their willingness to cooperate, their sense of enjoyment, what we will refer to later in this chapter as their "social capital"—has changed.

In explaining this scenario to my students, I often ask them which situation they would rather have their own children playing in. Nearly all prefer the situation of equality, even though the aggregate wealth (measured in M&Ms) is greater in the unequal room. The deterioration in the social environment is simply not worth the chance at a few more M&Ms. Their choice would no doubt be different if somehow the children could be trusted to realize that the simple transfer of three M&Ms from the bowl of the most well-off to the bowl of the least well-off would create the situation of complete equality, with a substantially improved social environment. However, human nature being what it is, that scenario is unlikely to occur. Figure 4.6 provides a graphic representation of the situation of the three children.

Figure 4.6 looks similar to Figure 4.5. Once again the solid line represents the hypothetical situation in which all children have the same number of M&Ms, while

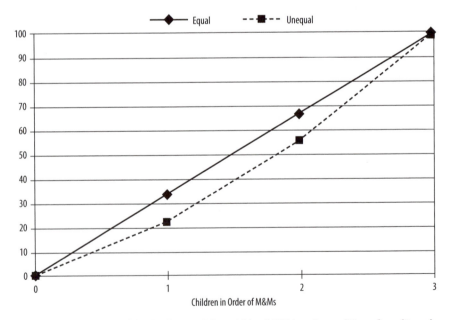

Figure 4.6. Comparison of the distribution of three children's M&Ms under conditions of equality and inequality.

the dashed line represents the condition of inequality. The unequal situation with three children encompasses a higher level of inequality than the previous situation with two children. With two children, complete equality would have been attained by redistributing one-and-a-half M&Ms; for three children one would have to redistribute three M&Ms. Note that the gap between the inequality curve and the line representing equality is wider in the situation of three children than it is with two children. This gap—the area between the line representing hypothetical full equality and the curve measuring actual inequality—represents the amount of resources being measured that would need to be redistributed to attain the situation of full equality. The wider the gap, the greater the degree of inequality represented.

Let us move from the situation of inequality in M&Ms among children to inequality in income among global populations. For this exercise, I ask you to imagine three hypothetical societies. For each society I will describe the distribution of income among families in that society, broken down into deciles. (A decile represents 10 percent of families. The deciles are rank-ordered, with decile 1 being the least well-off and decile 10 being the most well-off.)

Society 1: a society with full equality

- Each decile has the same share of income, with the rank ordering arbitrary

Society 2: a society with three well-defined classes

- Each of deciles 1–4 has 5 percent of aggregate income
- Each of deciles 5–9 has 12 percent of aggregate income
- Decile 10 has 20 percent of aggregate income

Society 3: a society with wide income inequalities and a small group (decile 10) with extremely high income

- Deciles 1–2: each has 2 percent of aggregate income
- Deciles 3–4: each has 4 percent of aggregate income
- Deciles 5–6: each has 7 percent of aggregate income
- Deciles 7–8: each has 10 percent of aggregate income
- Decile 9 has 15 percent of aggregate income
- Decile 10 has 39 percent of aggregate income

These societies are represented graphically in Figure 4.7.

The solid line represents a hypothetical society in which every family has the same level of income. The curve with long dashes represents a society with three well-defined classes. Forty percent of families are in the lower class, 50 percent are in the middle class, and 10 percent are in the upper class. The aggregate income of

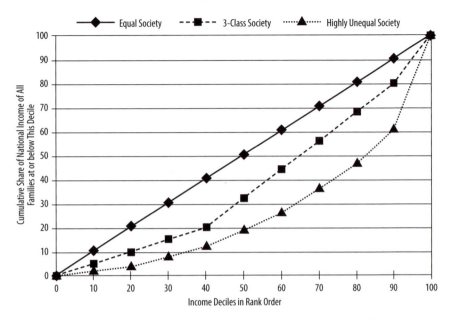

Figure 4.7. Comparing the distribution of family income in three societies with differing levels of inequality.

the upper class (representing 10 percent of families) is the same as that of the lower class (representing 40 percent of families). Thus, the most well-off families have income levels that are four times those of the least well-off families.

The curve in Figure 4.7 with the short dashes represents a society with extremely high levels of inequality. The top decile of families enjoys nearly 40 percent of all income, while families in the bottom six deciles have, in aggregate, only 26 percent of all income. In this society, the most well-off families have incomes that are nearly 20 times the income of the least well-off families. As was the case with M&Ms, the amount of aggregate income that would need to be redistributed to attain full income equality is represented by the gap between the straight line representing full equality and the curve representing the actual distribution: the higher the level of inequality in the society, the wider the gap.

Economists have created a numerical measure of the level of income equality within a society: the Gini coefficient. It represents the decimal fraction of the aggregate income within a society that would need to be redistributed to attain full equality. The curve that measures the actual distribution of income in a society is referred to as the Lorenz curve. The Gini coefficient is determined mathematically by (1) calculating the area between the line of full equality and the Lorenz curve, and (2) calculating the decimal ratio of that area to the area of the triangle under

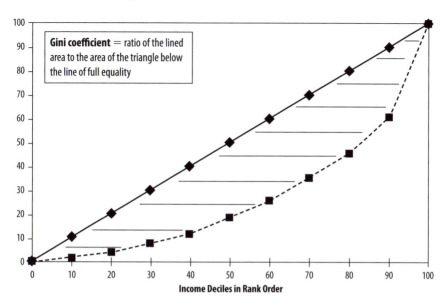

Figure 4.8. Graphic representation of the Gini coefficient.

the line of full equality. Figure 4.8 illustrates the Gini coefficient for the highly unequal society described above.

A number of researchers have suggested that the level of inequality within a society, as measured by the Gini coefficient or other similar measures, will have a consistent association with the health of that society. Kawachi and Kennedy (1997) did an analysis, comparing age-adjusted mortality rates within the states of the United States. Using data from the 1990 US census, they calculated the Gini coefficient for each state, and then graphed mortality rates by the Gini coefficient for each state. They found that mortality rates among states in the United States are generally associated with the Gini coefficient for that state: the higher the Gini coefficient, the higher the mortality rate.

Lopez (2004) used the Gini coefficient to compare health status within large metropolitan areas in the United States. He used self-reported health as his measure of health, and controlled for other factors such as differences in education, age, race, ethnicity, and gender. He also used a statistical adjustment to control for differences in actual levels of income among the metropolitan areas, to assure that he was measuring the effects of inequality rather than absolute levels of income. He concluded, "for each 1 point rise in the Gini index (on a hundred point scale) the risk of reporting Fair or Poor self-rated health increased by 4.0% (95% confidence interval 1.6–6.5%). Given that self-rated health is a good predictor of morbidity and mortality, this suggests that metropolitan area income inequality is affecting the health of US adults" (p. 2409).

In addition to the Gini coefficient, there are other measures of inequality within a society that are often used in comparing health status across societies. Some of the more common include:

- *"Robin Hood" index*: Represents the maximum vertical distance between the line of full equality and the Lorenz curve. It is similar to the Gini coefficient in measuring the amount of redistribution that would need to take place to attain equality.
- *Decile ratio*: Measures the ratio of the income earned by the top 10 percent of households to the income earned by the bottom 10 percent of households.
- *Income ratio*: Measures the ratio of the income of the highest-paid executive in a firm to the lowest-paid employee in that firm.
- *Poverty income ratio*: Measures the proportion of aggregate income earned by the bottom (50 percent, 70 percent, etc.) of households.

Social Capital: Explaining the Association between Inequality and Health

Why do communities, states, and national societies vary in their health status according to the level of inequality within them? Why would economic inequality affect health status independently of actual income levels? Answering these questions is key to understanding the social roots of health disparities.

Kawachi suggests that the answer lies in the differing levels of "social capital" inherent to societies of differing levels of economic or other forms of inequality. He defines social capital as "those features of social relationships—such as levels of interpersonal trust and norms of reciprocity and mutual aid—that facilitate collective action for mutual benefit" (Kawachi 1999, p. 120). He suggests that social capital can take many forms, including the material resources available within one's community as well as the strength of the social networks that tie together people in that community. He contrasts social capital to other forms of capital in the following way: "In contrast to financial capital, which resides in people's bank accounts, or human capital, which is embodied in individuals' investment in education and job training, social capital inheres in the structure and quality of social relationships between individuals" (p. 121).

Social capital within a community can exist at multiple levels. A tenants' association, formed to work with landlords to improve housing conditions in a development or on a city block, is one form of social capital. By relying on each other, the tenants are able simultaneously to contribute to improving their own living conditions as well as those of their neighbors. On a larger scale, social capital may reflect the extent to which one is tied into and participates in the political process. Having meaningful input into the political decisions that affect living conditions can enhance both one's material well-being and one's sense of self-efficacy.

Social capital can also exist at the level of the broader neighborhood or community. Neighborhoods will commonly develop common norms, sometimes formal and sometimes informal, that will affect both one's own behavior and one's sense of connectedness to his neighbors. These norms can be positive and supportive, giving one a sense of broad social support. They can also be negative, conveying the message that one would be unwise to trust in his neighbors or his community.

Scott and colleagues (2018) addressed the issue of whether the perceived characteristics of a neighborhood such as social cohesion, safety, aesthetic quality, and level of violence would be associated with the way people respond to stress physiologically. They followed a cohort of 233 adults between the ages of 25 and 65 and all living in the same socioeconomically, racially, and ethnically diverse zip code in The Bronx in New York City. While most of the subjects reported similar frequencies of stressful experiences, the way they perceived these stressors and the severity of their stress response and emotional impact varied among individuals.

In a nationally representative sample of men and women aged 50 years or more, Robinette and colleagues (2018) assessed how an individual's perception of the level of neighborhood cohesion and neighborhood disorder were associated with the risk of cardiovascular disease. They concluded that "people living in neighborhoods characterized as less cohesive engage in thoughts and behaviors that are related to greater physiological wear and tear" (p. 75), which in turn increase cardiovascular risk. In a similar study, Besser and colleagues (2018) found that the quality of the built environment, measured by such factors as building density and resources for walking around the neighborhood, was associated with cognitive abilities among older adults. Worse quality of the built environment was associated with more rapid cognitive decline, especially in African Americans.

Kawachi and colleagues (1997) used data gathered from a nationally representative survey of residents of 39 states. Respondents were asked whether they agreed with the following statements:

- Do you think most people would try to take advantage of you if they got a chance, or would they try to be fair?

- Generally speaking, would you say that most people can be trusted, or that you can't be too careful in dealing with people?
- Would you say that most of the time people try to be helpful, or are they mostly looking out for themselves?

From these questions they developed an index of the level of trust survey respondents expressed in their own communities. They then compared the average responses within a state with health data gathered for that state. For the 39 states in the study, they found a striking association between perceptions of trust in others within one's state and three separate measures of health status: death rates from heart disease, death rates from cancer, and infant mortality. The more respondents expressed trust in the people in their own community, the lower the chances of death within that state.

Wilkinson (1999) related the level of social capital within a community or a society with the level of status inequality within that community, suggesting that being in a position of low status will have important impacts on social capital by adversely affecting one's perceptions of the community in which they live. He suggests that "as social status differences in a society increase, the quality of social relations deteriorates . . . The combination of increasing social status differentials and deteriorating social relations could hardly be a more potent mix for population health . . . health and the quality of social relations in a society vary inversely with how hierarchical the social hierarchy is" (pp. 50–51).

Wilkinson goes on to suggest that those living in a position of social disadvantage in a hierarchical society will experience powerful negative forces related to social capital. These forces acting at the level of the neighborhood or the community include:

- high levels of violence
- high levels of social anxiety
- increased perceptions of discrimination

Marmot (1999) cited data comparing an aggregate score of the level of hostility within several large American cities with the annual death rate in that city. Honolulu, the city with the lowest hostility score, was also the city with the lowest death rate. Conversely, Philadelphia was the city with the highest hostility score and the highest death rate. Cities such as Cleveland, Chicago, Denver, and Minneapolis followed a consistent pattern: those cities with lower hostility scores also had lower death rates.

How might an increased level of violence and hostility within a city affect things such as rates of cancer and heart disease? The answer lies in the effects of chronically increased allostatic load. The constant stress created by living under these conditions will lead to chronically elevated levels of stressor hormones, which over time will lead to cellular damage, illness, and ultimately premature death. One's perceptions of their connection to, or alienation from, the surrounding community creates a form of social capital, which in turn is associated with allostatic load.

Nobel and colleagues (2017) followed more than 2,000 adults in two large urban centers in the United States who had been hospitalized for treatment of a heart attack or other acute coronary syndrome. All the patients had survived their hospital treatment and were discharged home. The authors were able to measure the level of neighborhood deprivation experienced by each patient during the first six months of their recovery. After controlling for individual SES, they found that the health of those living in more deprived neighborhoods declined more rapidly than those in less deprived neighborhoods. Increased allostatic load associated with a greater level of neighborhood deprivation was likely to play a role in this association.

Diez Roux and colleagues (2001) looked carefully at the characteristics of neighborhoods that contribute to the social capital of that neighborhood. They defined a neighborhood as containing about a thousand people living in the same block group as described by the US Census Bureau. They looked at neighborhoods in four metropolitan regions:

- Forsyth County, North Carolina
- Jackson, Mississippi
- Northwestern suburbs of Minneapolis
- Washington County, Maryland

To characterize the neighborhoods within these metropolitan regions, they looked at factors such as wealth, income, education, and occupation. From these characteristics, they created a composite score for the social environment of the neighborhood. They divided the neighborhoods into three groups:

Group 1: those neighborhoods having the worst social environment
Group 2: those neighborhoods having a middle-range social environment
Group 3: those neighborhoods having the best social environment

They then examined the medical records over a period of nine years for more than 13,000 adults between the ages of 45 and 64, looking for evidence of heart disease. Given significantly different rates of heart disease among whites and blacks and between men and women, they analyzed each group separately. Not surprisingly, they found that those living in neighborhoods with lower social capital scores had significantly more heart attacks and other cardiac events than those living in

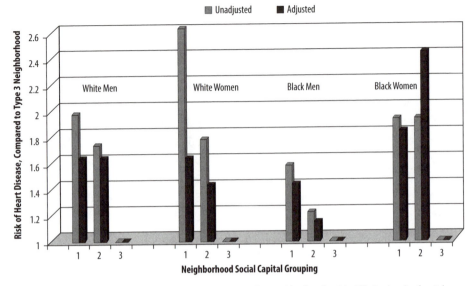

Figure 4.9. Comparing unadjusted risk of heart disease for neighborhoods with differing levels of social capital, and risk of heart disease adjusted for individual SES and medical risk factors. Shows risk compared to rates in Type 3 neighborhoods. *Source:* Based on Diez Roux et al. 2001.

neighborhoods with higher social capital. From what we have read, we would expect people with lower incomes, lower levels of education, or lower occupational status to have higher rates of heart disease.

The researchers carried their analysis one step further. Realizing that an individual's SES is a predictor of the risk of heart disease, they then asked whether the social capital of the neighborhood in which a person lives has an association with rates of heart disease that is independent of the SES of the individual. To do this, they recorded the income, educational level, and occupational category for each individual in the study. Using statistical methodologies, they first analyzed the risk of experiencing a cardiac event based only on the social capital score of the neighborhood, and then analyzed that risk a second time, controlling for the individual's SES characteristics. The results are shown in Figure 4.9.

For all the groups analyzed, the risk of heart disease was substantially higher in neighborhoods with low social capital or midrange social capital than in neighborhoods with high social capital. In nearly all cases, the risk of heart disease in these neighborhoods went down after adjusting for the SES characteristics and individual medical risk factors of the subjects.

It is interesting to note that the risk for black women in midrange neighborhoods actually went up after controlling for individual characteristics. What is perhaps more interesting is the continuing pattern of risk stratification among neighborhoods even after taking into account individual characteristics. One's own SES and medical risk factors are strong predictors of the risk of heart disease. However, the neighborhood in which one lives continues to have a powerful predictive effect on the risk of heart disease for the individuals living in that neighborhood. That neighborhood risk appears to be independent of the risk associated with individual SES and medical characteristics.

Diez Roux and colleagues then asked another important question comparing the impact of individual characteristics with neighborhood characteristics. Which situation has the higher risk of heart disease: having a high level of income but living in a neighborhood with low social capital or having a low level of income but living in a community with high social capital? They addressed this question by comparing the rates of heart disease for individuals at three income levels: less than $25,000, between $25,000 and $50,000, $50,000 or more. They did the analysis separately for white subjects and black subjects. They found that for whites, the risk of heart disease for a low-income subject living in a high-status neighborhood was the same as for a high-income individual living in a low-status neighborhood. For black subjects, the risk of heart disease for a low-income individual living in a high-status neighborhood was 24 percent greater than for a high-income individual living in a low-status neighborhood. The relative strength in predicting heart disease of one's own SES and the social capital of one's neighborhood differs for black subjects and white subjects. Results such as these raise the question as to whether low-income blacks face a different experience living in a higher-income community than do low-income whites, and whether the effect of neighborhood social capital may differ based on the race of the individual. (I address this question in greater depth in Chapter 6.)

As summarized by the researchers, "our findings point to the role of the broader social and economic forces that generate differences among neighborhoods in shaping the distribution of health outcomes. At a time of growing economic segregation of residential areas, differences among places may become even more relevant to explanations of disparities in health" (Diez Roux et al. 2001, p. 105).

Kind and Buckingham (2018) have summarized the importance of neighborhood quality as a factor affecting individual health status: "Poor and minority populations often live in socioeconomically disadvantaged neighborhoods, and neighborhood context directly affects access to food, safety, education, health behaviors, and stress levels. Living in a disadvantaged neighborhood has been linked to higher rates of diabetes, cardiovascular disease, and other diseases; increased utilization of health services; and earlier death" (p. 2456).

They have created a Neighborhood Atlas website that lists the Area Deprivation Index (ADI) for every nine-digit zip code in the United States and Puerto Rico. The ADI was originally developed by the US Health Resources and Services Administration, and is composed of 17 different variables included in the American Community Survey conducted by the Census Bureau. This database is maintained by the University of Wisconsin School of Medicine and Public Health (2018), and is available for researchers to access. They recommend that the ADI be used as a variable in future research on the association between neighborhood quality and health status.

A number of researchers have looked at the association between social capital and health status in countries outside the United States. Kim and colleagues (2011) evaluated survey data gathered from 167,000 adults in 64 different countries from all areas of the globe. Using social trust as a measure of social capital, they found consistent evidence that greater levels of social trust within a country were associated with better self-rated health status. Ahnquist and colleagues (2012) looked at survey data from a nationally representative sample of adults in Sweden and found that "measures of [low] economic capital and low social capital were significantly associated with poor health status" (p. 930). In a similar study of a nationally representative sample in the Netherlands, Mohnen and colleagues (2011) identified a consistent positive association between neighborhood social capital and individual health status.

A number of researchers have studied these questions within the United Kingdom. Giordano and colleagues (2012) examined longitudinal data in a representative data set gathered from 8,000 adults, initially in 2000 and again in 2007. They found that social capital (measured as perceptions of "generalized trust") reported in 2000 were positively associated with measures of self-rated health in 2007. In a study of 25,000 adults in England, Verhaeghe and Tampubolon (2012) evaluated the relationship between individual social capital and the characteristics of one's neighborhood and their effect on self-rated health status. They concluded that "generalized trust, participation with friends and relatives, and having salariat class people in the individual's network were associated with better self-rated health, after controlling for individual socio-demographic and socio-economic factors" (p. 355).

Addressing an issue discussed above in the US context, Stafford and Marmot (2003) used data from the Whitehall study to address two basic questions in the context of the United Kingdom:

1. Is it better for one's health to be poor living in a well-to-do neighborhood, or
2. Is it better to be affluent but living in a socially deprived neighborhood?

They used self-reported health status, recording the percent of respondents with a group reporting that they perceived their own health to be poor. They then compared

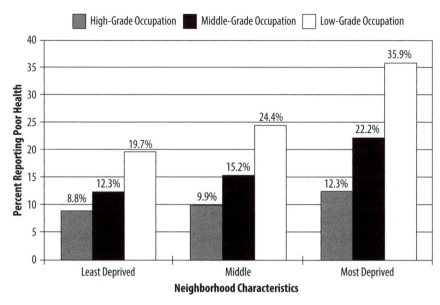

Figure 4.10. Association between neighborhood characteristics and rates of reporting poor health for workers at three levels of occupational status. *Source*: Based on Stafford and Marmot 2003.

the rate of reported poor health broken down by one's own occupational status and the characteristics of the neighborhood in which one lives. The results are shown in Figure 4.10.

It seems clear from the data that the type of person with the best health is the high-status worker living in one of the least-deprived neighborhoods, while the person with the worst health has a low-status occupation and lives in the most-deprived type of neighborhood. While the authors' analysis of these data did not reach statistical significance, it nonetheless appears again that both individual SES (here measured as occupational status) and neighborhood social capital have effects that are independent of each other, but that are additive for those experiencing the best or the worst of both. As to their original questions, it appears that for the population they studied the health of the high-grade worker living in the most-deprived neighborhood remains somewhat better than that of the low-grade worker who is fortunate enough to live in the least-deprived neighborhood. However, compared to a low-grade worker living in the most-deprived neighborhood, the low-grade worker living in the least-deprived neighborhood enjoys substantially better health.

The authors asked an interesting follow-up question that may clarify somewhat the factors that lead to the association between neighborhood social capital and individual health, even after controlling for the individual characteristics of neighborhood residents. They asked the study subjects to indicate where they saw themselves on the "ladder of society" by giving them a picture of a ladder with 10 steps and having them mark which step they perceived themselves as occupying. They again found some very interesting effects:

- Independent of neighborhood of residence, workers in low-status occupations placed themselves lowest on the ladder while workers in the high-status occupations placed themselves highest on the ladder.
- For workers in either medium-status or low-status occupations, those in the least-deprived neighborhoods placed themselves higher on the ladder than those in the most-deprived neighborhoods.
- Low-status workers in the most-deprived neighborhoods placed themselves lowest on the ladder.
- High-status workers placed themselves consistently higher on the ladder than any of the other groups, regardless of the type of neighborhood in which they lived.

Simandan (2018) published a commentary on the underlying importance of how an individual perceives their own position in the broader social hierarchy, focusing principally on their own SES as a determinant of what the author refers to as "status-based identity." As important as one's own current identity is the issue of the impact of transitioning from one social class to another. The author suggests that such a transition can produce "status-based identity uncertainty." As described by the author, "This happens because social class is an entrenched, difficult to overcome, aspect of identity fashioned over many years . . ." Even if the transition is upward in nature, "the status-based identity uncertainty triggered by social mobility increases one's allostatic load and decreases one's subjective well-being" (p. 259).

Measuring Subjective Social Status: Where Do I Stand on the Ladder of Society?

The "ladder of society" used by Stafford and Marmot was developed by a group of social scientists who came together in 1997 to establish the MacArthur Research Network on Socioeconomic Status and Health. Nancy Adler, at that time the Director of the Research Network, used a drawing of a ladder in a study of 57 otherwise healthy white women in the United States aged 30 to 46 years (Adler et al. 2000). As described by the authors (p. 587),

Participants were given a drawing of a ladder with 10 rungs that was described as follows: "Think of this ladder as representing where people stand in our society. At the top of the ladder are the people who are the best off, those who have the most money, most education, and best jobs. At the bottom are the people who are the worst off, those who have the least money, least education, and worst jobs or no job." They were then asked to place an X on the rung that best represents where they think they stand on the ladder.

This simple tool is commonly referred to as the MacArthur Scale of Subjective Social Status, and has been expanded to measure both perceived social status relative to other people in the United States, and perceived status relative to others in one's own community (Figure 4.11). The ladder is featured prominently in a published report titled *Reaching for a Healthier Life: Facts on Socioeconomic Status and Health in the U.S.* (MacArthur Research Network 2007).

In our imagined experiment with children and M&Ms described above, it might be interesting to have the children place themselves on the ladder when they had the same number of M&Ms, and then again when we had introduced inequality into the play environment. West and colleagues (2010) did use the ladder to ask

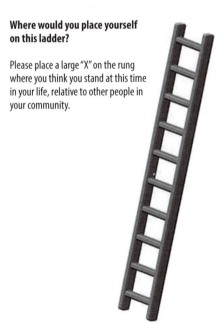

Where would you place yourself on this ladder?

Please place a large "X" on the rung where you think you stand at this time in your life, relative to other people in your community.

Figure 4.11. The MacArthur Scale of Subjective Social Status. *Source*: MacArthur Research Network on Socioeconomic Status and Health, Sociodemographic Questionnaire.

16-year-olds to place themselves within the perceived social hierarchy that is so common to the adolescent school environment (as any parent of an adolescent can tell you). They measured the level of cortisol present in each student using saliva samples obtained in the morning. While the researchers did not find an association between a student's SES at home and their cortisol level, they found consistent, inverse associations between a student's perceived social position at school and their level of cortisol.

The Other Face of Social Capital: Social Networks

Let us recall from Chapter 3 what we learned from Semenza's study of the factors associated with dying during the heat wave that occurred in 1995 in Chicago. Among those more likely to die from the heat were

- those who did not leave home each day
- those who lived alone
- those with fewer regular social contacts

For those facing the effects of the heat, especially those who were elderly with chronic medical conditions, having few regular contacts with family members, friends, or neighbors left many of them without help when the heat became overwhelming. There is growing evidence that weak social networks of this type have effects on health that go well beyond susceptibility to the heat. We are learning the many ways social networks can affect psychological health, cardiovascular health, and the ability to fight off communicable diseases.

Social capital as defined by Kawachi refers typically to the characteristics of a neighborhood or community. The level of social capital within a neighborhood is experienced by all those within the neighborhood. However, individuals within a neighborhood or community will each have their own level of social networks—the regular connections they have in a social context with family, friends, neighbors, or colleagues. As described by Kawachi and Berkman, "social networks are a characteristic that can (and most often have been) be measured at the individual level, whereas social capital should be properly considered a characteristic of the collective (neighbourhood, community, society) to which the individual belongs" (2000, p. 176).

Herzog and colleagues (2002) summarized the research showing the beneficial effects on the health of elderly people of what they refer to as "social engagement." They find that those people who have more regular social contacts tend to have lower mortality rates. These contacts may involve meeting with friends informally, attending church, or availing themselves of similar situations where they will have direct contact with other people. In addition to demonstrable effects on physical health, those with more regular social engagement also tend to display better mental health. Valtorta and colleagues (2016) reviewed the literature on the health impacts of loneliness and social isolation, and were able to confirm that those in such conditions of isolation were at an increased risk of developing coronary heart disease and stroke.

Michael and colleagues (2001) looked specifically at the association between the number of contacts with friends and relatives and the level of social engagement of more than 4,500 women between the ages of 60 and 72 who lived alone. They were able to demonstrate a significant protective effect for the strength of the women's social networks on their health status over a period of four years. Using scales derived from the SF-36, they found that those with stronger social networks maintained higher levels of mental health, vitality, and physical functioning. (See Chapter 2 for a description of the SF-36 health assessment instrument and its various subscales.)

Interestingly, the authors found that women living with a spouse tended to show a more rapid decline in the three health measures than women living alone, and that social network strength did not appear to affect the decline in health of the women living with a spouse. With the more rapid decline in health seen typically in men as compared to women, these results point to the question whether the strain of caring for a spouse with relatively poor health may place an added stress on older women that results in a more rapid decline in their own health.

It may be intuitive that those with stronger social networks and more frequent social contacts will demonstrate better mental health over time. Knowing what we do about the mechanisms through which psychosocial stress can lead to actual cellular damage and disease, we might ask whether social network strength might also affect diseases such as coronary heart disease.

Sundquist and colleagues (2004) studied this question in a sample of more than 6,800 men and women in Sweden. At the initiation of the study, none of the subjects showed signs of coronary heart disease. (Recall that coronary heart disease is caused by progressive damage to the blood vessels that supply the heart. The study of Yan and colleagues (2006) discussed earlier in this chapter demonstrated the association between lower social status and signs of early damage to those vessels in otherwise healthy adults.) They gathered data from the subjects about the level and type of their social engagement, using 18 questions developed as part of a wider social survey. The types of social activities included in the survey are shown in Table 4.1.

From these 18 types of activity, the authors constructed a single social participation index. They then examined the health of these subjects over a 10-year period, looking to see which subjects developed signs of coronary heart disease, such

Table 4.1. Types of Social Activity Used to Construct the Social Participation Index

1. Neighbors talk often in the area
2. Attend mutual activity in the neighborhood
3. Socialize with neighbors at least once every three months
4. Go to restaurant for pleasure
5. Go to disco or dance restaurant
6. Go to cinema
7. Go to theater
8. Go to concert
9. Go to art exhibition
10. Go to other exhibition or museum
11. Go to library
12. Attend divine service
13. Member of a choir
14. Active in a sports association
15. Take part in a study circle or an evening course
16. Member of a political party
17. Attend meeting of a local group (environmental for instance)
18. Know how to appeal against authorities

Source: Sundquist et al. 2004.

as a heart attack. In their analysis they took into account factors such as smoking or other behaviors known to be associated with heart disease. They found a significant association between the social participation score and the risk of developing heart disease: those with lower participation scores had an increased risk of developing heart disease. These findings suggest that a strong network of family and friends and more regular activities in a social context exert a protective physiologic influence, and are quite consistent with the model I developed above of allostatic load as a mediator of the health effects of relatively high or relatively low levels of psychosocial stress.

One further study provides substantial additional support for the concept of a physiologic benefit of strong social network ties. Cohen and colleagues (1997) set out to test the hypothesis that the diversity and strength of one's social network ties will have a protective effect against catching a cold. To do this, they recruited 276 healthy men and women between the ages of 18 and 55. In exchange for a payment of $800, each subject agreed to live for six days in a quarantined laboratory setting. After observing the subjects for 24 hours to be sure that they were not coming down with a cold before the study began, the researchers applied a solution containing a low dose of viruses known to cause the common cold onto the nasal membranes of each subject. (The nasal membranes are the principal route of entry into the body for cold viruses in a community setting.) They then followed each subject in the laboratory setting for five days more, recording which subjects came down with a cold. They assessed the presence of a cold in each of three ways:

1. Researchers looked for objective signs of a cold, such as an increase in antibody levels in the blood.
2. Subjects reported subjective symptoms of a cold, such as a fever or a runny nose.
3. Subjects had an increased score on the Jackson cold index, a previously validated means of detecting the presence of a cold.

The researchers asked each subject a series of questions about the frequency and number of social contacts they had with:

- spouse, parents, in-laws
- children and other close family members
- workmates, schoolmates, fellow volunteers
- members of social groups
- members of religious groups

From these reported social contacts, the researchers created an overall scale of social diversity, and divided the scale into three levels of social networks: low, moderate, and high. They then recorded how many subjects within each level developed a cold.

There is a problem we must first consider before deciding whether stronger social networks in and of themselves protect a person against getting a cold. We catch colds by being exposed to others in our social environment who have a cold. Each time we get a cold, we develop our own antibodies against the specific virus that caused the cold. Those antibodies then protect us from catching a cold from the same virus again in the future. It stands to reason that:

- the more people we are in contact with, the more colds we will get
- the more colds we get, the more we will have protective antibodies in our blood against future colds
- therefore, those with stronger social networks will be at a reduced risk of getting colds due to their higher level of antibodies from previous colds

To test for this, at the beginning of the study the researchers measured the level of antibodies against cold viruses in the blood of each subject, and then adjusted their subsequent analysis based on this preexisting level.

In their preliminary analyses, the researchers noted that those subjects who had completed a high school degree or less had the highest rate of getting a cold

(52 percent). Accordingly, they adjusted for educational level in their analysis of the association between social networks and cold susceptibility. They also adjusted for individual behaviors such as smoking or sleep patterns. After taking all these variables into account, they found a striking association between the subjects' social networks and their risk of developing a cold in response to the known exposure to a cold virus. Using any of the three ways of measuring the presence of a cold, those with low social network diversity had the highest chance of getting a cold and those with high social network diversity had the lowest chance.

How should we explain this association between the strength of one's social networks and one's likelihood of coming down with a cold? Something in the body of the subject with stronger social networks either blocks or impedes the virus in its attempt to begin growing in the subject's nasal tissues. The way our bodies allow us to get over a cold once we catch it is by mobilizing antibodies and white blood cells to kill the viruses. The more rapidly and more effectively our body can mount that immune response, the less likely the virus will have a chance to grow to the point where it causes illness. It appears that people with stronger and more diverse social networks also tend to have stronger and more responsive immune systems.

Cohen and colleagues also measured the levels of epinephrine, norepinephrine, and cortisol in their research subjects at the beginning of the study and found little association between the one-time level of these hormones and social network diversity. It is more likely that social networks exert their positive health effects over time. The beneficial effects of social networks on the immune system is gradual and cumulative.

Building a Causal Model of the Association between Low Social Status and Poor Health

Michael Marmot, one of the leading researchers into the nature and causes of disparities in health status, summarized the ways in which living in a position of social disadvantage results in reduced health status over time. He states, "My own view is that the mind is a crucial gateway through which social influences affect physiology to cause disease. The mind may work through effects on health-related behavior, such as smoking, eating, drinking, physical activity, or risk taking, or it may act through effects on neuroendocrine or immune mechanisms" (2001, p. 135).

Using what we have learned in this chapter about the physiologic processes by which chronic exposure to social and psychological stress leads to poor health outcomes, and combining it with what we learned in the previous chapter about the effects of low social status on health-related behaviors and exposure to environmen-

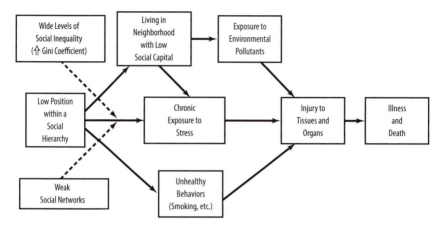

Figure 4.12. A model of the ways in which social inequality affects health status.

tal pollutants, we can now build a model illustrating the probable causal pathways through which low social status results over time in poor health or premature death. This model is illustrated in Figure 4.12.

In the model, the direction of the arrows suggests the direction of the causal relationship. When a person is in a position of low relative status within an established social hierarchy, there are immediate consequences.

First, the low-status person is more likely to engage in individual behaviors that, over the long term, are likely to result in adverse health consequences. Examples of these types of behavior include smoking, diet or physical inactivity with associated obesity, and alcohol or drug abuse. Over time, these behaviors contribute to cellular and tissue injury that leads to disease and/or death.

Second, the low-status person will likely live in a neighborhood or community with low levels of social capital. The lack of social cohesion and exposure to underlying hostility or violence within that community will result in three conditions, all with harmful health outcomes:

1. There will be an increased level of psychosocial stress for those who live there, adding to the more general stress of being in a position of low social status.
2. In addition, these neighborhoods and communities, often low-income and with little in the way of political power, are more likely to be exposed to high levels of environmental toxins or pollutants. These in turn contribute to the cellular inflammation and injury that result in illness and/or death.
3. Experiencing a position of low social status will lead to experiencing a variety of psychosocial stressors on a chronic basis. By elevating the individual's

allostatic load on a chronic basis, these stressors will eventually contribute to cellular inflammation and damage (for example, early calcification of the arteries of the heart), and eventually to illness and death.

In addition to this threefold effect of low social status (behavior, neighborhood environment, and stress), two forces enter into the model. These forces, indicated in Figure 4.12 by the dashed lines, appear to act on the general level of stress experienced by either increasing or decreasing the stress response.

The first force, the level of economic equality/inequality that is inherent to the society in which the individual lives, will either buffer (equality) or augment (inequality) the stress response to experiencing low social status. The level of inequality can be measured by such indices as the Gini coefficient or the "Robin Hood" index.

The second force is the individual's social networks and level of social support from friends, colleagues, and family. Those with more extensive social support networks will experience a buffering effect on the relationship between social status and stress response. They will likely experience lower levels of allostatic load and enhanced bodily defenses, such as the immune response.

A New Social Determinant of Health: Despair

At the conclusion of Chapter 1, I addressed a statistic that has raised considerable concern. For the first time in more than 50 years, life expectancy in the United States had fallen for two consecutive years. Life expectancy decreased from 78.9 years in 2014 to 78.7 years in 2016. This decrease was seen for both men and women (Kochanek et al. 2017). A year later, the bad news continued. Between 2016 and 2017, life expectancy in the United States fell for the third consecutive year, to 76.6 years (Murphy et al. 2018).

Case and Deaton (2015) had earlier reported "a marked increase in the all-cause mortality of middle-aged white non-Hispanic men and women in the United States between 1999 and 2013" (p. 15078). This increase in mortality, seen principally among people between the ages of 45 and 54, was seen only among non-Hispanic whites. Blacks and Hispanics at midlife had shown continued decreases in death rates. Among whites between the ages of 25 and 64, the highest death rates were among those living in rural counties (Stein et al. 2017). An editorial published in the journal *Annals of Internal Medicine* (Himmelstein and Woolhandler 2018) cited two principal causes of this outcome: suicide and substance abuse.

The federal Centers for Disease Control and Prevention reported that between 1999 and 2016, suicide rates nationally had increased by nearly 30 percent

(Stone et al. 2018). An earlier report (Ivey-Stephenson et al. 2017) compared suicide rates across three levels of urbanization: large metropolitan areas, medium/
small metropolitan areas, and rural/non-metropolitan areas. Across all three levels
of urbanization, suicide rates were highest among those aged 35–64 years. Suicide
rates were highest for two racial/ethnic groups: whites and American Indian/
Alaska Natives. Across all ages and racial/ethnic groups, suicide rates were highest
in rural areas.

Case and Deaton (2017) reported that these deaths were found principally among
whites with a high-school education or less, and were due largely to increases in two
factors: suicides and drug overdoses. They "propose a preliminary but plausible story
in which cumulative disadvantage over life, in the labor market, in marriage and
child outcomes, and in health, is triggered by progressively worsening labor market opportunities at the time of entry for whites with low levels of education" (p. 2).
It has largely been from Case and Deaton's description of the groups most at risk
that the term "deaths of despair" has arisen. In many rural areas, growing up among
working-class adults led many students to stop their education at high school, hop-
ing to go to work in the same factories and mills in which their fathers had worked.
In many areas, those jobs are no longer there. Factories and mills have closed or
moved, leaving young adults few options for finding a job with which they could
support their own family. Faced with this reality, many have turned to opioids and
other drugs to buffer this sense of despair.

In 2017 the *New York Times* published a story titled "Drug Deaths in America Are
Rising Faster Than Ever" (Katz 2017). Reporting data that staff from the *Times* had
gathered, they wrote, "Drug overdose deaths in 2016 most likely exceeded 59,000, the
largest annual jump ever recorded in the United States . . . Drug overdoses are now
the leading cause of death among Americans under 50." In 2018 the *Times* reported
that the number of deaths in 2017 due to drug overdose had risen to nearly 72,000
(Sanger-Katz 2018). An analysis by Hayes and colleagues (2018) estimated that
42 percent of the deaths of despair occurring in 2016 were due to drug overdose, with
31 percent due to suicide and 27 percent due to alcohol poisoning.

Hempstead and Phillips (2019) reported that the national rate of deaths from
unintentional opioid poisoning increased by 126 percent between 2005 and 2016.
They also found that, "While unintentional opioid overdoses have increased dramatically, rates of poisoning suicides have scarcely changed" (p. 29). While the national suicide rate increased by 23 percent over the period studied, the rate of suicide by opioid or other drug poisoning decreased. From these data they conclude
that "trends in intentional and unintentional drug poisoning mortality appear to
be unrelated" (p. 34).

There are two principal drugs responsible for these deaths: prescription opioid pills, and an illicit form of a drug called fentanyl that heroin users had injected, not realizing that it could be as many as 50 to 100 times more potent than heroin (Dowell et al. 2017). A study from the Centers for Disease Control and Prevention reported that use of illicit fentanyl was primarily responsible for the recent increase in deaths due to illicit drug use (O'Donnell et al. 2017).

In March 2017 President Donald Trump signed an Executive Order establishing the President's Commission on Combating Drug Addiction and the Opioid Crisis (Office of National Drug Control Policy 2017). The Commission issued its Final Report in November 2017 (President's Commission on Combating Drug Addiction and the Opioid Crisis 2017). In that report, the Commission officially acknowledged the growing opioid crisis as an "opioid epidemic," a term that is now commonly used.

Seervai and colleagues suggest that the United States does not have a single opioid epidemic—it has two: "The first is the prescription-drug epidemic—highly visible to the public, and more likely to occur among older adults in rural, white communities who misuse prescription painkillers. The second, more recently emerging epidemic, is among younger adults who are victims of illegally produced opioids such as fentanyl. Urban communities of color have recently witnessed a surge in deaths resulting from these illegally produced opioids" (2018, p. 1).

As is the case with suicides, the epidemic of deaths from prescription opioids is occurring largely in rural areas, and largely affecting middle-aged whites with low levels of education. An editorial in the *American Journal of Public Health* (Seth et al. 2018) supported this differentiation between deaths due to prescription opioids and those due to illicit opioids, such as heroin and illicitly manufactured fentanyl. "Although prescription and illicit opioid overdoses are closely entwined, it is important to differentiate the deaths to craft appropriate prevention and response efforts" (p. 500).

Distribution of Opioid Deaths by Age, Race/Ethnicity, and Geography

Gomes and colleagues (2018) looked at the national age distribution of those most affected by the increase in opioid deaths. They found that the age group with the highest burden of deaths was those between 25 and 34 years of age. In this age group, 20 percent of all deaths recorded in 2016 involved opioids. Huang and colleagues (2018) also evaluated the age distribution of opioid related deaths, while differentiating between those deaths related to prescription opioid use and those due to heroin and/or fentanyl overdose. In 2014 the group most at risk of prescription opioid deaths were those born between 1947 and 1964 (that is, aged 50–67 years), while those most at risk of illicit opioid deaths were those born between 1979 and 1992 (that is, aged 22–35 years).

Looking at opioid use and dependence rather than deaths, researchers from the University of Iowa's Children's Hospital and the University of Nebraska School of Medicine noted rising evidence of opioid use among patients between the ages of 18 and 21 who were treated in their emergency departments. When they compared their experience to national data, they found this increase in adolescent use of opioids to be widespread (Abbasi 2017).

Harrison and colleagues (2018) studied racial/ethnic differences in the rates of prescription opioid use between 2000 and 2015. They found that the rate of use had increased during this period for all racial/ethnic groups, with the greatest increase among non-Hispanic whites. While historically there had been a higher rate of opioid use among blacks, by 2015 the rates were approximately the same. Despite similar rates of using prescription opioids, in 2016 the death rate per 100,000 population due to opioid overdose was 17.5 in whites as compared to 10.3 in blacks (Kaiser Family Foundation 2018).

Zhou and colleagues (2018) looked at the records of 3.5 million individuals younger than 65 who had qualified for Medicare coverage due to a long-term disability. They were able to determine how many of them were receiving prescriptions for opioid medications as treatment for their disability. They found that the highest rate of long-term opioid use was among those aged 45–64. They found the highest rates of opioid use in areas of the South, Southwest, and Midwest, with "a strong negative correlation between various measures of opioid prescribing and county median household income, and a strong positive correlation between those measures and county unemployment rate" (p. 66).

Dwyer-Lindgren and colleagues (2018), using a combination of several national data sets, assessed changes at the county level in deaths due to drug use disorders between 1980 and 2014. Nationally, the death rate from drug use disorders increased by more than 600 percent. While death rates increased in every county in the United States, the magnitude of the increase varied substantially among counties and among regions of the country. The largest increases (of more than 5,000 percent) were seen in counties that were part of Kentucky, West Virginia, Ohio, Indiana, and eastern Oklahoma. As described by Warfield and colleagues (2019), "With the highest opioid overdose death rate in the United States since 2010, West Virginia is the center of the current opioid crisis" (p. 303).

In light of the outcomes of the 2016 presidential election, Goodwin and colleagues (2018) compared county-level rates of chronic use of prescription opioids among Medicare beneficiaries of all age groups and presidential voting patterns in the 2016 election. Consistent with the outcomes of the study by Zhou and colleagues, they found the highest rates of chronic opioid use among beneficiaries younger than 65 with a long-term disability. They found a significant association between the percent of the county that had voted Republican in the presidential election and the prevalence of chronic prescription opioid use. They also identified an association among differences in household income, educational attainment, and the rate of opioid use, leading the authors to conclude that "This association is related to underlying county socioeconomic characteristics that are common to both chronic opioid use and voting patterns, particularly characteristics pertaining to income, disability, insurance coverage, and unemployment" (p. 8).

Dasgupta and colleagues (2018) reviewed the development of the national opioid epidemic between 2000 and 2015 from a social as well as an economic perspective. From this review they reported that "the crisis is fundamentally fueled by economic and social upheaval, its etiology closely linked to the role of opioids as a refuge from physical and psychological trauma, concentrated disadvantage, isolation, and hopelessness" (p. 182). Voelker (2018) has described the impact of that crisis on one of the areas hardest hit by it. In August 2016, Cabell County, a small rural county in West Virginia, reported 20 opioid overdose cases within a period of 53 hours. Voelker interviewed Dr. Beth Toppins, a physician who works in the emergency department at Cabell Huntington Hospital in Huntington, West Virginia. She deals with overdose patients on a regular basis. As Dr. Toppins describes, "It's frustrating when you see the same patients that you've tried to help in any way you can over and over" (p. 1423).

Reporting in the *New York Times*, Goodnough (2018) described the experience of another physician who works in a rural area and deals with the opioid epidemic on a regular basis. Dr. Nicole Gastala is a family physician who moved to Marshalltown, Iowa, after finishing her residency training at the University of Iowa. Marshalltown is a town of about 27,000, mostly white residents, located about 60 miles from Des Moines. Rather than treating patients with life-threatening opioid overdoses, Dr. Gastala works with patients with opioid addiction to try and overcome their addiction. With little formal training in the treatment of opioid addiction, she has undergone what she described as "a complete evolution." She has been able to benefit by working with nurses and other staff who had grown up in Marshalltown, and who worked with opioid-addicted patients from an empathetic, non-judgmental basis.

Blendon and Benson (2018) reported the results of a nationally representative opinion poll regarding how we, as a country, should approach the opioid epidemic. From the perspective of the public, most of the blame for the epidemic goes to "doctors who inappropriately prescribe painkillers (33%) and people who sell prescription painkillers illegally (28%)" (p. 410). Blumenthal and Seervai (2017) have suggested that "Pharmaceutical companies have also been implicated. Several investigations have established that drug makers fueled the epidemic to increase their own sales."

Francis Collins, the Director of the National Institutes of Health, has reported on an NIH initiative called "Helping to End Addiction Long-term (HEAL)" (Collins et al. 2018). HEAL focuses on two principal means to address the crisis: improving treatments that are available for opioid misuse and addiction, and working to improve strategies for pain management without the chronic use of opioids. Wakeman and Barnett (2018) have argued that "there's a realistic, scalable solution for reaching the millions of Americans with opioid use disorder: mobilizing the primary care physician (PCP) workforce to offer office-based addiction treatment with buprenorphine, as other countries have done" (p. 1). Buprenorphine is an opioid derivative similar to methadone that can be used to prevent withdrawal symptoms from opioid addiction. In the same journal issue as the article by Wakeman and Barnett, Saloner and colleagues (2018) support the expanded use of buprenorphine, while also "expanding the pool of clinicians who treat opioid use disorder, improving measurement of treatment quality, and linking payment to outcomes" (p. 4).

In addition to training more physicians in the treatment of opioid addiction, Haffajee and colleagues (2018) report on the expansion among individual states in developing prescription drug monitoring programs (PDMPs). As of 2018 all states with the exception of Missouri had implemented PDMPs. These programs typically require physicians and other professionals who prescribe opioids to register with a state database. This allows prescribers or a delegated staff member both to check to see whether a patient has been prescribed opioids from another provider, and then, if a new prescription for opioids is provided to the patient, to enter that prescription into the database. They reported that in the states that had implemented PDMPs, "implementation was associated with sustained declines in the total opioid dosage prescribed and number of opioid fills" (p. 971).

Oquendo and colleagues (2018) underscore the difficulty that often arises in determining if a death due to opioid overdose might also have been a suicide. The authors point out that depression and opioid use are often concurrent. Most approaches to reducing opioid deaths do not also consider assessing suicide risk as part of the treatment. Accordingly, opioid-related deaths and suicides may simply be different forms of response for individuals confronting a life of despair due to the loss of job opportunities and weakening social support from family and community. As the authors conclude, "The significant increases in both opioid-overdose deaths and suicide rates in our country have contributed to reduced life expectancy for Americans. These two epidemics are intermingled, and solutions to address the opioid crisis require that we tailor interventions to preventing opioid-overdose deaths due to suicidal intent" (p. 1569).

Opioid-related deaths, suicides, and other forms of health disparities we have discussed so far are largely the consequences of being in a low social position based on SES. There are, of course, social hierarchies based on race/ethnicity in addition to those hierarchies of SES. Being a member of a minority racial or ethnic group often creates another form of social disadvantage. In the following chapters I explore the extent to which a position of racial/ethnic disadvantage carries with it the same type of physiologic and health consequences as a position of SES disadvantage. I also consider the corollary question of which form of disadvantage—racial/ethnic or SES—has the greater adverse impact on health.

CHAPTER FIVE

Race, Ethnicity, and Health

In reporting data for 2017 on overall birth rates and death rates for the US population, the federal government's National Center for Health Statistics reported separate data for the following categories:

- White (non-Hispanic)
- Black (non-Hispanic)
- American Indian or Alaskan Native
- Asian or Pacific Islander
- Hispanic

These reports combine categories of both race and ethnicity in describing changes in the population of the United States. In studying the health disparities that exist in our society and the potential means to reduce them, it is important to understand how the categories of race and ethnicity are used, and what they mean. Accordingly, I will clarify what I mean (and what I do not mean) by the terms *race* and *ethnicity*. To illustrate, I will describe some of the history of my family and the family of my wife.

In Figure 5.1 you will see two photographs. One is of a portrait of my great-great-grandfather. The second is of the great-great-grandfather of my wife—the older man with a mustache sitting with his family.

My great-great-grandfather was born in Boston in the late 1700s and trained as a minister in the Congregational Church. (The Congregational Church is a Protestant Christian sect that is descended from the New England Puritan community.) His ancestors came to New England on the *Mayflower*. He spent his career founding and leading churches on the edges of the wilderness of the New World—first in Maine, and then in Ohio.

My wife's great-great-grandfather was born in Russia and was Jewish. Throughout much of his life he suffered from the anti-Jewish pogroms that swept through

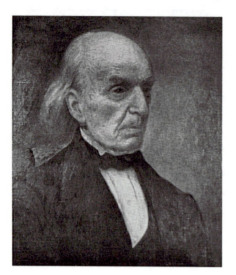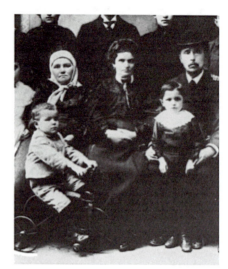

Figure 5.1. Ancestors of the author and the author's wife.

Russia and Central Europe. My wife's grandfather (the small boy on a tricycle in the photograph) finally fled Europe in the early 1900s, landing at Ellis Island and subsequently settling in New York City.

It is useful to ask two questions about my wife and myself. Are we of the same ethnicity? Are we members of the same race?

The answer to the first question is apparent. We certainly are not of the same ethnicity. A Russian Jew and a New England Protestant Christian (our respective great-great-grandfathers) are of quite different ethnicities. As descendants of these ethnic groups, my wife and I bring to our family very different ethnic traditions.

Are we members of the same race? The answer is yes. We are both white. When it comes time to check a box on a census form or a birth certificate, we each check "White." New England Protestants and Russian Jews, by both common perception and government policy, are white.

The disparate answers to these two questions raise a third question. Which category provides more information about an individual—race or ethnicity? In the case of my wife and me, our ethnicity will tell you quite a bit more about us than simply that we are white. This same question can be applied in the context of health. For a given individual, which category—race or ethnicity—will provide more information about an individual's health status? As we will see in this chapter and the one that follows, it is crucially important to answer this question, and to do so using scientific data rather than tradition or popular perception.

What Are Race and Ethnicity?

The *Oxford English Dictionary* offers two definitions of the word *race* that capture the two most common ways the concept is used. Under one concept, race implies common ancestry. This definition states that race is "a group of people belonging to the same family and descended from a common ancestor." The second concept approaches race as categorizing people based on differences in physical appearance. This definition states that a race is "any of the (putative) major groupings of mankind, usually defined in terms of distinct physical features or shared ethnicity, and sometimes (more controversially) considered to encompass common biological or genetic characteristics."

It is interesting to note that the editors of the *Oxford English Dictionary* chose to qualify this second definition, informing readers that the concept of race "in early use usually applied to groups of people with obviously distinct physical characteristics such as skin colour, etc. . . . Now often used more generally to denote groups of different cultural or ethnic origin." It appears that, from a lexicological perspective, the two historical meanings of the word now overlap.

The US Census Bureau is the federal agency charged with measuring and categorizing the US population. In preparing for the national census to be conducted in 2020, it has published a document titled "Race & Ethnicity," in which it defines the categories of race and ethnicity it plans to use (US Census Bureau 2017). In introducing the categories used for measuring race and ethnicity, it states, "The U.S. Census Bureau considers race and ethnicity to be two separate and distinct concepts" (p. 1). It then goes on to provide the following two definitions that reflect government policy: "The Census Bureau defines race as a person's self-identification with one or more social groups . . . Ethnicity determines whether a person is of Hispanic origin or not."

In gathering data for the 2020 census, the Census Bureau will ask the same questions about race and ethnicity it included in the 2010 census (US Census Bureau 2018).

1. Is this person of Hispanic, Latino, or Spanish origin?
2. What is this person's race?

The census divides responses to the second question into the five racial groups listed and defined as follows:

- "White" refers to a person having origins in any of the original peoples of Europe, the Middle East, or North Africa.

- "Black or African American" refers to a person having origins in any of the Black racial groups of Africa.
- "American Indian or Alaska Native" refers to a person having origins in any of the original peoples of North and South America (including Central America), and who maintains tribal affiliation or community attachment.
- "Asian" refers to a person having origins in any of the original peoples of the Far East, Southeast Asia, or the Indian subcontinent.
- "Native Hawaiian and Other Pacific Islander" refers to a person having origins in any of the original peoples of Hawaii, Guam, Samoa, or other Pacific Islands. (In the 1990 census, this category was included in the "Asian" category of race.)

While offering a number of Asian categories as possible choices in response to the question about race (Chinese, Filipino, Asian Indian, Vietnamese, Korean, Japanese), each respondent who checks one of these boxes is categorized as Asian by race, while those who check one of the Pacific Island boxes is categorized as Native Hawaiian or Other Pacific Islander.

Contrast the approach to race used by the US census with that used by the Canadian census. Canada conducts its national census every five years, the most recent being in 2016. In establishing the standards for categorizing Canadians, Statistics Canada (the analogue of the US Census Bureau) defined the term *race* as, "based primarily upon genetically imparted physiognomical features among which skin colour is a dominant, but not the sole, attribute." However, the following statement precedes this definition. "This standard is no longer recommended for use and is not to be used."

Instead, the Canadian census gathers data on "the population group or groups to which the person belongs." It divides these population groups into two categories, based on the following questions (Statistics Canada 2016):

Question 17: What were the ethnic or cultural origins of this person's ancestors? An ancestor is usually more distant than a grandparent. For example, Canadian, English, Chinese, French, East Indian, Italian, German, Scottish, Cree, Mi'kmaq, Salish, Métis, Inuit, Filipino, Irish, Dutch, Ukrainian, Polish, Portuguese, Vietnamese, Korean, Jamaican, Greek, Iranian, Lebanese, Mexican, Somali, Colombian, etc.

Question 18: Is this person an aboriginal person, that is First Nations (North American Indian), Métis or Inuk (Inuit)?

While the Canadian census categorizes people into the two broad groups of Aboriginal / Not Aboriginal, with further subdivision of the latter group, the US
Census Bureau divides people into the categories of Hispanic/Non-Hispanic, with
further subdivision by race. The Canadian census places primary emphasis on the
ancestral origins of its population, without using the concept of race.

The *Oxford English Dictionary* defines *ethnic* as "of or relating to national or cultural origin or tradition." From this definition, ethnicity can be based on factors
such as the use of a common language. This is the approach the US Census Bureau
takes regarding ethnicity. With "Hispanic" and "Non-Hispanic" as the two principal ethnic categories, it differentiates those whose ancestors came from a Spanish-
speaking country from those whose ancestors did not. While Spanish-speaking
countries include Spain, for practical purposes in the United States, Hispanic means
having ancestors who came from the Spanish-speaking countries of Central America, South America, or the Caribbean.

Thus, the United States categorizes its population along two independent axes:
race and Hispanic ethnicity. A white person can be either Hispanic or non-Hispanic.
Similarly, a Hispanic person can be any race. While the list of possible ethnicities
is extensive in Canada, it is limited in the United States. Anglo-Saxon Protestant
and Russian Jew are not categories that are recorded by the US Census Bureau. Despite the potential wealth of information regarding health risks that ethnicity often contains, it is not a category that receives much attention in either population
data or health data in the United States.

The Overlap between Race and Ethnicity

Despite being approached as separate categories by the US Census Bureau, a close
examination of the way race and ethnicity are defined and used reveals substantial
overlap between the two categories. Recall that one of the dictionary definitions of
race cited above sees it as identifying people with a common ancestry. Similarly, the
definition of ethnicity includes "relating to national or cultural origin or tradition."
Common ancestry can be used to define either race or ethnicity.

Earlier we saw that the US Census Bureau defines black as "people having origins in any of the Black racial groups of Africa" and white as "having origins in any
of the original peoples of Europe, the Middle East, or North Africa." The racial
categories defined by the US Census Bureau are based largely on ancestry. How does
the use of ancestry in defining race differ from the use of ancestry in defining ethnicity? A group of genetics researchers has reviewed the distinction between race

and ethnicity. While acknowledging that both categories are derived from a person's ancestry, they "define racial groups on the basis of primary continent of origin" while they define ethnicity as "a self-defined construct that may be based on geographic, social, cultural, and religious grounds" (Risch et al. 2002, p. 3). Race uses the continent from which one's ancestors originated to define its categories; ethnicity uses the geographic region from which one's ancestors originated (for example, Anglo-Saxon or Russian) coupled with commonalities of religion or language to create its categories.

If race refers to one's continent of origin and ethnicity refers to one's narrower geographic roots coupled with religious or cultural roots, which category should we use in evaluating the health status or health risks of the US population? This question receives a great deal of attention in both scientific and policy contexts. Despite decades of research, the answer remains contentious. By knowing a person's race (as defined by the US Census Bureau), do we gain useful information about their health risks? Will we learn more by knowing that person's ethnicity? If there are certain health risks associated with a certain racial or ethnic group, what is the basis of those risks? Are they due to biologic factors, or are they due to social or cultural factors? Is there a biologic basis by which we can separate people into consistent racial or ethnic groups? These are some of the questions around which the discussion of race, ethnicity, and health revolves.

To illustrate this discussion and the different perspectives that are part of it, let us consider the results of a study of the way people respond to a particular medication for heart failure. The medicine is called angiotensin-converting enzyme inhibitor (ACE-I). It has been shown to be effective in the treatment of a condition called congestive heart failure (CHF), in which the heart muscle is weakened and unable to pump the blood effectively. By acting on the kidney to reduce the amount of fluid in the body, ACE-I can reduce the strain on the heart and reduce the symptoms caused by CHF.

To determine if ACE-I treatment is equally effective in blacks and whites, Exner and colleagues (2001) treated about 2,000 patients drawn from these two racial groups, each having CHF. After following these patients for about three years, the researchers were able to identify two principal findings:

1. The death rate was not reduced by treatment with ACE-I in either blacks or whites.
2. The frequency with which patients were hospitalized for treatment of CHF was reduced in whites taking ACE-I, but was not reduced in blacks taking ACE-I.

From these results the authors concluded that "therapeutic recommendations may need to be tailored according to racial background" (p. 1357). The authors suggested that a person's race (as distinct from ethnicity) can be used to predict that person's response to a specific treatment such as ACE-I therapy.

Realizing that such a conclusion was controversial, the editors of the journal in which the study was published asked two different authors, representing two different perspectives, to respond. Wood responded by stating, "Racial and ethnic differences in drug responses have now been well described for a range of drugs and reflect genetic differences, environmental differences (including shared cultural and dietary habits), and fundamental differences in the pathogenesis of diseases. . . . Thus, racial differences in the response to drugs not only have practical importance for the choice and dose of drugs but should also alert physicians to the important underlying genetic determinants of drug response" (2001, pp. 1394–95).

It is interesting to note that Wood first ascribes differences in drug responses to a combination of race and ethnicity, but concludes by suggesting that race alone, independent of ethnicity, can be used effectively to predict response to a drug. Wood suggests that there are clear genetic differences between races, and that these genetic differences are tied directly to differences in the body's response to certain drugs. In tying racial groups to underlying genetic differences, Wood reflects one side of the debate over what does (or does not) distinguish a race.

In response, Schwartz argued that "race is a social construct, not a scientific classification" and suggested that the use of racial categories in medical care is both inaccurate and dangerous. "A racial designation in the context of medical management not only defies everything we have learned from biology, genetics, and history but also opens the door to inequities in medical care. . . . Instruction in medical genetics should emphasize the fallacy of race as a scientific concept and the dangers inherent in practicing race-based medicine" (2001, pp. 1392–93).

The article by Exner and colleagues and the editorial responses by Wood and Schwartz contributed to a growing controversy in the medical literature about whether, in the context of medical care, different races should be seen as having predictable genetic differences that are tied to differences in the way the body reacts to certain treatments.

To address this and related questions, in 2003 the federal government sponsored a conference at which genetic and medical researchers from around the country were brought together and asked to address the following question: "What does the current body of scientific information say about the connections among race, ethnicity, genetics, and health?" (Patrinos 2004). A series of researchers contributed papers to this national conference, which were published in 2004 in a special issue of the journal *Nature Genetics*. In an introduction to that issue, the representative of the federal agency that sponsored the conference commented that "the term 'race' does not describe most of us with the subtlety and complexity required to capture and appreciate our genetic diversity. . . . Oversimplified concepts of race don't work in any objective realm. It's bad medicine and it's bad science" (Patrinos 2004, pp. S1–S2).

There appears to be general consensus among the authors of the papers coming out of the conference that there are identifiable genetic differences among people whose ancestors came from different continents. After reviewing the genetic evolution of the human species from its origins in East Africa, Tishkoff and Kidd conclude that "populations do, generally, cluster by broad geographic regions that correspond with common racial classification (Africa, Europe, Asia, Oceania, Americas)" (2004, p. S26). However, the amount of genetic variation that occurs among groups with differing continental origins is tiny compared to the amount of genetic similarity that exists among all people, regardless of ancestry. Jorde and Wooding (2004) estimate that less than 1 percent of the DNA structure of humans differs across individuals. Of this 1 percent of difference, 85 to 90 percent occurs at the level of the individual in ways that have no association with ancestral continent. Only 10 to 15 percent of the less than 1 percent of difference occurs in ways that can be tied to continent of origin. Thus, it is certainly true that a person of European ancestry and a person of sub-Saharan African ancestry will have clear differences in appearance, and these differences will be due to underlying genetic differences. A person with light skin and light hair will have differences in the structure of the genes for skin color and hair color from a person with dark skin and dark hair. The same will be true for facial structure. The genes that create these differences in surface appearance are so few compared to the genes that create the structural and functional similarity among all humans that they have little association with important biologic characteristics.

This is not to say that people of different races (that is, differing continent of origin) will not, as a group, have differing frequencies of certain genes. It is simply that the differences in underlying frequencies are insufficient to define the group as a race. Take, for example, the genetic mutation that is associated with sickle cell disease. This mutation is found in a higher frequency among individuals whose ancestors came from Africa than in individuals whose ancestors came from Europe. Yet the presence of the sickle cell mutation does not define a person as belonging to a certain race. There are subpopulations among those of European ancestry (for example, those of certain Mediterranean ancestral groups) that also have an increased frequency of the sickle cell mutation. As summarized by Jorde and Wooding, "[Genetic] clustering of individuals is correlated with geographic origin or ancestry. These clusters are also correlated with some traditional concepts of race, but the correlations are imperfect" (p. S28).

Part of the problem in deriving genetic associations from racial classifications appears to come from the different ways in which the concept of race has been approached by different scientific disciplines. Keita and colleagues (2004) argue that there is a scientifically accurate way to approach race—by categorizing variations that occur in animal species that create genetically different groups without creating a new species. Using race in this context is scientifically valid. However, dividing the human species into subgroups based on continent of origin is not scientifically consistent with dividing the human species based on clear genetic differences. Using race to separate groups based on continental origin has little scientific basis. Rather, this use of the concept of race is a social construction—that is, it is based on a common understanding that evolves over time among a particular social group, and that is not grounded in science. In describing this concept of race, Keita and colleagues conclude: "'Race' is 'socially constructed' when the word is incorrectly used as the covering term for social or demographic groups. Broadly designated groups, such as 'Hispanic' or 'European American' do not meet the classical or phylogenetic criteria for subspecies or the criterion for a breeding population. . . . 'Race' is a legitimate taxonomic concept that works for chimpanzees but does not apply to humans" (pp. S18–S19).

The History of the Use of "Race" as a Category in the United States

Recall from our discussion above that race is an explicit category used to categorize the population of the United States but that it is not used by the Canadian government to categorize its population. Similarly, the national census of Japan asks each resident to identify their nationality, but asks no questions about race (Japan, Statistics Bureau 2006). Why does the United States use the category of race, while other industrialized countries, both Western and Eastern, do not?

The concept of race as it is used in the United States has its origins in Western Europe. As European explorers were able to visit new parts of the globe, they recognized that the people they encountered often had a very different physical appearance than themselves. Since these physical differences were most striking when people from different continents were compared, the explorers came to distinguish human groups based on their continent of origin. Africans appeared quite distinct from Europeans. Those from Central and East Asia had their own distinct physical appearance, as did the native inhabitants of the Americas. Each time European explorers experienced the people of a new continent, they identified these people as a group distinct from their own.

The racial categories used by the United States have their origins in the eighteenth century. A Swedish naturalist named Carl Linnaeus made an exhaustive study of both plants and animals, seeking to establish a taxonomy of all animal life. In 1735 he first published *Systema Naturae*, a small pamphlet describing his understanding of the divisions of life on earth. Over a period of several years he gradually expanded this work into a multivolume publication. In it, he identified what he believed to be the four subspecies of humans:

1. *Afer niger* (African black): impassive, lazy, crafty, slow, foolish
2. *Americanus rubescus* (American red): ill-tempered, subjugated, obstinate
3. *Asiaticus luridus* (Asian yellow): melancholy, greedy, severe, haughty
4. *Europaeus albus* (European white): serious, strong, active, very smart, inventive

It should be apparent that the categories of subspecies identified by Linnaeus are nearly identical to the racial categories used by the US government. For much of the twentieth century, before 1997 when the "Native Hawaiian and Other Pacific Islander" category was separated from "Asian," the US system of racial categorization was identical to that proposed by Linnaeus.

Linnaeus did not stop at naming the subspecies of *Homo sapiens*. He also ascribed predominant behavioral characteristics to them. American reds (that is, American Indians) he described as "obstinate, and regulated by custom"; Asians were "severe, ruled by opinion"; Africans were "crafty, governed by caprice"; Europeans were "gentle, governed by law" (Marks 1995; Lee and colleagues 2001, p. 38).

It is interesting to note that another scientist who was a contemporary of Linnaeus differed somewhat in his human taxonomy. Writing in 1781, Johan Blumenbach suggested that, in addition to the four categories identified by Linnaeus, there was a fifth category—the Malay, now often referred to as the people of Oceania and corresponding largely to the Native Hawaiian and Other Pacific Islander category used by the US Census Bureau (Marks 1995). However, Blumenbach created these categories based purely on physical appearance. He ascribed no behavioral or psychological characteristics to these groups.

While Linnaeus and Blumenbach were in substantial agreement regarding most of the system of racial classification, they differed as to whether to include the peoples of Oceania as a separate racial category. How many human races were there: four or five? The answer depended on whether one adopted Linnaeus's view or that of Blumenbach. The view proposed by Linnaeus came to predominate, and it was the system of racial categorization used by the US government for most of the twentieth century. In the US census conducted in 1990, there were four racial categories from which to choose: white, black, Asian/Pacific Islander, or Native American. In 1997 the government officially changed its policy of racial categorization, decreeing that Native Hawaiian and Other Pacific Islander was the fifth race (Lee 2001). They did not do so because of Blumenbach—they did so for a set of reasons specific to the late twentieth century. It is interesting to note that, in making that change, the government was switching from the racial categories proposed by Linnaeus in 1758 to the categories proposed by Blumenbach in 1781.

Is There a Genetic Basis for Race?

While the consensus of the geneticists contributing papers to the federally sponsored conference discussed above is that race as a social category is very imprecise, they consistently acknowledge that there are genetic differences among population groups with differing continents of ancestral origin. In 2015 the *Annals of the American Academy of Political and Social Science* published a special issue titled "Race, Racial Inequality, and Biological Determinism in the Genetic and Genomic Era." In the introduction to the papers in the issue, Byrd and Hughey (2015) describe a continued debate regarding belief systems among scientists—a debate intensified by the scientific successes of the Human Genome Project. Some believe that race is genetically inherited, while others believe that biological differences among humans are due principally to behavioral differences. As described by Byrd and Hughey, these differing belief systems "form the 'ideological double helix' that intertwines to shape beliefs about race and inequality and influence the theoretical approaches, analytic strategies, and interpretations taken by scholars conducting biomedical and social scientific research" (p. 8).

A paper by Rosenberg and colleagues (2002) has addressed these issues, and has added substantially to our understanding of the genetic similarities and differences of different ancestral groups. They were able to obtain DNA samples from 1,056 individuals, representing 52 distinct populations around the globe. Each population had remained geographically stable for a number of generations. They tested each sample to determine the genetic structure of 377 different microsatellites—small segments of DNA without any known function. They asked themselves the following question: Without knowing the geographic origin of the samples, is it possible to sort the samples into groups based on genetic similarities that correspond to the geographic regions commonly associated with race as the concept is used in the United States?

To undertake this task, a computer was programmed to look at minute differences in microsatellite structure (sometimes as small as a single nucleotide), and to use an algorithm contained within a computer program to sort the samples into groups, such that the sorting maximized the overall difference in genetic structure among the groups. A key aspect of this sorting algorithm is that the computer does not determine the number of groups into which the samples will be sorted—a human selects this number and enters it into the computer. Based on this arbitrary number of groups, the computer groups the samples so as to maximize the genetic differences among the groups. The scientists ran this test five times, first sorting the samples into two groups, then three groups, and so on up to a maximum of six groups.

Once the DNA samples had been sorted into the specified number of groups based on genetic structure, the scientists looked at the geographic locations from which the samples within a group had been drawn. They wanted to know if the locations associated with a genetic group were also associated in some larger geographic area. They found that there was a fairly clear geographic patterning to the groups, and that the patterning overlapped substantially (but not completely) with the recognized continents. As stated by the authors, "Genetic clusters often correspond closely to predefined regional or population groups" (p. 2384). In fact, when the computer was programmed to divide the samples into four groups, the resulting groups corresponded largely to the four racial categories originally identified by Linnaeus.

Group 1: Europe, Middle East, Central Asia, and South Asia
Group 2: Sub-Saharan Africa
Group 3: East Asia and Oceania
Group 4: Americas (American Indians and other people indigenous to the Americas)

It is interesting to note what happened when the scientists programmed the computer to identify five genetic groups rather than four. When so instructed, the computer split East Asia and Oceania into separate groups, thus essentially recreating the five racial groups identified in 1781 by Linnaeus's contemporary, Blumenbach.

Who was more accurate in their classification scheme, Linnaeus or Blumenbach? Do humans exist as four inherent groups or five? The answer to this question is entirely arbitrary. The peoples of Oceania are both genetically similar to, and genetically distinct from the peoples of East Asia. Do we focus on their similarity or their difference?

Rosenberg and colleagues were able to reproduce the findings summarized above by Jorde and Wooding: of the small amount of genetic variation that was identified among the samples (most of the DNA structure was identical), 93 to 95 percent of that variation occurred at the level of the individual, with no association with the group from which the individual is drawn. Only 3 to 5 percent of the variation they found in genetic structure occurred among geographic groups. Nonetheless, this tiny amount of genetic variation was enough for the computer to do its task of sorting the samples into groups. Instructing the computer in how many groups to use will change the outcome of that sorting process. Unless there is a scientific basis for selecting that number of groups, the number will be arbitrary.

What if the computer is instructed to sort the samples into two groups? We get the following results:

Group 1: Sub-Saharan Africa, Europe, Middle East, Central Asia, and South Asia
Group 2: East Asia and Oceania and the Americas

This division has sorted the human population into two recognizable groups: Westerners and Easterners. It has essentially cleaved the globe in two along a line of longitude. By this sorting, sub-Saharan Africans are more genetically similar to Europeans than they are genetically different, analogous to the Asia/Oceania situation discussed above.

What happens when we ask the computer to sort the samples into three groups? Sub-Saharan Africa is separated out from its previous group, and we have:

Group 1: Sub-Saharan Africa
Group 2: Europe, Middle East, Central Asia, and South Asia
Group 3: East Asia and Oceania and the Americas

Instructed to sort the samples into six groups, how will the computer respond? What will be the sixth group, and will it correspond to any racial category? (After all, the US Census Bureau stopped at five categories.) What we find is very interesting.

Group 1: Europe, Middle East, Central Asia, and South Asia
Group 2: Sub-Saharan Africa
Group 3: East Asia
Group 4: Oceania
Group 5: Americas
Group 6: Kalash

The sixth group identified by the computer is the Kalash, a tribal group of about 4,000 people living in northwestern Pakistan. There is a small amount of genetic difference between the Kalash and the surrounding peoples of Central Asia that is sufficient for the computer to distinguish the two groups as different, once the remainder of the world's population has been sorted into five groups. Do the Kalash constitute a race? Of course not! They are a distinct ethnic group with their own culture and geography, but are nearly identical on a genetic basis to other groups surrounding them.

Many who read the Rosenberg study focused on only the sorting that took place when the computer was programmed to identify four groups. They argued that these results confirmed that there is a biologic basis for the historical racial categories of white, black, Asian, and American Indian. There is enough similarity within these groups and enough difference among these groups to consider them genetically distinct. What are we to make of this assertion? To answer this question, let us imagine what might happen if, instead of sorting human DNA samples, we asked the computer to sort a deck of cards into groups based on similarities and differences among the cards.

As in the Rosenberg study, we would first program the computer to sort the cards into two groups. Using digital analysis of color scans of the cards, we would expect the computer to sort the deck into the red cards and the black cards. If we program the computer to sort the deck into three groups, we might get something like this: one group containing all the face cards, one group containing all the red-numbered cards, and one group containing all the black-numbered cards. Instructing the computer to sort the deck into four groups will likely result in groups made up of the four suits: spades, hearts, diamonds, and clubs.

Which is the most scientific way to sort the cards? There is no single answer to this question. The science in the sorting process was in the way we scanned the cards into digital images and the protocol we instructed the computer to use in analyzing those images. Each result—two groups, three groups, or four groups—is equally scientific, as each used the same sorting process.

However, in playing a game of cards, we are not principally concerned with the scientific nature of the cards. We are concerned primarily with understanding the rules of the game. For most card games played in the Western world, the cards are sorted according to suits. Why don't we play the same games using two suits, or three? Simple—because the rules say there are four suits. Where did the rules come from? In the case of card games, many of the rules came from an Englishman by the name of Edmond Hoyle, who lived in the eighteenth century. As described on the website playingcards.wikidot.com, Hoyle "was best known as an expert on the rules and strategies behind card games and board games including chess and backgammon, memorializing the common phrase 'According to Hoyle.'" In 1770 Hoyle published his book, *Hoyles Games*, describing the rules by which card games were to be played. The 2001 version of the book is titled *Hoyle's Rules of Games*.

Why do we play card games with four suits rather than two? Because that's what the rules say. Over a period of several centuries we have come to a widely accepted consensus to play the game with four suits. Playing a game of cards with four suits rather than three is a social convention. In the words of sociologists, the suits in a deck of cards have been "socially constructed."

Let us use this same reasoning to ask which of the results of the Rosenberg study we should focus on. Should we consider the peoples of Oceania to be similar to or distinct from the peoples of East Asia? Should we consider the peoples of sub-Saharan Africa to be similar to (the result when sorting into two groups) or distinct from (the result when sorting into more than two groups) the peoples of Europe? Few would argue that sub-Saharan Africans should be considered to be of the same race as Europeans. However, this argument is not based on science, but on the social construction of racial categories that developed in much of Europe in the eighteenth century and before. Why are there four races rather than two? Because that's what the rules say. Just as people have come to agree on the rules of a card game, people (at least in the United States) also have come to agree on the "rules" of our society. Approaching the world's population as containing four races, as we did in the United States prior to 1997, was a social convention, just as dividing a deck of cards into four suits rather than two is a social convention. Changing from four races to five, as the US government elected to do in 1997, simply changed the rules, adopting the categories originally suggested by Blumenbach as compared to those suggested by Linnaeus.

There are other examples in history of ethnic groups—people linked by a common language, culture, and ancestry—having been assigned to one racial group by social convention, only to have their perceived race change as the social convention changes. To provide an example of this phenomenon, I offer again some history from my own family. Figure 5.2 shows photographs of my mother and father when they were young. It should be apparent that, by today's standards, my mother and father are members of the same race—white.

My father was born in 1897, and his father was Irish. His father's family had emigrated to Nova Scotia at the time of the potato famine, and eventually settled in British Columbia. My mother was of Anglo-Saxon descent, with ancestors dating to the *Mayflower*. In the 1890s many in a position of power and authority in the United States did not consider a person of Irish ancestry to be a member of the white race (Roediger 1999). Among these were Senator Henry Cabot Lodge, of Massachusetts, who in the same year my father was born argued on the floor of the US Senate

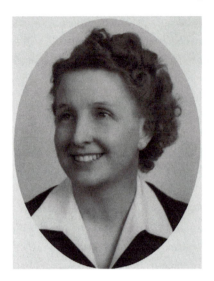 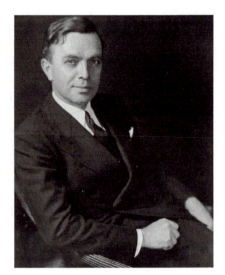

Figure 5.2. The author's mother and father.

that the immigration of Irish and other European groups to the United States was becoming a threat to the white race and should be limited. "Surely it is not too much to sift now the hordes that pour out of every European steamship unsifted, uncounted, unchecked. . . . The races that built up this country come in diminishing numbers. New races, utterly alien, come in ever increasing numbers. What we now seek to accomplish by the pending bill is to sift this immigration and restrict it" (Lodge 1897, p. 1432). Based on these comments, Senator Lodge and many others like him would have considered my mother, whose ancestors were members of "the race that built up this country," to be white by race, but my father, whose ancestors fled Ireland in the nineteenth century, to be members of a "new race, utterly alien," and therefore not part of the white race.

To categorize the race of a child of Irish Canadian and English American descent (that is, the author's race) as anything other than white would be very unusual today. When my father was born a common social convention excluded those of Irish ancestry from the white race. Today that same convention includes the Irish within the white race. The social construction of race—the rules of the game—has changed in regard to the Irish, as it has for Jews, Italians, and other immigrant groups.

We should recognize some additional questions raised by the genetic data presented by Rosenberg and colleagues. The 1,056 subjects of their research were all from distinct population groups that had remained geographically stable for multiple generations. Rosenberg also looked at the genetic structure of certain populations in which there had been substantial geographic migration and resulting "admixture"—intermarriage and interbreeding. The genetic structures of many ethnic groups living in the Middle East, for example, are so heterogeneous that it was impossible for the computer to make any type of reliable separation. Similarly, a number of geographic groups were excluded from the study because they represented populations that were transitional between regions. For example, individuals from Ethiopia and Somalia have a genetic structure that is midway between that of Europeans and sub-Saharan Africans. Similarly, much of the African American and Hispanic population of the United States has experienced high levels of admixture over time, making it very difficult to reliably assign individuals to a specific geographic group.

Finally, we should recognize that some of the population groups sorted in one way by the computer in the Rosenberg study are typically sorted in a different way when the concept of race as a social construction is applied. In particular, the subjects drawn from South Asia sort into a different group based on genetics than they do based on social convention. Subjects from India and Pakistan are typically considered to be Asian by race. The US Census Bureau explicitly identifies those from the Indian subcontinent as Asian. However, in the Rosenberg study, South Asians such as Indians and Pakistanis are more genetically similar to Europeans than they are to East Asians, and are included in the European group in all the iterations of the sorting process. Thus, South Asians are Asian by social convention but white by genetic sorting.

As a second example of the difference between social convention and genetic structure, let us imagine what might have happened if Othello had been included as a subject in the Rosenberg study. As Shakespeare described him, Othello was a superb military commander—so successful that the Duke of Venice hired him to lead the Venetian army into battle against an invasion by the Turks. Othello of course was not Venetian. He was a Moor from the historical area of Mauritania (an area of North Africa that includes present-day Algeria and Morocco). Because he was a Moor, Othello had a skin color that was considerably darker than that of his Venetian hosts. His skin color, and the cultural difference it signified, was to get Othello into trouble when he first fell in love with and then (secretly) married Desdemona, the daughter of Barbantio, one of Venice's leading citizens.

When Barbantio learns that his daughter has chosen to marry Othello, he goes in search of him. On finding Othello, he assails him with the following words (act 1, scene 2):

> O thou foul thief, where hast thou stow'd my daughter?
>   Damn'd as thou art, thou hast enchanted her . . . to [thy] sooty bosom.

Barbantio is extremely upset that his daughter has married a man with a "sooty bosom" (that is, with dark skin). At the time Shakespeare was writing *Othello*, Moors were considered to be black—in the same group as sub-Saharan Africans. Well into the twentieth century, this social convention persisted throughout much of Europe and the United States.

It turns out that Barbantio had less to worry about than he thought. Data from the Rosenberg study confirm that, genetically, Moors and other ethnic groups from North Africa cluster with Europeans, having more genetic similarity to Europeans than to sub-Saharan Africans. If we insist on dividing the Western hemisphere into two racial groups based on genetic similarities and differences, then Othello was white. Interestingly, the US Census Bureau would also consider Othello to be white, as it includes North Africans and those from the Middle East in the white racial category.

If we consider the evolution of the human species, it makes sense that North Africans are more similar genetically to Europeans than they are to sub-Saharan Africans. The origins of the human species were in the area of the Horn of Africa— currently Ethiopia, Somalia, and Eritrea. Gradually the new human species migrated north into the regions of the Middle East and North Africa, and south to the regions south of the Saharan Desert. The presence of the Sahara as a geographic barrier meant that there was little admixture over time between the northern migrants and the southern migrants. Each group gradually developed its own set of genetic markers. The people of Europe have their evolutionary origins in the northern group of migrants—those inhabiting North Africa and the Middle East. It thus makes sense that modern-day North Africans have more in common genetically with Europeans than they do with sub-Saharan Africans.

There is, however, an important caveat about the above discussion of the genetic clustering of individuals from South Asia or from the Middle East / North Africa. The genetic clustering of these population groups with Europeans was based on Rosenberg and colleagues' study of microsatellites—segments of DNA containing multiple nucleotides. As an alternative, Li and colleagues (2008) analyzed the same genetic material studied by Rosenberg, only instead of using microsatellite structure they evaluated single nucleotide polymorphisms (SNP). As its name suggests, an SNP looks at which nucleotide is present in a specific location on a DNA molecule. By doing this at 650,000 different DNA locations, they were able to repeat the sorting into groups. Using SNPs and sorting the genetic material into five groups, they came up with the same grouping as Rosenberg. However, when the computer was then asked to sort the material into six groups based on SNPs, the sixth group was South Asians. (The Kalashi were no longer identified as a separate group.) Sorting the material into seven groups identified populations from the Middle East and North Africa as the seventh group. Thus, determining whether South Asians and North Africans differ genetically from Europeans depends on whether we use SNPs or microsatellites as our basis for comparison.

Problems in the Continued Use of Race to Measure Health Outcomes

As discussed above, the four (or five) racial categories that have been identified in the United States are based largely on a social construction of what constitutes race. The common social convention is to distinguish races such as white and black, and to report health outcomes separately, with the expectation that the racial differences identified will be important in identifying those individuals who are at highest risk of adverse health outcomes. Such an approach, however, has inherent problems. I illustrate these problems in a discussion of three important medical conditions: low birth weight, heart disease, and high blood pressure.

Low Birth Weight

In 2016 infants born to black mothers in the United States died before their first birthday at the rate of 11.1 for every 1,000 live births. For the same year, the infant mortality rate for babies born to white mothers was 4.9 per 1,000 live births. One of the main contributors to this difference in infant mortality is the much higher frequency with which babies born to black mothers are underweight—either low birth weight (LBW) (weighing less than 2,500 grams) or very-low birth weight (VLBW) (weighing less than 1,500 grams). Babies born at these weights are much more likely to die before their first birthday than babies with a normal birth weight. In 2016 13.1 percent of black infants weighed less than 2,500 grams, while 2.8 percent weighed less than 1,500 grams. In the same year, 7.1 percent of white infants were less than 2,500 grams while 1.1 percent were less than 1,500 grams (CDC 2018).

In 1997 David and Collins reported on a study of babies born in the state of Illinois between 1980 and 1995. They compared the weights of 44,000 babies born to white mothers and 46,000 babies born to black mothers. They separated the data on black infants based on whether the mother had been born in the United States or in Africa. When they did this, they found that the distribution of birth weights of the babies of African-born black mothers was nearly identical with that of US-born white mothers, while the distribution of birth weights for the US-born black mothers was significantly lower. The distribution of birth weights for the three

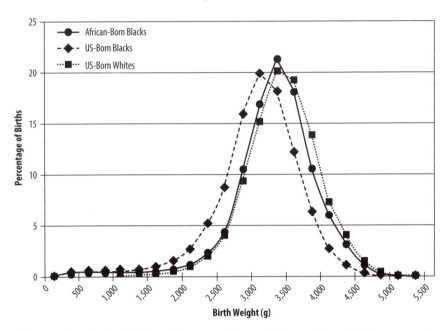

Figure 5.3. Distribution of birth weights among infants of US-born white and black women and African-born black women in Illinois, 1980–95. *Source*: R. J. David and J. W. Collins, "Differing Birth Weight among Infants of U.S.-Born Blacks, African-Born Blacks, and U.S.-Born Whites," *New England Journal of Medicine* 337 (1997):1209–14. Copyright © 1997 Massachusetts Medical Society. All rights reserved. Reprinted with permission.

groups is shown in Figure 5.3. The average birth weight and frequency of birth weight categories are shown in Table 5.1.

While the rate of VLBW infants was higher among the African-born black mothers than the US-born white mothers (2.3 percent as compared to 0.7 percent), the rate of LBW infants was similar (4.8 percent compared to 3.6 percent) and the average birth weight was only 3 percent lower (3,333 grams for African-born black mothers, 3,446 grams for US-born white mothers). US-born black mothers, on the other hand, had both VLBW and LBW infants at a higher rate than whites—2.6 percent and 10.6 percent, respectively—and had infants that weighed on average 3,089 grams, or more than 10 percent less than white infants.

Comparing rates of LBW and the associated risk of infant mortality only by the race of the mother may yield inaccurate information and lead to inappropriate treatment decisions. If a doctor assumes that, because black mothers have many more tiny infants than white mothers, a black mother is therefore at increased risk of giving

Table 5.1. Average Birth Weight and Frequency of Low and Very Low Birth Weight among White, African-Born Black, and US-Born Black Mothers in Illinois

	White	African-Born Black	US-Born Black
Average birth weight (grams)	3,446	3,333	3,089
Low birth weight (1,500–2,500 grams), as a proportion of all births	3.6%	4.8%	10.6%
Very low birth weight (<1,500 grams), as a proportion of all births	0.7%	2.3%	2.6%

Source: R. J. David and J. W. Collins 1997.

birth to a tiny child, that doctor would have inappropriately looked at the patient's race rather than her ethnicity. A US-born black mother is in the same race as an African-born black mother. However, the ethnic characteristics of these two women is likely to be very different. In the David and Collins study, the African-born black mothers, when compared to the US-born black mothers, were:

· older
· more likely to be married
· more highly educated
· less likely to have been late in starting prenatal care

The social and economic differences between these two ethnic communities of black women are substantial. To know her risk of having a premature or underweight baby, you would have to know to which ethnic group a black woman in Illinois belongs.

Elo and Culhane (2010) found similar differences in a comparison of pregnant black women in Philadelphia. They compared behaviors associated with birth outcomes in women born in the United States, Africa, or the Caribbean. The foreign born women were less likely to engage in risky behaviors, and in addition had better self-reported health status, with the difference somewhat more pronounced in African-born women as compared to those born in the Caribbean. These ethnic differences persisted after controlling for SES.

Heart Disease

Using nationally representative data and established cardiovascular risk metrics, Mainous and colleagues (2018) were able to measure changes in cardiovascular disease risk for individuals aged 40–79 for the period 1999–2014. Looking at the population overall, they found no change in the risk an individual faces of dying from

Table 5.2. Age-Adjusted Annual Death Rates from All
Causes, New York City, 1988–92

	Male	Female
United States, all races	680.2	387.9
New York, all races	878.9	456.8
New York, white	721.4	393.1
New York, black	1,224.8	593.7

Source: Fang et al. 1996.
Note: Deaths per 100,000 population.

cardiovascular disease within the next 10 years. When looking at risk according to gender and race, they found that black men had the highest risk of death and were the only group that showed a change in risk over time. The 10-year risk of a black male dying of cardiovascular disease went from 53.5 percent in 1999–2002 to 65.2 percent in 2011–14. Does this mean that physicians should treat every black male patient they encounter as being at increased risk of early death from cardiovascular disease?

Fang and colleagues (1996) published a study comparing the risk of death from cardiovascular disease among white and black residents of New York City. Overall, New York City had a substantially higher rate of death from all causes than the rest of the country at that time. In addition, the overall death rate among blacks in New York was substantially higher than the rate for whites. These data are shown in Table 5.2.

Cardiovascular disease was the most common cause of death, accounting for 34 percent of deaths among blacks in New York and 52 percent of deaths among whites. Imagine that you are a doctor and two new adult male patients have come to see you, one white and the other black. You reason that, because the death rate for cardiovascular disease is higher among blacks than among whites, your new black patient will be at a higher risk of death than your white patient. However, in arriving at such a conclusion, you would have made a fundamental error. Because the average death rate for black males is higher than that for white males, it does not necessarily follow that any black man will be at a higher risk of death than any white man.

The black community of New York City represents a variety of distinct ethnic groups, each with unique cultural characteristics. Three of the largest groups are blacks who were born in the Southeast of the United States, blacks born in the Northeast of the United States, and blacks born in the Caribbean. The diet, educational levels, behaviors, and other cultural characteristics of these three ethnic communities may have important differences. These ethnic differences may contribute to health status and to death rates. This is precisely what Fang and colleagues found. When they compared the cardiovascular death rates for these three ethnic groups

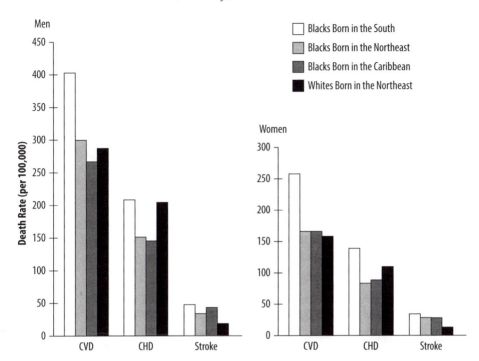

Figure 5.4. Age-adjusted annual rates of death from selected cardiovascular diseases in non-Hispanic blacks and whites in New York City, according to birthplace, 1988–92. CVD = cardiovascular disease; CHD = coronary heart disease. *Source*: J. Fang, S. Madhavan, and M. Alderman, "The Association between Birthplace and Mortality from Cardiovascular Causes among Black and White Residents of New York City," *New England Journal of Medicine* 335 (1996):1545–51. Copyright © 1997 Massachusetts Medical Society. All rights reserved. Reprinted with permission.

with that of whites in New York, they found a very interesting pattern, as illustrated in Figure 5.4.

The cardiovascular death rate for blacks born in the Southeast was by far the highest of all the groups, for both men and women. Among men, the *lowest* cardiovascular death rate was among blacks born in the Caribbean. For women, rates for blacks born in the Northeast, blacks born in the Caribbean, and whites born in the Northeast were almost indistinguishable. Looking only at deaths from coronary heart disease (for example, heart attacks), the rate among blacks born in the Southeast remained substantially higher than that of whites, but the rates for northeastern blacks and Caribbean blacks were substantially lower than for whites. For deaths from stroke, all three black groups had higher rates than whites.

Kaufman and colleagues (2015) undertook a comprehensive review of 68 research articles published over more than a decade that studied genome-wide associations between genetic variation among races and associated variation in cardiovascular disease. From this review they concluded that "Despite the rapid increase in the number of genomic studies over the past decade that covered many outcomes, the accumulated evidence for a genetic contribution to CVD disparities in blacks versus whites has been essentially nil" (p. 468).

In assessing the risk of death from cardiovascular disease in general, or coronary heart disease in particular, for any individual, it is not sufficient to know that the person is black. The physician must know the patient's ethnicity and individual patterns of behavior before being able to accurately predict and treat the risk of disease. As was the case in the genetic sorting of global populations in the Rosenberg study, and the distribution of birth weights in the David study, these authors found that there is more variation within races than there is between races. Race alone provides relatively little information about an individual's health risks.

High Blood Pressure

The CDC reported that in 2016, 31 percent of the adult population in the United States had high blood pressure (CDC 2018). However, the prevalence of high blood pressure is quite different among different racial and ethnic groups (Table 5.3).

The highest rate of high blood pressure is among black women—a rate that is more than 50 percent greater than the comparable rate for white women. The rate for black men is 34 percent greater than that of white men. The lowest rate is for Mexican American men, with Mexican American women having the second lowest rate among these groups. The report also included the rate of high blood pressure for "Hispanic or Latino" men and women, which includes all sectors of the Hispanic population. The rates are comparable to those of Mexican Americans. Prior to 2010 the National Center for Health Statistics (NCHS) only reported rates of high blood pressure for Mexican Americans. In light of the heterogeneity of the category "Hispanic or Latino," the NCHS now includes rates for both categories.

Table 5.3. High Blood Pressure in the US Population Over Age 20, by Race, Ethnicity, and Gender, 2016

	Male (percent)	Female (percent)
All races	31.5	29.3
White (not Hispanic)	31.1	27.0
Black (not Hispanic)	41.8	42.9
Mexican Americans	27.9	30.1
Hispanic or Latino	27.9	29.8

Source: National Center for Health Statistics—Health, United States, 2017.

Given the strikingly different prevalence of high blood pressure between blacks and whites in the United States, it is crucially important to approach the treatment of high blood pressure in a manner that is supported by scientific data. In 2003 a national panel of high blood pressure researchers studied the scientific literature and published a consensus statement on the optimal approach to treating high blood pressure in African Americans (Douglas et al. 2003). They noted that two drugs often used as first-line treatment for high blood pressure in whites—beta-blockers and ACE-I—"may produce less blood-pressure lowering effect in African Americans than in whites" (p. 537). An accompanying editorial went somewhat further, stating that "these drugs should not be used as initial single-drug therapies for African Americans" (Materson 2003, p. 522). This recommendation—that these two drugs be used as first-line treatment in whites but not in blacks—has been echoed in a number of other publications and adopted by many physicians as best medical practice.

In 2014 the Joint National Committee, a federally sponsored advisory group on the treatment of high blood pressure, issued its guidelines for the treatment of high blood pressure (James et al. 2014). The Committee reviewed extensive research on the optimal treatment of blood pressure in adults and issued recommended treatment protocols based on that research. It issued the following guideline regarding the optimal use of blood pressure medications: "There is moderate evidence to support initiating drug treatment with an angiotensin-converting enzyme inhibitor, angiotensin receptor blocker, calcium channel blocker, or thiazide-type diuretic in the nonblack hypertensive population, including those with diabetes. In the black hypertensive population, including those with diabetes, a calcium channel blocker or thiazide-type diuretic is recommended as initial therapy" (p. 507).

This guideline recommends that physicians approach treating black patients as if they were a homogeneous group sharing common biological traits that affect response to blood pressure medications.

From the discussion above, we might want to question the assumption that all people who are black by race will have the same response to certain medications. This is precisely the question Mokwe and colleagues (2004) posed in a study of the use of one particular ACE-I drug in treating comparable samples of blacks and whites with high blood pressure. When they looked only at each subject's race without considering individual characteristics such as obesity, kidney function, and the presence of diabetes, they identified a lesser response to treatment among the blacks compared to the whites. However, when they took into account differences between the black subjects and the white subjects in the rates of these confounding conditions, they found that most of the difference in blood pressure response went away, leading them to conclude that "a large source of variability of blood pressure response to treatment is within, not between, racial groups, and that factors that vary at the level of the individual contribute to apparent racial differences in response to treatment" (p. 1202). These authors went on to caution physicians about using race to decide treatment choices.

> Our results question the wisdom of using black race, per se, as a major criterion on which to base decisions regarding ACE inhibitor monotherapy because of their presumed lack of effectiveness for lowering BP. Race differences in *group* BP responses to monotherapy with ACE inhibitors are an inaccurate means of predicting the magnitude of BP-lowering with an ACE inhibitor in individual patients of either race because of the near-complete overlap of the BP response distributions of blacks and whites, and because a significant portion of the race difference in BP response is attributable to factors that vary at the level of the individual. (p. 1206)

Sehgal mirrored this conclusion in his review of 15 different studies comparing a variety of drugs for the treatment of high blood pressure in blacks and whites. He found that, while the average change in blood pressure was statistically lower in blacks than in whites, the difference in average response for the two groups was very small (between 0.6 mm and 3.0 mm out of a typical systolic blood pressure of 140–160), and that this difference in average group response was due to differences in response by a small subset of blacks. He found that "80% to 95% of whites and blacks have similar responses to commonly used antihypertensive drugs" (p. 569). After reviewing these 15 different scientific studies Sehgal concluded that "race has little value in predicting antihypertensive drug response, because whites and blacks overlap greatly in their response to all categories of drugs. These findings are consistent with other work demonstrating that most genetic diversity exists within and not between races and that race is a poor predictor of drug-metabolizing enzymes (which in turn influence drug response)" (p. 570).

In following birth weight and associated infant mortality, in comparing death rates from cardiovascular disease, and in selecting a treatment for high blood pressure, we find a consistent sequence of conclusions that are supported by scientific evidence.

- In comparing blacks and whites as racial groups, it is often possible to document significant differences in the mean (average) outcome.
- Once individual characteristics of group members are taken into account (for example, ethnicity, rates of other illness) most of the observed difference goes away.

- There is consistently more variation in these outcomes within racial groups than there is between racial groups.
- A person's race taken alone provides little information about and acts as a poor predictor of health outcomes.

Can We Use Hispanic Ethnicity to Predict Health Status?

In its report on death rates in the US population for 2016, the federal government's National Center for Health Statistics reported that the age-adjusted death rate per 100,000 population was 749 for the non-Hispanic white population and 526 for the Hispanic population. From these data it would be technically accurate to state that the death rate for Hispanics is 30 percent lower than that of whites. However, as was the case with race as a category, simply knowing that a person is Hispanic will tell you little about their risk of death relative to whites. Recall from the discussion of the US census above that, for those who indicate that they are of Hispanic ethnicity, they are then asked to indicate to which subgroup within Hispanic they belong, with the largest three groups identified: Mexican, Puerto Rican, and Cuban.

Looking again at the data on deaths in 2016, we find that the age-adjusted death rate for these three groups was quite different:

- Mexican, 544
- Puerto Rican, 629
- Cuban, 523

While the death rate for all three groups was less than that of whites, there was substantial variation among the groups. It appears that, as with race, there is substantially more variation in health status within the Hispanic ethnicity than there is between Hispanics and non-Hispanic whites.

What Race Is and Isn't

When I was a medical student in the 1970s, I learned what most medical students at the time learned: sickle cell disease was a black disease. It was a genetic mutation that only appeared in black patients, with ancestral roots in Africa. In the early years of my clinical practice, I also learned the fallacy of this belief. The genetic mutant of sickle cell disease appears in ancestral populations historically exposed to high rates of malaria. The heterozygous mutation of sickle cell trait protected individuals from the ravages of malaria. As described by the American Society of Hematology (2018), "Sickle cell trait can also affect Hispanics, South Asians, Caucasians from southern Europe, and people from Middle Eastern countries. More than 100 million people worldwide have sickle cell trait."

Most African Americans have a mixture of African and European ancestry, which includes a mixture of genetic traits that are found more commonly in one ancestral group or the other. It is the presence or absence of a specific genetic trait, not one's assigned race, that affects one's risk for disease. As described by Moises Velasquez-Manoff (2017), a science writer for the *New York Times*, "there is variation in the human family, but there are few sharp divides where one set of traits ends and another begins. Rather, traits exist in gradients, reaching high frequency in some populations and lower frequency in others."

In an article also published in the *New York Times* a few months after that by Velasquez-Manoff, Harvard geneticist David Reich (2018a) described how recent genetic research has enabled scientists to identify specific mutations that have strong associations with disease rates, and which are found with differing frequencies among ancestral groups. Reich and his colleagues were able to identify a group of genetic mutations located in a small section of the genome that were shown to be risk factors for the development of prostate cancer. These mutations were found at a higher rate among African Americans than among whites, thus accounting for a higher rate of prostate cancer among blacks in the Unites States than among whites. However, among African Americans who had inherited the genetic pattern more commonly found in those of European ancestry, their risk of developing prostate cancer was about the same as that of whites of European ancestry.

Reich posed a question for his readers: "So how should we prepare for the likelihood that in the coming years, genetic studies will show that many traits are influenced by genetic variations, and that these traits will differ on average across human populations?" In a follow-up article published a week later in the *Times*, Reich (2018b) answers his question. "[W]e have known for almost a half-century that for the great majority of human traits shaped by genetics, there is far greater variation among individuals than populations . . . 'Race' has trivial predictive power about an individual person's biological capabilities . . . 'Race' is fundamentally a social category—not a biological one—as anthropologists have shown."

If, as Reich suggests, race is a social category and not a biologic one, how do we explain the consistent disparities in disease rates, mortality rates, and life expectancy among black Americans and white Americans? How do race, ethnicity, and SES interact to affect these disparities? I address these questions in the following chapter.

CHAPTER SIX

Race/Ethnicity, Socioeconomic Status, and Health

Which Is More Important in Affecting Health Status?

In the previous chapter I explored the concept of race, distinguishing it from that of ethnicity. I looked at the ways in which perceptions of race have evolved over time, concluding that the commonly used racial categories are based on social convention and do not represent inherent biological division of the human species. However, saying that racial categories are socially constructed and that the number of races is somewhat arbitrary is not to say that there is no association between race and health. Quite the contrary, as there has been a consistent association between race/ethnicity and health throughout much of the history of the United States. Looking at data from the period 2010–16, we can see these associations (Figure 6.1).

Figure 6.1 shows the changes in age-adjusted death rates for the four largest racial groups in the United States for this period. For each group, there has been a gradual decline in the death rate over this period, generally in the range of one to seven percent. Despite these declines, the rank ordering of the races has remained the same, and the gap between races has stayed fairly constant. In 2016 the death rate for black Americans was 18 percent greater than that for white Americans, while that for Asian Americans was 47 percent lower than the rate for whites.

Cunningham and colleagues (2017) followed changes in age-adjusted death rates for the period 1999–2015. They found that the black death rate declined by 25 percent over this time, while the white death rate declined by 14 percent. While black death rates remained higher than white death rates for all ages less than 65, they did find an important change for those aged 65 or greater. "Among persons aged ≥65 years, there was a black-white mortality crossover, whereby blacks had slightly lower age-adjusted deaths than whites beginning in 2010" (p. 447).

Sloan and colleagues (2010) also looked at changes in black/white mortality rates over time, but did so over the period of nearly a century. They were able to obtain records of black and white veterans of the Civil War who were still alive in 1900. They tracked the death rates of these men over the period 1900–14, and then compared the relative death rates by race to black and white men followed between 1992

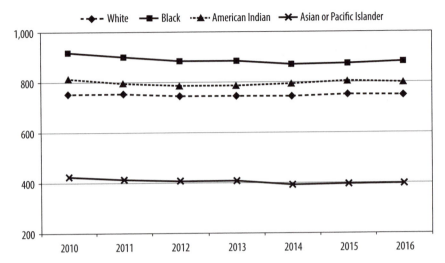

Figure 6.1. Age-adjusted annual mortality rates in the United States, by race, 2010–16. Deaths per 100,000 population. *Source*: CDC—National Center for Health Statistics; Deaths: final data for 2016.

and 2006 as part of a large national study. While the overall death rate for both groups fell dramatically over the period of a century, the relative death rates did not change. The black death rate among Civil War veterans was 18 percent higher than the white rate, while the black death rate in the latter group was 17 percent higher than the white rate.

Figure 6.2 shows the life expectancy at birth for the period 2006–16. These data are separated both by race and by gender. The life expectancy for Hispanic females is consistently the highest of all groups measured, with white females second highest. Similarly, the life expectancy for Hispanic males is somewhat greater than that for white males at a point midway in the distribution. However, the life expectancy for black males in 2016 was nearly five years lower than that of white males, while the life expectancy of black females was more than three years lower than that of their white counterparts.

In comparing life expectancy and death rates among the racial and ethnic groups identified in these federal data, it is important to understand the characteristics of the American Indian / Alaska Native (AI/AN) population. Of the approximately 3.7 million AI/AN individuals in the United States, approximately 2.2 million live on or near tribal land, while 1.5 million live in urban areas or rural areas not adjacent to tribal lands. The United States Indian Health Service (IHS) provides health care services and maintains health data on those AI/AN individuals living in tribal lands. For the period 2009–11, the IHS reported that the overall age-adjusted death rate

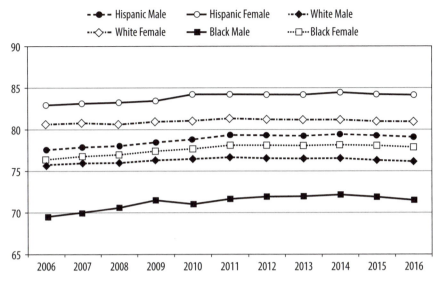

Figure 6.2. Life expectancy at birth, by race and sex, 2005–16. *Source:* CDC—National Center for Health Statistics—Health, United States, 2017.

for tribal-affiliated AI/AN individuals was 1.3 times greater than that of the overall United States population (Indian Health Services 2018).

During the period 2007–09, life expectancy for AI/AN males was 68.0 years, as compared to 76.0 for white males and 70.5 for black males. Life expectancy for AI/AN females was 74.3 years, as compared to 80.7 for white females and 77.0 for black females (Arias et al. 2014). While heart disease and cancer are the leading causes of death for both AI/AN and non-AI/AN groups in the United States, accidents (principally motor vehicle accidents), suicides, diabetes, and alcohol-related liver disease are among the top causes of death among AI/AN who live within tribal communities (Sancar et al. 2018).

Evidence of these disparities affecting the AI/AN population led Sequist (2017) to publish a commentary in the *Lancet*, one of the leading British medical journals, in which he argued that "key steps are needed to substantially reduce the health inequities experienced by AI/AN people. First, a public health approach to addressing the social determinants of health is needed to target the root causes and ultimate consequences of unhealthy and risky behaviours" (p. 1379).

Beyond death rates and life expectancy, rates of infant deaths also differ substantially among racial and ethnic groups. Figure 6.3 shows the infant mortality rate from 2007 to 2016 for the largest racial and ethnic groups in the United States. (Note that the federal government rarely reports separate health data for

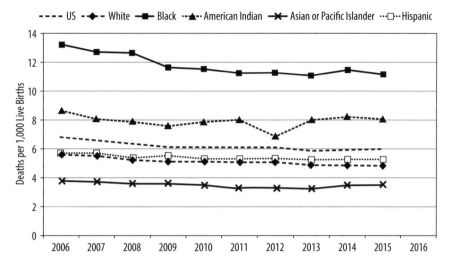

Figure 6.3. Infant mortality in the United States, by race/ethnicity, 2007–16. *Source*: Kids Count Data Center.

Native Hawaiians and Other Pacific Islanders, though being separated out as a race in 1997.) The infant mortality rate has remained nearly flat during this period, except for a gradual decline in the black rate. Once again we see a rank ordering among the racial/ethnic groups. In 2016 the infant mortality for babies born to black mothers was more than twice that of babies born to white mothers, while the rate for babies born to Asian mothers was 33 percent lower than that for white mothers. It is interesting to note that the infant mortality rate for babies born to Hispanic mothers has remained nearly identical to the rate for babies born to white mothers.

LaVeist (2000) attempted to quantify the burden of illness experienced by disadvantaged racial and ethnic groups in the United States. Using data gathered by the federal government, he estimated the increased mortality rate among blacks and Hispanics compared to whites, doing separate analyses for age groups 15–24, 25–44, and 45–64. Comparing Hispanics to whites, he found little difference in overall death rates for any of the three age groups. While the death rate among young Hispanics (ages 15–24) was approximately 12 percent higher than that of whites, the death rate among Hispanics ages 25–44 was 4 percent lower than that of whites, and the rate among the oldest group of Hispanics was 22 percent lower than that of whites.

The death rate of blacks, however, was 1.8 times that of whites for the youngest age group, 2.2 times that of whites for the middle age group, and 1.9 times that of whites for the older age group. Some of these disparities are due to differences in socioeconomic status (SES) between blacks and whites. Some are due to social and economic disadvantages associated with being black that are not experienced by Hispanics to the same degree. As described by LaVeist, "Disparities in morbidity and mortality among racial and ethnic groups can be viewed as the added burden of living in America as a racial minority expressed in terms of life and death" (p. 9).

Linking Race and Ethnicity to Socioeconomic Status

If race is a socially constructed category with few meaningful biological differences among races, why do we see such consistent patterns in fundamental measures of group health status such as death rates, infant mortality, and life expectancy? What differences can we identify among racial/ethnic groups that can be linked to these health disparities? The answer to these questions becomes readily apparent when we look at the average socioeconomic status for members of these racial/ethnic groups.

Figure 6.4 shows the highest level of education attained by adults in the United States age 18 or older, broken down by race/ethnicity. The graph indicates the percentage within each group with the indicated level as of 2017. It is clear that non-Hispanic whites and Asians have substantially higher levels of educational attain-

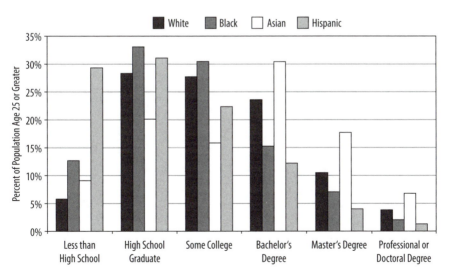

Figure 6.4. Educational attainment of the US population age 18 or over, by race/ethnicity, 2017. *Source*: US Census Bureau.

ment than blacks and Hispanics: 14 percent of whites and 24 percent of Asians have attained graduate or professional degrees; 9 percent of blacks and 5 percent of Hispanics have these degrees. Comparably, 13 percent of blacks and 30 percent of Hispanics never finished high school; 6 percent of whites and 9 percent of Asians failed to graduate from high school.

From the discussion in Chapter 3, we know that educational attainment is a principal measure of SES, and is strongly associated with other measures of SES, such as income, and with health status. In 2017 the median income for full-time workers with only a high school diploma was $39,005; for those workers who never finished high school the median income was $31,121. As an indication of the economic value of higher education, the median income in 2017 of a full-time worker with a bachelor's degree was $62,100 and with a master's degree was $77,685 (see Figure 3.1). Given the lower level of education of blacks and Hispanics on average, their household income is correspondingly lower. In 2017 the median income of black households was $41,064 and of Hispanic households was $37,377. In the same year, the median income of white households was $55,250 and of Asians was $62,153 (US Census Bureau 2018).

As a caveat to this discussion, we should be aware that these data pertain only to year-round full-time workers. A higher percentage of black and Hispanic adults are either unemployed or employed on a part-time basis than whites or Asians (US Department of Labor). The racial/ethnic differences in median income for full-time workers understate the difference in annual income for all members of a racial/ethnic group.

A question arises as to whether racial/ethnic differences in educational attainment can fully explain racial/ethnic differences in earnings. Will all people with a given level of educational attainment have approximately the same income? Alternatively, will there continue to be racial/ethnic differences in income for workers with the same level of education? The answer to these questions is shown in Figure 6.5.

For both high school graduates and those who never finished high school, the median annual earnings of a full-time white worker is several thousand dollars higher than that of workers from other racial/ethnic groups. For those with a bachelor's degree or master's degree, both white and Asian workers have substantially higher incomes than black or Hispanic workers. (Note that for those with a master's degree, the income of an Asian worker is several thousand dollars higher than that of a white worker.) Black and Hispanic workers find themselves lower on the SES hierarchy than whites and Asians for at least two reasons: they have substantially lower levels of average educational attainment, and for a given level of educational attainment they earn lower average incomes.

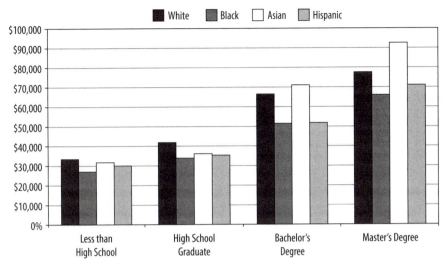

Figure 6.5. Median annual income of year-round, full-time workers aged 25–64, by educational attainment and race/ethnicity, 2017. *Source*: US Census Bureau, Current Population Survey.

Does Race/Ethnicity Still Affect Health Status after Taking into Account Socioeconomic Status?

We would expect that the resulting lower SES of blacks and Hispanics in the United States would be associated with worse health status. Compared to whites and Asians, blacks do have higher death rates and infant mortality rates and a shorter life expectancy. The principal cause of this association is not the fact that a person is black. Rather, the person is lower on the SES hierarchy in association with lower levels of educational attainment.

There is a similar association between race/ethnicity and SES in affecting disease rates. Beginning in 1985–86, Bancks and colleagues (2017) were able to follow a diverse cohort of more than 4,000 individuals aged 18–30 years, none of whom had diabetes at the time of enrollment. By 2015–16, 12 percent of the study population had developed diabetes. Both black men and black women were more likely to have developed diabetes than white men and white women. After adjusting for a series of biological factors such as body mass index, behavioral factors such as diet and smoking, and SES factors such as employment, there was no longer a disparity in diabetes risk. Differences in adult diabetes rates are not innately racial.

The relationship between race/ethnicity, SES, and health is illustrated in Figure 6.6. The situation with Hispanics is more complex, as discussed below.

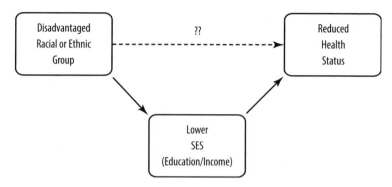

Figure 6.6. The association between race/ethnicity, SES, and health.

The association between being in a disadvantaged racial or ethnic group and having worse health status involves two steps:

1. Being in a disadvantaged group is associated with both a higher level of behavioral risk factors and having a lower level of educational attainment.
2. Having a lower level of educational attainment is associated with worse health status, for reasons discussed in Chapter 4.

Figure 6.6 includes an arrow going directly from "Disadvantaged Racial or Ethnic Group" to "Reduced Health Status." The arrow is dashed rather than solid, indicating that it poses a question rather than illustrating an established relationship. After taking account of differences in SES, is the health of blacks and Hispanics (the two groups with clear disadvantages in educational attainment and income) worse than that of whites and Asians (the groups with an advantage in both education and income)?

This question was addressed in a study by Wong and colleagues (2002). Using nationally representative data for the period 1986–94, they measured the death rate for the 30 most frequent causes of death in the United States, comparing deaths in the black population with those in the white population. (Their study did not include data on other racial/ethnic groups.) Using data about the race and educational attainment of the US population, they used statistical modeling to predict the impact on life expectancy in the hypothetical situation of eliminating deaths from each of 30 different causes of death. They did this in two hypothetical situations: comparing a population with high levels of education and a population with low levels of education, with each population having the same black/ white racial distribution; and comparing a black population and a white population, with each population having the same distribution of educational attainment. The results of this analysis are illustrated in Figure 6.7.

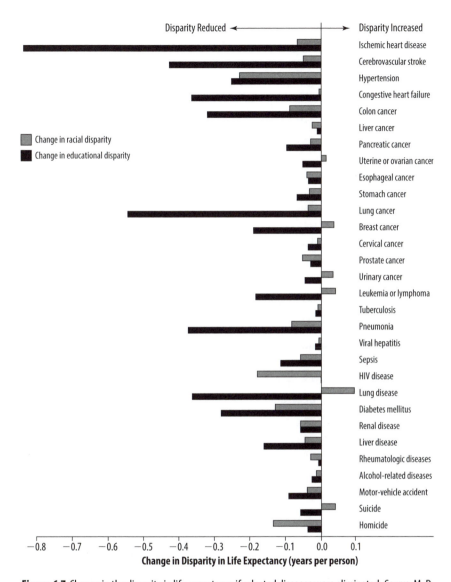

Disparity Reduced ◄———————————► Disparity Increased

Ischemic heart disease
Cerebrovascular stroke
Hypertension
Congestive heart failure
Colon cancer
Liver cancer
Pancreatic cancer
Uterine or ovarian cancer
Esophageal cancer
Stomach cancer
Lung cancer
Breast cancer
Cervical cancer
Prostate cancer
Urinary cancer
Leukemia or lymphoma
Tuberculosis
Pneumonia
Viral hepatitis
Sepsis
HIV disease
Lung disease
Diabetes mellitus
Renal disease
Liver disease
Rheumatologic diseases
Alcohol-related diseases
Motor-vehicle accident
Suicide
Homicide

■ Change in racial disparity
■ Change in educational disparity

−0.8 −0.7 −0.6 −0.5 −0.4 −0.3 −0.2 −0.1 0.0 0.1

Change in Disparity in Life Expectancy (years per person)

Figure 6.7. Change in the disparity in life expectancy if selected diseases were eliminated. *Source*: M. D. Wong, M. F. Shapiro, W. J. Boscardin, and S. L. Ettner, "Contribution of Major Diseases to Disparities in Mortality," *New England Journal of Medicine* 347, no. 20 (2002):1585–92. Copyright © 1997 Massachusetts Medical Society. All rights reserved. Reprinted with permission.

In the figure the darker shaded bars indicate the extent to which the measured disparity in overall life expectancy would have been reduced for the group with unequal levels of education if deaths from the identified disease were eliminated. The lighter shaded bars indicate the extent to which the measured black/white disparity in life expectancy would have been reduced among populations with equal levels of education. A bar to the left of the vertical zero-line indicates that the disparity would have been reduced; a bar to the right of the vertical zero-line indicates that the disparity would have increased.

For nearly every condition listed:

- the darker shaded bar is longer than the lighter shaded bar, indicating that most of the black/white disparity in life expectancy for a specific cause of death can be explained by educational differences that are independent of race
- a lighter shaded bar remains, indicating that part of the black/white disparity remains even after equalizing educational attainment

For a number of the major causes of death, the increase in black life expectancy compared to that of whites would be substantial if educational levels were equalized. For ischemic heart disease, cerebrovascular disease (for example, stroke), congestive heart failure, and lung cancer, nearly all the disparity in life expectancy can be explained by educational differences. The authors point out that the most likely explanation for the finding in regards to lung cancer is the strikingly higher levels of smoking seen in population groups with lower levels of education (National Center for Health Statistics 2018).

It should also be pointed out that, for a few diseases—including breast cancer, urinary cancer, leukemia, suicide, and certain forms of lung disease—the death rate among blacks would be increased and the life expectancy correspondingly reduced if educational levels were equalized. These conditions tend to be more common in people with higher educational levels than those with lower education.

I should emphasize the implications of the second conclusion—that black/white disparity remains even after equalizing educational attainment. For nearly all the conditions studied by Wong and colleagues, a racial disparity in death rates and life expectancy would continue to exist even if we were able to equalize the educational attainment of the black population and the white population in the United States. This persistent racial disparity is most noticeable for four conditions: hypertension, diabetes, HIV disease, and being a victim of homicide. From the study of Wong and colleagues, it appears that the causal arrow linking being a member of a disadvantaged racial/ethnic group (in this case, black) is directly linked with worse health status in a manner that is independent of educational attainment.

Louie and Ward (2011) reported data from a study of a nationally representative sample of US adults aged 60 or older. Rather than looking at racial differences in death rates, they examined the functional limitations reported by these subjects, analyzing the association with SES and with race/ethnicity. They found consistently higher levels of disease burden among those reporting lower SES (measured as education and income). After controlling for SES, they found blacks to have worse physical functioning than whites or Hispanics. Most of this residual racial difference was due to a higher rate of conditions such as diabetes and cardiovascular disease among blacks. After further controlling for this disease burden, they found that most of the disparity between blacks and whites went away. Interestingly, after controlling for both SES and disease burden, the health of Hispanics was better than that of either whites or blacks on several of the functional measures.

Farmer and Ferraro (2005) explored whether the magnitude of the residual association between race and health after accounting for SES is the same for all levels of SES. They used data gathered from a survey of a nationally representative sample of 5,968 white adults and 873 black adults who were followed for a total of 20 years. They measured SES in four ways: educational attainment, income, occupational status, and employment status. They measured health status in two ways: the presence of chronic medical conditions, and self-reported health status on a 5-point scale from "excellent" to "poor."

The authors found that black subjects reported a higher prevalence of chronic medical conditions at all levels of SES, indicating a residual effect for race. The results of their analysis of self-reported health status showed a very interesting finding. Despite having higher rates of chronic medical conditions, blacks at lower SES levels perceived their health status to be higher than that of whites at lower levels of SES. However, as the SES of the respondents increased, the self-reported health status of the white subjects increased, while that of the black subjects remained fairly constant, with the result that the widest gap in self-reported health between black and white subjects was at the highest levels of SES. The authors referred to this effect as the "'diminishing returns' hypothesis; as education levels increased, black adults did not have the same improvement in self-rated health as white adults" (p. 191).

Gornick and colleagues (1996) came to a similar conclusion. They compared the death rates among more than 26 million Medicare beneficiaries, using the median

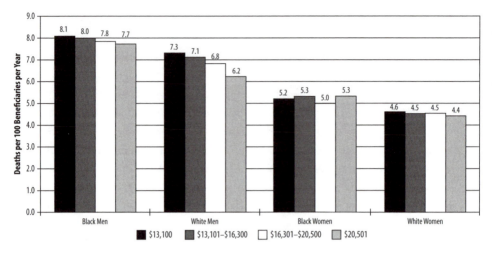

Figure 6.8. Death rates among Medicare beneficiaries age 65 or older, according to race, gender, and SES, 1993. *Source*: Based on Gornick et al. 1996.

income in 1990 for the census tract within which a beneficiary lived as an approximation of the individual beneficiary's income. As SES (measured by income) increases, the death rate decreases substantially more for white men than for black men, suggesting that the benefits of rising SES differ by race (Figure 6.8). A similar but smaller effect was seen for women.

Colen and colleagues (2018) studied both the health and the SES trajectories of a nationally representative sample of young adults followed over a period of 33 years. They measured changes over time in health status and in self-reported experiences of discrimination. They found that the black/white gap in health status was larger for those in higher levels of SES as older adults than for those at lower SES. They conclude that blacks who move into higher levels of SES over time experience greater levels of discrimination than those who remain at lower levels of SES, with the increased experience of discrimination largely responsible for the widened gap in health status.

In a study published in 1993, Guralnik and colleagues compared the magnitude of the association between SES and health status, using education as their measure of SES, while also taking both race and gender into account. They analyzed data on 2,219 black subjects and 1,838 white subjects, all over the age of 65 and all living in the Piedmont region of North Carolina. They measured health status both as total life expectancy and as life expectancy without significant physical limitations (which they referred to as "active life expectancy"). I describe below the differences they reported in active life expectancy. (See Chapter 2 for additional discussion of the difference in using life expectancy or life expectancy adjusted for quality of life as outcome measures.)

The first analysis compared the association between gender and life expectancy, doing the analysis separately for black and white subjects. Among black subjects, women enjoyed an additional 5.9 years in life expectancy compared to men. For white subjects, women had an advantage of 4.8 years.

The authors then looked at the comparable differences in active life expectancy due specifically to differences in education. They divided educational status into two categories: of the 3,992 subjects on whom they had data about level of education, 77 percent had not finished high school and were classified as "lower education," and 23 percent had completed high school and were categorized as "higher education." Among black subjects, men with higher education had an additional 2.9 years of active life expectancy, while women with higher education had an additional 3.9 years. The comparable statistics for white subjects was an additional 2.4 years for men and 2.8 years for women.

The authors then looked at the effect specifically of race. They reported this analysis separately for men and women, and within those categories separately for those with higher education and those with lower education.

Among men, they found that

- whites with lower education lived 0.9 years longer than blacks with lower education
- whites with higher education lived 0.4 years longer than blacks with higher education

Among women, they discovered that

- whites with lower education lived 0.4 years less than blacks with lower education
- whites with higher education lived 1.5 years less than blacks with higher education

Differences in life expectancy unadjusted for level of disability were comparable. Based on the relative magnitude of these increments in active life expectancy, it is possible to conclude three things from this study:

1. Gender has a larger influence on life expectancy than race or education.
2. Education has a larger influence on life expectancy than race alone.
3. Race still has an association with life expectancy, even after taking into account gender and education.

Race/Ethnicity, Socioeconomic Status, and Geography

In Chapter 4 we considered the rising death rates from deaths of despair, due principally to opioid overdose and suicide. Rates for both these causes of early mortality were higher in rural counties than in urban counties. Recent research from the United States Centers for Medicare and Medicaid services provides data indicating that the health disparities in rural counties go substantially beyond these deaths of despair (James et al. 2018).

Racial and ethnic minorities living in rural counties exhibit worse health behaviors and report worse health status than whites. The largest minority groups living in rural counties are blacks and Hispanics. Historically, blacks represented the largest minority population in rural areas. The 2010 Census indicated that Hispanics had grown to be the largest rural population. The health status of the rural American Indian/Alaska Native (AI/AN) population is also lower than that of whites. All three groups have lower income and lower levels of education than rural whites. The rates of obesity are also greater among these rural minorities than among rural whites. The rates of binge drinking were higher among whites than among the minority populations.

Responding to the report by James et al., Kozhimannil and Henning-Smith (2018) point out that the geographic distribution of the three principal rural minority populations are somewhat skewed. Blacks are more likely to live in what they refer to as the "Black Belt" within southern states, Hispanics are more likely to live in southwestern and western states, and AI/AN live in the West and upper Midwest. They also underscore the historical fact that "racism has shaped the history of rural communities," and they argue that "interventions should be community-driven" (p. 38).

Roth and colleagues (2017) looked specifically at variation in cardiac death rates among counties in the United States, comparing rates in rural and urban counties. While rates of specific cardiac conditions vary by geography, the authors reported that "The largest concentration of counties with high cardiovascular disease mortality extended from southeastern Oklahoma along the Mississippi River Valley to eastern Kentucky" (p. 1976). While these authors did not report differences in cardiac death rates by race or ethnicity, it is important to note that the area with the highest cardiac death rates coincides largely with the "Black Belt" identified by Kozhimannil and Henning-Smith.

Mensah and colleagues (2017) published an editorial response to the report by Roth et al., in which they argue that "Geographic variation in the social determinants of cardiovascular health is a compelling explanation for much of the variation described by Roth and colleagues" (p. 1955). They identify social determinants such as poverty, income, education, occupation, and health-related behaviors as the principal factors contributing to these disparities.

With financial support from the Bill & Melinda Gates Foundation, the Institute for Health Metrics and Evaluation (IHME), a private, nonprofit organization based at the University of Washington, has been publishing a series of reports on "The Global Burden of Disease" (Institute for Health Metrics and Evaluation 2018). In the most recent report analyzing data through 2016, the authors reported that three specific health-related behaviors—tobacco use, obesity, and drug or alcohol use—accounted for the largest share of premature deaths (US Burden of Disease Collaborators 2018). These three risk factors tended to cluster in certain geographic areas of the United States. Koh and Parekh (2018) published an editorial response to the report, underscoring that "Mississippi, Alabama, Kentucky, Louisiana, and West Virginia have among the highest age-standardized death rates and YLLs [Years of Life Lost]" (p. 1438). Overall, approximately 60 percent of the county-level variation in mortality and life expectancy is due to "socioeconomic and race/ethnicity factors" (p. 1439).

Dwyer-Lindgren and colleagues (2017), using data compiled by the National Center for Health Statistics, looked at changes in life expectancy for the period 1980–2014 among counties in the United States. Consistent with the findings of the Global Burden of Disease study, they concluded that "Geographic disparities in life expectancy among US counties are large and increasing. Much of the variation in life expectancy among counties can be explained by a combination of socioeconomic and race/ethnicity factors . . ." (p. 1003). In our discussions of the causes of racial and ethnic disparities in health status, it is important to consider geographical differences.

Race/Ethnicity, Socioeconomic Status, and Infant Mortality

In August 1963 the nation joined President John F. Kennedy and First Lady Jacqueline Kennedy in mourning the death of their newborn son, Patrick Bouvier Kennedy. Patrick had been born about five weeks prematurely, weighing 2,112 grams (4 pounds, 10 ounces). At that time there was little that medicine could offer. His lungs were too premature to function properly, and Patrick died two days after he was born of what was then referred to as hyaline membrane disease.

The last 30 years of the twentieth century saw numerous advances in the medical care available to newborn infants. Newer antibiotics for infections, respirators and pharmaceutical treatments for immature lungs, and advanced electronic monitoring allowed more and more of the tiny babies such as Patrick Kennedy to survive.

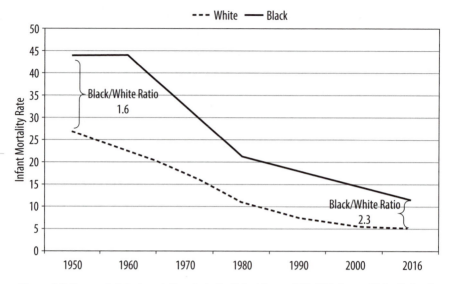

Figure 6.9. Changes in infant mortality rate in the United States, 1950–2013. *Source*: CDC—National Center for Health Statistics, User Guide to the 2016 Period Linked Birth / Infant Death.

The infant mortality rate (measured as the number of infants per thousand live births who die before their first birthday) plummeted in the United States, from 29.2 deaths per 1,000 in 1950 to 5.8 deaths per 1,000 in 2017 (CDC 2018).

The decline in infant mortality has not been the same for all racial groups. The death rate among infants born to white mothers declined from 26.8 per 1,000 in 1950 to 4.9 per 1,000 in 2016 (a decline of 81 percent), while the death rate among infants born to black mothers declined from 43.9 per 1,000 to 11.4 per 1,000 over the same period (a decline of 74 percent) (Figure 6.9). While the mortality rate for both races declined substantially, the steeper decline in white infant deaths resulted in a widening ratio between black deaths and white deaths. In 1950 black infants died at 1.6 times the rate of white infants; in 2010 they died at 2.3 times the rate of white infants.

To understand the source and the complexity of the worsening black/white disparity in infant mortality, we must first appreciate the association between the weight at which a baby is born and the chances that baby will die. To be considered to have a normal birth weight (NBW), a baby must weigh at least 2,500 grams (about 5.5 pounds). Babies weighing less than that are classified either as low birth weight (LBW) for those weighing between 1,500 and 2,500 grams or very low birth weight (VLBW) for those weighing less than 1,500 grams. As you might imagine, the mortality rate for infants born in these differing weight categories will be strik-

Table 6.1. Comparing Infant Deaths in 2016 for Whites, Blacks, and Hispanics

Birth Weight	White	Black	Hispanic	Black/White Ratio	Hispanic/White Ratio
	Infant Mortality Rate (deaths per 1,000 live births)				
2,500 grams or more (NBW)	2.0	3.4	1.6	1.7	0.8
Between 1,500 and 2,500 grams (LBW)	13.7	14.0	13.8	1.0	1.0
Less than 1,500 grams (VLBW)	199.0	228.5	208.3	1.1	1.0
	Percent of All Births				
Between 1,500 and 2,500 grams (LBW)	5.9	10.7	6.1	1.8	0
Less than 1,500 grams (VLBW)	1.1	3.0	1.2	2.7	1.1
	Percent of All Infant Deaths				
Between 1,500 and 2,500 grams (LBW)	16.8	13.3	16.9	0.8	1.0
Less than 1,500 grams (VLBW)	44.7	60.8	52.8	1.4	1.2

Source: CDC—National Center for Health Statistics. User Guide to the 2016 Period Linked Birth / Infant Death.

ingly different. In 2016 the overall infant mortality rate in the United States was 5.9 deaths per 1,000 live births. In that same year the mortality rate was 2.1 deaths per 1,000 for NBW infants, 13.4 deaths per 1,000 for LBW infants, and 212.2 deaths per 1,000 for VLBW infants (CDC 2018).

Table 6.1 compares the pattern of birth weights and infant mortality rates in 2016 for babies born to white, black, and Hispanic mothers in the United States. The top section of the table compares the infant mortality rate by race/ethnicity for babies born at NBW, LBW, or VLBW. The middle section compares the proportion of all births that occurs among LBW and VLBW infants. The bottom section of the table compares the proportion of all infant deaths that occurs among LBW and VLBW infants.

The first thing to note is that for infants born at either LBW or VLBW, there is relatively little difference in infant mortality among whites, blacks, and Hispanics. The black/white ratio and the Hispanic/white ratio is 1.0 or close to it—indicating that babies of all three groups born at these weights have about the same chance of surviving. However, for NBW infants there are striking differences between the death rate of black infants and either white or Hispanic infants. For these babies, the black mortality rate is 1.7 times that of white infants, while the Hispanic rate is only 0.8 times that of whites. While LBW and VLBW infants have about the same chance of surviving regardless of race/ethnicity, NBW infants are substantially more likely to die before their first birthday if they are black.

This difference in the black/white mortality rate for NBW infants—a ratio of 1.7—accounts for much, but not all, of the 2.3 ratio in overall infant deaths shown in Figure 6.9. The balance of this disparity in infant mortality comes not because of the mortality rate of infants at a specific birth weight, but rather because of differences in the rate at which infants are born at LBW and VLBW—the groups with the highest risk of infant death.

As seen in the middle section of Table 6.1, both LBW and VLBW infants account for a substantially larger percentage of overall births among black infants than among either white or Hispanic infants. Black infants are born in the LBW group at a rate that is 1.8 times that of white infants. Black infants in the VLBW group are born at this weight at a rate that is 2.7 times that of white infants. The same is not true of Hispanic infants. They are born in these two weight groups at essentially the same rate as whites—a ratio of 1.0 for LBW and 1.1 for VLBW.

Looking at the bottom section of Table 6.1, we can see the contributions to the disparities in infant mortality rate attributable to these disparities in birth weight. While VLBW infants account for 44.7 percent of all deaths among white infants, they account for 60.8 percent of deaths among black infants—a ratio of 1.2. Interestingly, even though there are more births among black LBW infants than among white LBW infants as a percentage of all births, the black LBW deaths account for a smaller percentage of all infant deaths—due largely to the huge percentage of black infant deaths accounted for by VLBW infants. As with the distribution of birth weights, the percentage of infant deaths attributable to LBW and VLBW infants is nearly identical for white and Hispanic infants.

From these data, we can draw three important conclusions:

1. Approximately half of the disparity in infant mortality between black infants and white infants is due to the higher rate of death among black infants born at NBW.
2. The other half of the black/white disparity in infant mortality is due mostly to the higher rate at which black infants are born at either LBW or VLBW, even though the chance of survival at these weights is nearly the same for both racial groups.
3. The mortality rate for Hispanic infants, the distribution of birth weights among Hispanic infants, and the contribution of LBW and VLBW deaths to the overall infant mortality rate are about the same as that of white infants.

From these three conclusions, three questions come immediately to mind:

1. Why do black infants born at NBW die more often than white infants— because of their race or because of differences in SES?

Table 6.2. Infant Deaths for White and Black Mothers with a College Education

Birth Weight	White	Black	Black/White Ratio
	Infant Mortality Rate Overall		
All birth weights combined	5.4	10.2	1.9
	Infant Mortality Rate by Birth Weight		
2,500 grams or more (NBW)	2.6	2.6	1.0
Between 1,500 and 2,500 grams (LBW)	32	25	0.8
Less than 1,500 grams (VLBW)	384	368	1.0
	Proportion of All Births		
Between 1,500 and 2,500 grams (LBW)	2.6%	5.4%	2.1
Less than 1,500 grams (VLBW)	0.5%	1.6%	3.2

Source: Schoendorf et al. 1992. Data from 1985.

2. Why are black infants born more often at an abnormal birth weight than white infants—because of their race or because of differences in SES?

3. Given the striking differences in SES between whites and Hispanics in the United States (Figure 6.4), why are the infant mortality rates and birth weight distributions for these two groups nearly the same?

An answer to the first question is provided by a study by Schoendorf and colleagues published in 1992. Though it uses infant mortality data from the years 1983–85, the findings from this study are still relevant. The authors were able to identify 865,128 white infants and 42,230 black infants, all born to mothers who had completed a college education. Thus, using education as an indicator of SES, all of these infants were born to mothers in approximately the same socioeconomic position. Table 6.2 presents the distribution of infant deaths and birth weights for these two groups.

The range of infant mortality rates in 1983–85 was quite different than it is today. In 1990, for example, the overall white infant mortality was 7.6 deaths per 1,000, while in 2016 it was 4.8. Comparable figures for black infants were 18.0 in 1990 and 11.1 in 2016. Similarly, the mortality rates for LBW and VLBW infants reported in this study are quite a bit higher than comparable rates today.

The top section of Table 6.2 shows the overall infant mortality rates for black and white infants in the Schoendorf study. We see that, overall, black infants in this study were nearly twice as likely as white infants to die. The middle section of the table shows the infant mortality rates broken down by birth weight. What we see is that the mortality rate of black infants born to a college-educated mother is nearly identical to that of comparable white infants for all three birth weight groups. For black infants born in the LBW category, the rate is even lower than that of whites.

Despite the comparable mortality rates within birth weight groups, the substantially higher rate at which black mothers with a college education had LBW and VLBW infants, combined with the much higher mortality rates within these groups, resulted in the disparity in overall infant mortality identified by the study. When we control for SES (that is, compare subjects with comparable SES) by looking at only college-educated mothers, we see that the disparity in infant mortality for NBW infants goes away. From this study it is reasonable to conclude that as much as half of the black/white disparity in infant mortality seen in 2016—that among NBW infants—is attributable to differences in SES between black and white mothers. However, it is also reasonable to conclude that a substantial portion of the remaining half of the disparity—that associated with the higher frequency among black mothers of LBW and VLBW births—remains after holding SES constant and is therefore due to some factor other than SES that differs between black and white mothers.

Shaw and colleagues (2018) provide a well-supported explanation of the factors leading to higher rates of preterm births among some groups. They conclude that "the etiology of preterm birth is increasingly understood to be linked to psychological, physical, and environmental stressors, with maternal-fetal impacts varying by time of exposure. Various pathways have been hypothesized, including immunological, vascular, or neuroendocrine alterations triggered by such stressors or via stress-related health behaviors" (p. 687). Shaw et al. were not comparing racial or ethnic differences, however. They were comparing US Army soldiers who gave birth while on active duty. They compared the rates of preterm births (defined as giving birth before 37 weeks of gestation) between soldiers who had been on overseas deployment during the 12 months prior to giving birth and those who had not had overseas deployment. While there were no racial differences in preterm births among these soldiers, those who gave birth within six months of returning home had a preterm birth rate of 6.4 percent, while those who were not on deployment during their pregnancy had a preterm birth rate of 3.1 percent. There were no black/white differences in the rate of preterm births. The authors noted that the overall rate of preterm births among these soldiers was lower than the national rate of preterm births during that period, "which is consistent with the expectation that soldiers represent a healthy, low-risk population" (p. 691).

Research has shown that, in addition to serving on active overseas military duty, living in a highly racially segregated community also exposes women to the "psychological, physical, and environmental stressors" identified by Shaw et al. as contributing to the rate of prematurity and low birth weight. Mehra and colleagues (2017) reviewed 42 previously published articles that examined the association between racial segregation and birth outcomes. They identified a consistent association between the level of segregation experienced by black women and both preterm birth and low birth weight, with greater degrees of segregation associated with greater disparities in birth outcomes.

Instead of looking at the level of residential segregation, Orchard and Price (2017) evaluated the association between the level of self-expressed racial prejudice within a county and the black/white differences in birth outcomes. They extracted data from the Implicit Association Test website (Project Implicit 2018). Those who log into the site are asked to identify their relative preference for European Americans and African Americans on a 7-point scale. The authors calculated an average racial preference score for nearly 2,400 counties in the United States. As described by the authors, "We find that counties with the highest levels of racial prejudice also have the largest black-white gaps in adverse birth outcomes . . . [T]he high prejudice counties have a black-white gap in low birth weight deliveries that is 14% larger than in low prejudice counties" (p. 196).

A study by McLemore and colleagues (2018) confirmed that perceived racial discrimination in the process of obtaining prenatal care creates an additional stressor for pregnant women of color already at increased risk of preterm birth. The researchers analyzed focus group transcripts of 54 low-income, high-risk black or Hispanic women in which the women discussed the process of obtaining prenatal care. The subjects described experiencing disrespect, racial discrimination, and stressful interaction with staff. This added stress may further increase the risk of preterm birth among the black women, though not necessarily for the Hispanic women due to the Latina paradox.

The "Latina Paradox": Reduced Infant Mortality Despite Reduced Socioeconomic Status

Despite the markedly lower levels of SES seen in the US Hispanic community, the rate of LBW and VLBW among Hispanic infants is nearly identical to that of white infants, and the Hispanic infant mortality rate is nearly the same as the white rate. The association of low SES and increased infant mortality seen in the black community does not seem to hold for the Hispanic community. For more than a decade researchers have recognized that the infant mortality rate for Hispanics is substantially below that of blacks, despite the relatively low levels of SES in both communities.

Studying Mexican and Cuban subgroups of the Hispanics, Singh and Yu (1996) noted that a principal source of the reduced infant deaths among Hispanic women was the large number of recent immigrants within this group. They noted that Hispanic women who had immigrated to the United States had a level of infant mortality that was 20 percent lower than Hispanic women who were born in this country.

In a more comprehensive analysis, Acevedo-Garcia and colleagues (2005) were able to confirm this finding. They identified a substantially reduced incidence of low birth weights, both LBW and VLBW, in infants of black women who had immigrated to this country, consistent with the findings of David and Collins discussed in the previous chapter. They also found this strong association between foreign nativity and reduced incidence of low birth weights in Hispanic women. They were able to identify an additional aspect of this association that appears important to our discussion. The protective effect of foreign nativity, with substantially reduced rates of low birth weights for women born elsewhere who have immigrated to the United States, seems strongest among the women with the lowest education. With the high rate of foreign nativity among Hispanic women in the United States, and with the relatively low levels of educational attainment among these women, it is understandable that the frequency of low birth weights and infant mortality is often lower in the Hispanic community than it is in the white community.

McGlade and colleagues (2004) reviewed the literature addressing this association between Hispanic ethnicity and reduced infant mortality. They refer to this association as the "Latina paradox"—the fact that "Latina mothers in the United States enjoy surprisingly favorable birth outcomes despite their social disadvantages" (p. 2062). They conclude that there are cultural aspects unique to women who have immigrated to the United States from Mexico and other Latin American countries, and that these cultural factors exert a protective effect when a woman becomes pregnant. Much of the protection stems from the especially strong family and social support networks that are available to these women. "Protective factors include a strong cultural support for maternity, healthy traditional dietary practices, and the norm of selfless devotion to the maternal role (*marianismo*). These protective factors are believed to provide a healthy normative and behavioral context for maternity, and they enable immigrant mothers to resist adopting the negative risk behaviors of the new host society, particularly those related to smoking, alcohol abuse, and diet" (p. 263). A similar study by Elo and Culhane (2010) compared health behaviors among US-born, African-born, and Caribbean-born pregnant black women in Philadelphia, concluding that the foreign-born women were significantly less likely to engage in alcohol use, smoking, or marijuana use while pregnant.

Ironically, McGlade and colleagues found strong evidence for the loss of these protective factors for the daughters and granddaughters of Latina immigrants. With each successive generation growing up in the United States and experiencing the influences of the predominant US culture, the protective effect is eroded, leading the authors to conclude that "this loss of advantage in birth outcomes is caused in part by the process of acculturation to the norms of mainstream American society" (p. 2063).

There is evidence that the health benefits associated with emigrating to the United States from one's country of birth extend beyond birth outcomes. Both Hispanic and Asian immigrants show improved health status for a range of measures as compared to those born in the United States. This immigrant benefit also tends to reduce the educational gradient among these immigrant groups (Kimbro et al. 2008). Similar results were found in a comparison of blacks in the United States born in the United States, in Africa, or in the Caribbean (Griffith et al. 2011).

It is important to acknowledge an important caveat to our understanding of the health benefits associated with immigration. In the years leading up to and following the 2016 national elections, many states as well as the federal government have adopted aggressive policies to identify and to exclude undocumented immigrants. A review by Philbin and colleagues (2018) described the multiple ways these policies might affect birth outcomes: "through stress related to structural racism; by affecting access to beneficial social institutions, particularly education; by affecting access to healthcare and related services; and through constraining access to material conditions such as food, wages, working conditions, and housing" (p. 29). Close scrutiny of potential changes in Hispanic birth outcomes is an important public health policy goal.

Sources of the Persisting Association between Race and Health Status

For infant mortality, life expectancy, and many other measures, those who are black by race have worse health on average than those who are white. This is due mostly to black/white differences in SES, but a disparity in health status persists even after taking SES into account. It is important for us to identify the possible causes for this persistent racial difference in health status.

If there were consistent biological differences between those in the black race and those in the white race, these differences might explain at least part of the residual difference. However, as I discussed in Chapter 5, racial categories reflect historical distinctions that were based on social convention and not on science. As shown by the research of Rosenberg and colleagues discussed in Chapter 5, population groups in sub-Saharan Africa are more similar genetically to European population groups than they are to Asian population groups. The amount of genetic difference that permits these distinctions is tiny compared to the full human genome. In addition, the extent of historical admixture between white and black populations in the United States is substantial, further complicating attempts to identify consistent genetic differences between black and white racial groups.

While meaningful genetic differences may not exist, the social circumstances experienced by black and white populations in the United States differ substantially, both historically and currently. We have all studied the history of the slave trade; we are all familiar with the social roots of the American Civil War. The history of overt racial discrimination against blacks in this country is one of the deepest stains on our society.

The emergence and growth of the "Black Lives Matter" movement in the wake of repeated police killings of black individuals underscores the persistence of discriminatory treatment of black Americans. We must ask whether the history of racial discrimination in this country, and the many residual effects of that discrimination, may contribute to the racial difference in health status that persists after taking into account SES.

Phelan and Link (2015) propose a model that links racial discrimination, socioeconomic inequality, and health outcomes in a stepwise manner. Under their model, "(a) Racism is a fundamental cause of racial differences in SES; (b) SES is a fundamental cause of inequalities in health and mortality; and (c) racism is a fundamental cause of racial differences in health and mortality independent of SES" (p. 313). The model proposed by Phelan and Link offers a clear answer to the question I addressed in Figure 6.6. From their perspective, racial discrimination has a clear adverse impact on the health of black Americans even after controlling for the effects of SES disadvantage.

The association between poor health and experiencing racial discrimination identified by Phelan and Link raises some of the same issues I addressed in Chapter 4 concerning the mechanisms by which low SES is associated with poor health. In those discussions I considered low SES as a position of social disadvantage relative to high SES, and I identified a number of ways this position of disadvantage may translate into poor health status. I now reexamine those same issues in the context of racial, rather than SES, disadvantage.

Figure 4.11 identified two specific pathways by which those who occupy a low position within a social hierarchy may experience worse health outcomes over time:

1. Occupying a low position in a social hierarchy results in chronic exposure to stress (recall the M&M experiment described in Chapter 4). Chronic stress leads to a chronic elevation in allostatic load, with damage to tissues and organs resulting over time. As a consequence of this damage, those in the low-status position develop illnesses earlier and experience more severe consequences from those illnesses.

2. Those in a low-status position end up living in neighborhoods that have lower social capital, and as a result experience both more environmentally related illness and additional stress related to the characteristics of their neighborhoods.

Both of these mechanisms are possible explanations for the worse health outcomes black Americans experience that persist after taking into account black/white differences in SES.

I should of course acknowledge that another factor independent of SES may directly contribute to racial health disparities. It may be that, independent of SES, blacks have less access to health care than whites, or that blacks receive lower-quality health care when that care is available. Certainly, for much of the twentieth century, there was explicit racial segregation in the health care system in many areas of the country. I address that issue in Chapter 8. The discussion below looks only at possible explanations for persisting racial health disparities that do not pertain to the availability of health care.

Race as a Form of Low Social Status

Clearly, experiencing overt racial discrimination can be expected to lead to chronic stress of the type that will result in tissue damage and resultant illness. The types of blatant racism that were common during the early and middle twentieth century have been outlawed, the result of a series of landmark civil rights laws first enacted in the 1960s. Yet, as I discuss in more depth in Chapter 9, racial bias continues to exist in forms that have little to do with overt, conscious racism. Many of these biases exist in ways of which the person holding them is not fully conscious. Upon seeing a black face on a computer screen, a person may have a different, unconscious emotional reaction from what they might have if the face on the screen had been white.

A person experiencing racial bias may not perceive unconscious bias to be different from overt, conscious racism. The stress level of a person experiencing repeated bias that was not consciously intended may be no different than the stress level that would be induced had the race-based discrimination been intended. Din-Dzietham and colleagues (2004) examined this relationship in a study of black adults living in Atlanta, Georgia. The average age of the 356 study participants was 49 years; 85 percent had graduated from high school; 60 percent had at least some college education.

The researchers asked the study participants the extent to which they had experienced race-based discrimination at work (RBDW). Of the participants, 137 (39 percent) reported that they had not experienced RBDW; 197 (55 percent) reported that they had experienced RBDW that originated from other workers who were not black. The remaining workers (6 percent) reported only having experienced RBDW from other workers who were also black.

Using multivariate analysis to control for SES (measured both as education and income) as well as other pertinent characteristics such as gender and age, the researchers asked whether there was an association between having experienced RBDW and two measured outcomes: the level of stress the subject reported having experienced as a result of RBDW, and the level of the subject's blood pressure. They found significant correlations between having experienced RBDW and the reported level of stress, and between the level of stress and the level of blood pressure. (These associations were only found when the reported RBDW originated from other workers who were not black. They were not found when the only reported RBDW was on the part of other black workers.) Those subjects who had experienced the highest level of RBDW tended also to have the highest blood pressure readings and the highest prevalence of hypertensive disease.

A follow-up analysis of these data (Davis et al. 2005) suggested that, rather than the experience of discrimination itself, it is the level of personal stress that resulted from the discrimination that had the strongest association with blood pressure. One's coping mechanism—the way one has learned to respond to and adapt to the experience of discrimination—appears to be an important mediator of the association between race-based discrimination and elevated blood pressure.

Krieger and Sidney (1996) came to a similar conclusion in a study of 1,974 black subjects and 2,112 white subjects, all between the ages of 25 and 37. The subjects were asked if they had experienced racial discrimination in a variety of settings, including at school, at work, in housing, while getting medical care, on the streets, or from the police. The subjects who reported having experienced discrimination in one or more of these contexts were then asked how they responded to this discrimination. Did they keep it to themselves, or did they try to do something about it? As in the previous study, the researchers used multivariate analysis to look for an association between the experience of racial discrimination and the level of the subject's blood pressure, while controlling for other factors such as age, gender, and SES (measured as education, income, and whether the subject owned or rented his or her dwelling).

The results of these analyses both support and contradict the findings of Din-Dzietham and colleagues. While their study identified a clear association between the experience of racial discrimination and the level of a subject's blood pressure, this study by Krieger and Sidney did not find as strong an association between the experience of discrimination itself and blood pressure levels. Rather, they found that the subject's reported response to discrimination when it occurred was the stronger predictor of blood pressure, even when the subjects reported not having experienced discrimination in the specific settings enumerated by the researchers. As described by the authors: "Blood pressure was highest among those reporting having experienced no racial discrimination and lowest among those reporting discrimination in one or two of the specified contexts. It is unlikely that these results mean that experiencing moderate discrimination is desirable; more plausibly, individuals belonging to groups subjected to discrimination may be at lower risk of elevated blood pressure if they are able to articulate, rather than internalize, their experiences of discrimination" (pp. 1375–76).

Dunlay and colleagues (2017) reported similar findings in their study of the association between perceived racial discrimination and cardiovascular disease. They analyzed data from the Jackson Heart Study, a collaborative longitudinal study of the health outcomes of about 5,000 African Americans between the ages of 21 and 94, first recruited into the study in the period 2000–04. All subjects were free of known cardiovascular disease (CVD) at the time they entered the study. The authors followed the health of these subjects over a 10-year period, looking for evidence of new CVD. Participants were also asked about the level of racial discrimination they had experienced, both on an everyday basis and over the course of their lifetime.

The authors found a clear and direct association between the level of discrimination reported and the SES metrics of respondents. Those with higher levels of education and income also reported experiencing higher levels of discrimination. Those who reported higher levels of discrimination were also younger than those reporting lower levels of discrimination. Given the younger age and higher SES of those reporting discrimination, the authors found no association between the level of discrimination reported and the risk for CVD. They did identify an inverse association between the level of discrimination reported and the risk of death from all causes.

Leitner and colleagues (2016) accessed the Project Implicit database of county-level racial bias described above in the study of birth outcomes by Orchard and

Price. Using this same measure of county-level explicit racial bias, they identified an association between the level of bias in a county and both greater death rates due to CVD as well as decreased access to health care for blacks living in the county.

The authors of these studies seem to be suggesting that racial discrimination is so widespread in our society that nearly all black Americans will experience it in one way or another—a message reiterated by President Barack Obama in his remarks to the press following the verdict in the Trayvon Martin case (Landler and Shear 2013). Those who report not having experienced discrimination may have a tendency to accept unfair treatment without challenging it, while others both acknowledge the presence of discrimination and have developed active coping mechanisms to address it.

Social epidemiologist Sherman James refers to this active coping with discrimination as "John Henryism" (James 1994). James concurs that blacks, especially those in lower SES, are chronically exposed to a range of stressors. Dealing with this stress on a day-to-day basis requires considerable effort. As James argues, "not all individuals so exposed will respond to these noxious conditions with high-effort coping. Some will, while others will not; or, perhaps, more accurately, some will respond with effortful active coping for a time, and then give up, while others—encouraged by their success—will persist" (p. 168). James references the nineteenth century legend of John Henry, the Steel Driving Man, who was able to defeat the new steam engine in driving steel railroad spikes, but then died after doing so. Under James' theory of John Henryism, those members of the black community "who persist with effortful active coping under difficult circumstances" will experience even greater levels of chronic stress as well as the adverse health outcomes related to this level of stress. The concept of John Henryism adds support to the concept that racial discrimination experienced by blacks will frequently be associated with higher levels of stress-related allostatic load, and over time with increased rates of illness.

Recall from our discussion in Chapter 4 that chronically elevated allostatic load can result in injury to the cells lining the arteries and arterioles, with consequent elevation in the biomarkers of cellular injury and evidence of scarring of the blood vessels. Will the chronic stress of experiencing racial discrimination contribute to this type of cellular injury among African Americans? A number of researchers have looked specifically at this question.

Adam and colleagues (2015) measured salivary cortisol levels in a sample of 62 white adults and 50 black adults with an average age of 32 years who were part of a longitudinal study that began when the subjects were 12 years old. Subjects were asked about their perceived level of racial discrimination over the 20 years of the study. As might be expected, black subjects reported both greater levels of perceived discrimination and lower levels of SES than the white subjects. Those reporting greater levels of perceived discrimination had greater levels of disruption of their diurnal cortisol levels at age 32, a pattern "that has been associated with numerous health risks" (p. 289).

Geronimus and colleagues (2006) created an aggregate measure of allostatic load, and then compared this measure among a nationally representative sample of black and white adults aged 18–64. They found higher scores among the black subjects, particularly those in the 35–64 age range, that were not explained by having experienced poverty. In a similar manner, Crimmins and colleagues (2007) compared white, black, and Hispanic adults aged 40 and older on a measure of inflammation that combined blood levels of C-reactive protein (CRP), fibrinogen, and albumin. Blacks had significantly higher levels of these inflammatory biomarkers than either whites or Hispanics, even after controlling for SES.

Das (2013) looked at a nationally representative sample of black, white, and Hispanic men between the ages of 57 and 85. Among this age group, black men had significantly higher rates of diabetes and hypertension than white men. The author asked which of four factors best explains this disparity: low social support, poor health behaviors, obesity, or cellular inflammation. Inflammation was measured as the level of CRP in the blood. The author found a significantly higher level of CRP among the black men, and this factor was most strongly associated with the health problems, leading the author to conclude that "these outcomes seem to derive most consistently from . . . chronic inflammation, arguably a biologic weathering mechanism induced by older black men's cumulative and multidimensional stress. In other words, these problems seem at least in part to be directly rooted in the systems of social stratification in which these men have lived their lives" (p. 82).

Gruenewald and colleagues (2009) undertook a similar study, comparing black and white men and women between the ages of 37 and 55. They measured inflammation using both CRP and an inflammatory marker called interleukin-6. They found consistently higher levels of the inflammatory biomarkers in both black men and women as compared to their white counterparts, although much of the difference was attributable to differences in SES and health behaviors.

Using the same database analyzed by Gruenewald, Matthews and colleagues (2011) looked at the level of coronary artery calcium (CAC), a measure of scarring in the lining of the arteries that supply the heart, in blacks and whites. They found the strongest predictor of CAC to be low levels of educational attainment and low occupational prestige, and that these associations were strongest in black men and women.

The carotid artery is the main artery in the neck that supplies blood to the brain and sensory organs of the head. Narrowing and scarring in the carotid artery are risk factors for an increased likelihood of suffering a stroke, and is reflective of more generalized scarring in the arterial circulation that can be a major contributor to hypertension and other problems. Heffernan and colleagues (2008) measured the thickness and stiffness of the lining of the carotid artery in otherwise healthy black and white men with an average age of 23 years. They found no significant differences in other risk factors for cardiovascular disease, such as elevated cholesterol, diabetes, hypertension, or obesity. Nonetheless they found that the black men had greater thickness and stiffness of the lining of their carotid artery.

Thurston and Matthews (2009) performed a similar study comparing the thickness and stiffness of the carotid lining in black and white teenagers with an average age of 18. They found the same results—the black teenagers were already showing evidence of damage associated with chronic inflammation in the lining of their arterial circulation, making them at increased risk of subsequent cardiovascular illness. Low SES was a significant contributor to the carotid thickness and stiffness found in black teenagers.

This finding—that even young African Americans show evidence of vascular injury associated with the stress of having experienced racial bias as they were growing up—raises an important question pertaining to the finding described above that even college-educated black women in the United States have a higher rate than college-educated white women of having low-birth weight infants, with the associated increased rate of infant mortality. The uterus is one of the most richly vascular organ systems in the body, allowing the mother to provide the developing fetus with necessary nutrients. If a college-educated black mother were to have thickening and stiffening of the arteries and arterioles supplying blood to the uterus and to the fetal placenta, would that not make her at higher risk of delivering a low- or very-low birth weight infant? I have not seen studies exploring this specific question, but I can only imagine that the micro-vascular changes occurring in the carotid artery would simultaneously be taking place in the uterine circulation.

Beyond increasing the risk of cardiovascular and other diseases, the experience of racial discrimination has also been shown to be associated with deterioration in mental health. Gee and colleagues (2006) were able to demonstrate an association between the mental health status of a group of black and Hispanic residents of New Hampshire and the degree to which they reported having experienced racial or ethnic discrimination. Similarly, Subramanyama and colleagues (2012), as part of a study of African American adults aged 21–95 living in the Jackson, Mississippi, metropolitan area, looked at self-reports of perceived social status and the risk of depression. Perceived status was measured using the "ladder of society" instrument described in Chapter 4. They found lower perceived social status to be associated with a greater risk of reporting symptoms of depression.

Might these patterns of discrimination and associated poor health outcomes also exist in Canada? Siddiqi and colleagues (2017) examined data from the Canadian Community Health Survey, a nationally representative survey of Canadians conducted annually. In the 2013 version of the survey, subjects were asked to rate their experiences of everyday discrimination using a previously validated scale. Subjects were also asked about their health status. The authors reported that "racial minorities in Canada differed significantly in their experiences of discrimination. While Blacks were the most likely to experience discrimination, followed by Aboriginals . . . [A]fter controlling for demographic and socioeconomic covariates, in a Canadian population, experiencing frequent discrimination was associated with nearly twice the odds of having a chronic condition . . ." (p. 139).

It is important to note the levels of discrimination experienced by Aboriginals in Canada. This group is analogous to the American Indian / Alaska Native (AI/AN) population in the United States. Citing data regarding the increased illness and mortality rates among AI/AN populations, Browne (2017) argues that "Racism and intersecting forms of discrimination therefore must be considered determinants of health for Indigenous peoples, and strategies are required to mitigate their negative impacts on health" (p. 24).

There appears to be consistent evidence to support the concept that those identified as members of the black race in the United States as well as Canada experience a form of social disadvantage that is analogous to the disadvantage associated with low SES. Braveman (2012) reviewed current health disparities research in an article titled "Health inequalities by class and race in the US: What can we learn from the patterns?" She concludes that "psychological disadvantages related to racial discrimination may contribute to racial or ethnic inequalities in health that persist after considering socioeconomic measures" (p. 666). The stress associated with being in a racially disadvantaged group is separate from, and in addition to, the stress associated with being in an economically disadvantaged group. I illustrate this relationship in Figure 6.10.

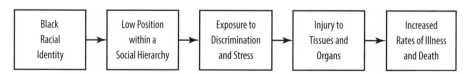

Figure 6.10. The association between race, social disadvantage, stress, and health for black Americans.

In an article published in the *New York Times*, Khullar (2017) reminded readers that, "Long before the Rev. Dr. Martin Luther King declared health inequity the most shocking and inhumane form of injustice, W.E.B. Du Bois wrote that 'the Negro death rate and sickness are largely matters of condition and not due to racial traits and tendencies.' . . . Research suggests that discrimination is internalized over a lifetime, and linked to a variety of poor health markers and outcomes."

Harvard Professor David R. Williams (2017) has echoed Khullar's perspective. "African-Americans live sicker and die sooner than whites in America . . . A large and growing body of research shows that day-to-day experiences of African-Americans create physiological responses that lead to premature aging . . . the first thing we have to do is acknowledge that the everyday racial discrimination embedded in our culture is sickening and killing African-Americans, and make a new commitment to work together to make America a healthier place for all." Whether conscious or unconscious, and whether it originates in individual behavior or the institutional structure of our society, racial discrimination and its adverse impact on health status are continuing realities for many Americans.

Race, Residential Segregation, Social Capital, and Health

The second association I would like to examine is whether the neighborhood characteristics experienced by black Americans carry with them aspects of social disadvantage that also are analogous to disadvantage associated with low SES. If we were to find systematic differences in the characteristics of the neighborhoods in which black and white Americans live, then we will have identified another pathway by which racial disadvantage leads to worse health, even for those at comparable levels of SES.

Following the Civil War and subsequent freedom for former black slaves, living in a highly segregated community was the norm for black Americans. Using data from the US census conducted in 1880 coupled with follow-up data on death rates in 1900–10, Logan and Parman (2017) were able to determine that, while the overall death rate among blacks was substantially greater than that among whites, those blacks living in highly segregated urban communities had lower death rates than blacks living in less segregated communities.

By the end of the twentieth century, this pattern was reversed. A growing body of research provides evidence that the racial composition of neighborhoods is associated with disparities in a range of health outcomes, with these disparities affecting blacks disproportionately. A study by Subramanian and colleagues (2005) found that racial differences in health status, measured at the neighborhood level, persist after taking into account neighborhood SES. Studying census tract data in Massachusetts, they concluded that, especially in low-income neighborhoods, "the consequences of neighborhood deprivation may be particularly exacerbated for Blacks, compared to Whites" (p. 263).

Data from LeClere and colleagues (1997) clarify the issue of whether harmful neighborhood conditions are associated with the SES composition of the neighborhood, the racial/ethnic composition of the neighborhood, or both. They analyzed census tract data from a nationally representative data set and found a strong association between the concentration of blacks within a neighborhood and the death rate in that neighborhood. The higher the percentage of blacks, the higher the death rate, for neighborhoods at all SES levels. This association was especially strong in low-income neighborhoods, and was largely explained by the conditions within the neighborhood and the level of hardship experienced by the residents of the community, especially women.

Data reported by Cullen and colleagues (2012) replicate this finding. The authors looked at county-level data, looking for factors associated with the black/white disparity in survival to the age of 70. They found the survival rates for black men and women to be consistently lower than those of white men and women. This was true in both the most advantaged as well as the most disadvantaged counties. Included in the variables that were associated with these disparities were both the SES characteristics of the county (measured as education and income), as well as the percent of the county's population that is black. The higher the black population in the county, the worse the disparity was, after controlling for SES.

Whitman and colleagues (2012) reported a similar study, in which they compared black/white death rates from breast cancer. As I describe in Chapter 10, while breast cancer occurs at about the same rate in white women and black women in the United States, the death rate from breast cancer is consistently higher among black women. Whitman compared the black/white breast cancer death rates in the 25 largest cities in the United States and found the black death rate to be higher in 22 of them, with the difference reaching statistical significance in 13 cities. In an examination of the characteristics of the cities that were correlated with a higher black death rate, the authors found that the extent of black/white residential segregation was the only significant predictor of a higher breast cancer death rate for black residents of the city.

A study by Do (2009) looked at both individual and neighborhood characteristics of a nationally representative sample, assessing the factors associated with self-rated health. The author found that long-term measures of neighborhood poverty, rather than individual measures of SES, were more strongly associated with adverse health outcomes. She was able to confirm a disproportionate exposure among blacks to this type of long-term poverty. The author concluded that "chronic exposure to neighborhood poverty helps explain the black/white health disparity. . . . The enduring effects of segregation and neighborhood poverty in perpetuating racial health disparities become even more salient when we consider the strong likelihood for black families of residing in impoverished neighborhoods across successive generations" (p. 1374).

Do and colleagues (2017) followed up on this earlier study with a study that compared self-rated health status of individuals living in high poverty neighborhoods with those of individuals living in low poverty neighborhoods. Consistent with their earlier study, they found that "Segregation was positively associated with poor health for blacks in high poverty neighborhoods, but not for those in lower poverty neighborhoods. Hence, the self-rated health of blacks clearly suffers as a result of black-white segregation" (p. 85).

Working with the same database as that used by Bancks and colleagues (2017) as described earlier in this chapter, Kershaw and colleagues (2017) followed the change in blood pressure over time in 2,280 black subjects. They found that a subset of these subjects who were living in high poverty, highly segregated communities at baseline were able to move to communities with lower levels of both poverty and segregation. Among these subjects, they found a decrease in systolic blood pressure over time. By contrast, those who started out in less segregated neighborhoods but moved to neighborhoods with higher levels of segregation experienced an increase in systolic blood pressure. Given the important role of hypertension as a risk factor for cardiovascular disease, residential racial segregation plays an important role in the disparities seen in black Americans.

Debbink and Bader (2011) asked whether the frequency of low birth weight in metropolitan areas of Michigan was associated with the extent of racial segregation in those areas. They found that the likelihood of having a low birth weight infant was higher for women living in a racially segregated black neighborhood. Consistent with the potential for vascular injury due to chronically elevated allostatic load discussed earlier in this chapter, the authors suggested that "chronic stress associated with the circumstances of racially isolated neighborhoods might affect placental vascular function, creating an oxygen-nutrient insufficiency that leads to intrauterine growth restriction" (p. 1717).

Hayanga and colleagues (2013) examined the association between the degree of residential segregation within US counties and the lung cancer death rate within that county. They found that (a) blacks overall had a higher rate of lung cancer mortality than whites, and (b) the most racially segregated counties had the highest death rates, even after controlling for per-capita income within the county. These findings are not surprising in light of other studies showing consistently higher rates of air pollution experienced by blacks living in racially segregated communities (Abel and White 2011; Hackbarth, Romley, and Goldman 2011).

If the neighborhoods in which blacks live have harmful effects on health, we would expect that whites who live in predominantly black neighborhoods would also suffer those adverse health consequences. This is precisely the conclusion of a study by Deaton and Lubotsky (2003). They examined national data that was broken down by metropolitan statistical areas (MSAs)—geographic regions that are larger than neighborhoods identified by census tract. They found that the higher percentage of the residents within an MSA that were black, the higher was the mortality rate within that MSA *for all residents, black or white.* Even when MSAs are matched for measures of SES such as income or education, a higher percentage of black residents is associated with a higher mortality rate.

By contrast, LaVeist and colleagues (2011) compared the health of low-income black and white residents living in a racially integrated neighborhood in Baltimore. The authors "found that the racial disparity we normally see in national samples was attenuated or completely erased when white and black Americans live under similar conditions. . . . When social factors and medical care are equalized, racial disparities are minimized" (p. 1884).

These results take on special significance in light of data presented by Massey (2004). He looked at the residential racial composition of several large metropolitan areas in the Midwest and Northeast. Using a measure of racial segregation called the dissimilarity index, which measures several aspects of racial integration or segregation, he identified three categories of residential racial segregation: low or moderately segregated, highly segregated, and hypersegregated. He found that about one-third of blacks lived in conditions of low to moderate segregation. Nearly half of blacks lived in hypersegregated communities. In addition, he found that the levels of racial segregation had changed relatively little over the period 1980–2000, and that the level of residential segregation changes relatively little as income levels rise. Even among blacks with 1990 incomes over $50,000, the segregation index remained high. Further, he found that the more segregated a community was, the higher its level of crime, violence, and other forms of social disorder. He tied a chronic exposure to reduced social capital within a residential community to reduced health status.

The foregoing review suggests a biosocial model of stratification that connects elements of social structure (racial segregation and income inequality interacting to produce concentrated poverty and its correlate, spatially concentrated violence) to

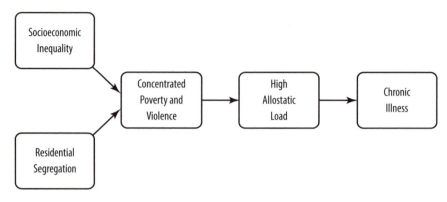

Figure 6.11. Massey's biosocial model of racial stratification. *Source*: Based on Massey 2004, p. 21.

distinctively high allostatic loads among African Americans (through their involuntary confinement in areas of concentrated poverty and violence) to an elevated risk of coronary heart disease (hypertension, thrombosis, atherosclerosis, diabetes, and obesity), a greater likelihood of inflammatory disorders (asthma, multiple sclerosis, arthritis), and impaired cognition (memory loss, reduced learning ability, and nerve damage in the brain). Massey offers a model of these relationships (Figure 6.11).

In Massey's model, socioeconomic inequality and persisting residential segregation by race within SES categories combine to create concentrations of poverty and violence that impact blacks more than whites. The chronic stress of these living conditions and the associated chronically elevated allostatic load experienced by blacks, even blacks with higher levels of SES, result in a range of poor health outcomes from chronic illnesses such as cardiovascular disease, to kidney disease, to inflammatory conditions such as arthritis.

Williams and colleagues (2010) have provided a comprehensive review of the many factors that contribute to health disparities associated with race and SES. They concluded that differences at the neighborhood and community level are a major contributor to these disparities, and that "differences in neighborhood quality and community conditions are driven by residential segregation by race" (p. 78). From the data they reviewed, they were able to identify six principal ways in which residential segregation affects the health of black Americans (p. 79).

1. Segregation limits socioeconomic mobility by limiting access to quality elementary and high school education, preparation for higher education, and employment opportunities.
2. The conditions created by concentrated poverty and segregation make it more difficult for residents to adhere to good health practices.

3. The concentration of poverty can lead to exposure to elevated levels of economic hardship and other chronic and acute stressors at the individual, household, and neighborhood level.

4. The weakened community and neighborhood infrastructure in segregated areas can also adversely affect interpersonal relationships and trust among neighbors.

5. The institutional neglect and disinvestment in poor, segregated communities contributes to increased exposure to environmental toxins, poor quality housing, and criminal victimization.

6. Segregation adversely affects both access to care and the quality of care.

An editorial published in 2018 by the editors of *JAMA* summarized the root causes of much of the existing inequality in health status in the United States: "The discussion of race and medicine in the United States is challenging and emotionally charged. Substantial disparities in health outcomes, based on race, ethnicity, and socioeconomic status, continue to exist . . . The history of racism in the United States and in medicine and health care is long and painful" (Fontanarosa and Bauchner 2018, p. 1539).

In this chapter we have looked at many of the factors contributing to the reduced health status experienced by many black Americans. While SES may have the most powerful influence in determining health disparities, experiencing racial bias and facing the concentrated poverty that often exists in racially segregated communities contribute to disparities based on race that persist after taking into account SES.

Our discussion so far has focused mainly on the ways social and racial/ethnic inequality affect the health status of adults. What, though, of the health of children? Do children experience the same types of health disparities based on social inequality? I address this issue in the following chapter.

CHAPTER SEVEN

Children's Health Disparities

Up to this point, our discussion has focused on health disparities experienced by adults of differing SES and differing race/ethnicity. Typical measures of these inequalities include death rates, illness rates, rates of disability, and life expectancy. In the previous chapter we considered disparities in birth weight distribution and associated infant mortality. While the death of an infant is tragic under any circumstances, we usually use comparative rates of infant mortality as a measure of the health of women.

If we instead focus our attention on children in the United States, and ask how the health of these children varies based on factors such as SES and race/ethnicity, we need to use different measures of health status. Certainly childhood death rates are an important topic. Thakrar and colleagues (2018) compared death rates among children in the US for the period 1961–2010 with those children from 19 countries who were members of the OECD. The good news was that child mortality rates declined consistently for both US children and OECD children. The concerning news was that, for the period 2001–10, "the risk of death in the U.S. was 76 percent greater for infants and 57 percent greater for children ages 1-19" than for other children in the OECD (p. 140).

Singh and Kogan (2007) evaluated changes in the United States between 1969 and 2000 in the rates of childhood deaths from the most common causes of death. They grouped children into quintiles of SES, based on an aggregate measure of deprivation in the county in which a child lived.

There was a progressive reduction in the childhood death rate for each quintile of deprivation for each time period (Figure 7.1). Nonetheless, the clear stepwise increase in death rates with each step of worsening deprivation changed little over the period examined. When the authors looked at some of the most common causes of childhood deaths—unintentional injuries, homicides, and cardiovascular disease—they found similar patterns. (Interestingly, the SES gradient was not as apparent in their evaluation of deaths due to cancer and birth defects.) Consistent with data from the

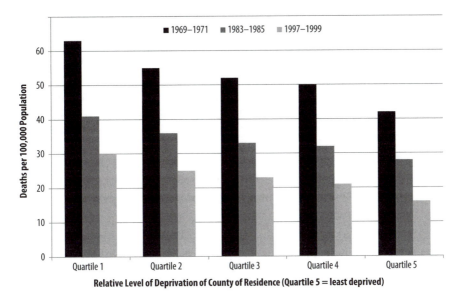

Figure 7.1. Changes in death rates among US children age 0–14, based on relative level of deprivation. *Source*: Based on Singh and Kogan 2007.

previous chapter, when the authors controlled for a child's level of socioeconomic deprivation, they found that "Black children experienced approximately 50% higher mortality throughout the study period than did White children" (p. 1660).

Death rates, however, do not provide a nearly complete picture of the relative health status of children from differing socioeconomic and racial/ethnic backgrounds. To gain a full understanding of the well-being of children, we also need to consider the overall health status of children, measured on a comprehensive scale such as we discussed in Chapter 2 (see Figure 2.1). Mehta and colleagues (2013) used a combination of indicators of child health in looking at recent trends in racial and ethnic health disparities in children. For the period 1998–2009, the authors "found little evidence that racial/ethnic disparities in child health have changed over time. In fact, for certain illnesses such as asthma, black-white disparities grew significantly larger over time" (p. 6).

In considering the implications of persisting health disparities among children, we should also consider the future consequences for adult health status of behaviors and exposures experienced by the children. As described by Stoll and colleagues (2013), "New perspectives about pediatric origins of adult disease, social determinants of health, and long-term effects of early exposures and interactions suggest that the poor health of children (reflected in rates of prematurity, obesity, behavioral and developmental problems, etc.) can be a harbinger of poor adult health" (p. 1780).

It is important to underscore the authors' inclusion of "behavioral and developmental problems" as a "harbinger of poor adult health." Especially in children, early childhood development and subsequent patterns of behavior play fundamental roles in affecting lifelong health status. Thus, in this chapter on disparities in children's health, I will include a discussion of the complex early roots of behavior and their effect on outcomes such as educational attainment and associated socioeconomic well-being.

The Changing Demographics of Children in the United States

Established in 1994, the Federal Interagency Forum on Child and Family Statistics publishes annual updates on the status of America's children. Their 2017 report provides an important perspective on the changing demographics of young Americans: "Racial and ethnic diversity have grown dramatically in the United States in the last three decades. This growth was first evident among children. This population is projected to become even more diverse in the decades to come. In 2020, less than half of all children are projected to be White, non-Hispanic. By 2050, 32 percent of U.S. children are projected to be Hispanic (up from 25 percent in 2016), and 39 percent are projected to be White, non-Hispanic (down from 51 percent in 2016)" (p. vii).

In 2015 20 percent of all children ages 0–17 lived in poverty; 59 percent of children lived in counties with air pollution above national standards; and 39 percent of children lived in substandard housing, based either on housing quality or affordability. In 2014 18 percent of children ages 6–11 and 21 percent of adolescents ages 12–17 were obese, with higher rates among Mexican American (25 percent) and black (23 percent) children. In 2015 13 percent of children had been diagnosed with asthma at some time in their lives, while 8 percent of children were reported to currently have asthma. The rate of current asthma was higher among black (13 percent) and Puerto Rican (14 percent) children. It thus seems clear that health disparities among children differ among socioeconomic and racial/ethnic groups.

An important part of the changing demographics of children is the growing number of children with one or more parents who were born elsewhere and immigrated to the United States. The percentage of US children with at least one foreign-born parent grew from 15 percent in 1994 to 25 percent in 2016. Twenty-three percent of babies born in 2016 in the United States were born to a mother who was Hispanic. In California, 47 percent of all babies born in 2016 were Hispanic (Martin and colleagues 2018).

In 2009 the National Population Council of Mexico and the University of California, working in close collaboration, released a study of the heightened challenges faced by children of Mexican immigrants in the United States. At that time, immigrant children with parents from Mexico made up 37 percent of all immigrant children in the United States. As one of the fastest growing groups in the United States, these children nevertheless face a series of challenges. For 60 percent of these children, neither parent was a US citizen. For 49 percent, neither parent finished high school—by far the highest percentage among immigrant groups.

One of the principal consequences of having noncitizen, immigrant parents with low levels of education and associated low levels of English language proficiency is the likelihood that a Mexican immigrant child will not have health insurance, and as a consequence will have reduced access to health care. This often happens even if the child is fully eligible for publicly sponsored insurance such as Medicaid or the Children's Health Insurance Program (CHIP). At that time, 19 percent of Mexican immigrant children under age 6 were uninsured, while 27 percent of those aged 6–17 were uninsured. This compared to uninsured rates among US-born black children of 7 percent for those under 6 and 9 percent for those 6–17. The lack of health insurance means that many Mexican and other Hispanic immigrant children have no regular source of medical care. As a consequence many parents delay care for their child, and then rely on the hospital emergency room for care. In addition, many of these children do not get needed prescription medicines, glasses, or dental care.

The percentage of children without health insurance has decreased since that time, with 4.3 percent of white children, 4.9 percent of black children, 4.6 percent of Asian children, and 7.7 percent of Hispanic children lacking health insurance in 2017 (Berchick et al. 2018). However, of the 3.3 million children who were uninsured in 2016, 57 percent were eligible for either Medicaid or CHIP but had not been enrolled by their parents or caregivers. Among children eligible for Medicaid or CHIP, 7.3 percent of white children, 3.9 percent of black children, 5.2 percent of Asian children, and 6.5 percent of Hispanic children remained un-enrolled despite their eligibility for these programs (Haley et al. 2018).

The Importance of Early Child Development as a Source of Health Disparities

From an evolutionary perspective, it is essential for a baby giraffe on the day of its birth to be able to stand up, begin to walk, and soon be able to run. Without these capabilities, the infant would be vulnerable to predators. Accordingly, the neural pathways and connections within the giraffe's brain and between the brain and the extremities are largely formed on the day of birth, having largely developed *in utero*.

A human infant is certainly not able to do any of these on the day it is born. It typically takes two months for an infant to begin to move its arms and legs in a coordinated manner, and 12–18 months to begin to walk (CDC 2013). The neural pathways and connections in a human infant's brain have only partially developed at the time of its birth. If a human infant were to remain in the mother's womb long enough to develop its neural connections sufficiently to walk, the infant's head would be too large to fit through the human pelvic birth canal. Accordingly, there is a critical period of further neural development during the initial months of life. Understanding the complex neural and physiologic control mechanisms that develop during this initial critical time period, and how they can be affected by the social and psychological circumstances in which an infant is raised, are essential to gaining a full understanding of the early roots of child health disparities.

In May 2013 the journal *JAMA* (*Journal of the American Medical Association*) published a special issue on child health. In one of the leading articles, Brent and Silverstein (2013) summarized our current understanding of the association between early childhood adversity and subsequent health and well-being. "There is overwhelming evidence that early childhood adversity—related to parental psychiatric disorder, poverty, abuse, loss, neglect, or trauma—has protean effects on children's physical and mental health and ultimately on their ability to become competent and productive adults. . . . Early child adversity . . . has been linked to myriad chronic conditions associated with premature mortality: smoking, substance abuse, obesity, cardiovascular disease, depression, and attempted suicide" (p. 1777).

In 2012 the American Academy of Pediatrics (AAP) issued a policy statement describing our growing understanding of the importance of adopting an "ecobiodevelopmental" (EBD) approach to understanding how genetics, molecular biology, and the impact of the social environment can combine to affect child and adult health. The AAP policy statement describes how "Applying this EBD framework to the challenges posed by significant childhood adversity reveals the powerful role that toxic stress can play in disrupting the architecture of the developing brain, thereby influencing behavioral, educational, economic, and health outcomes decades and generations later" (p. e225).

One of the leading researchers in the area of the impact of early childhood development has been Dr. Jack Shonkoff of Harvard University. In 2000 Shonkoff was coeditor of a report published by the Institute of Medicine titled *From Neurons to*

Neighborhoods: The Science of Early Childhood Development (Shonkoff and Phillips 2000). In their summary of the report, the editors identified three central conclusions of the study (p. 5):

1. From birth to age five, children rapidly develop foundational capabilities on which subsequent development builds. In addition to their remarkable linguistic and cognitive gains, they exhibit dramatic progress in their emotional, social, regulatory, and moral capacities. All of these critical dimensions of early development are intertwined, and each requires focused attention.

2. Striking disparities in what children know and can do are evident well before they enter kindergarten. These differences are strongly associated with social and economic circumstances, and they are predictive of subsequent academic performance.

3. Early child development can be seriously compromised by social, regulatory, and emotional impairments. Indeed, young children are capable of deep and lasting sadness, grief, and disorganization in response to trauma, loss, and early personal rejection.

The authors of the report called on researchers to focus increased attention on the ways that social and environmental factors can influence the neurologic development of the infant brain and physiologic control mechanisms. "Enormous potential exists at the intersection of child development research, neuroscience, and molecular and behavioral genetics to unlock some of the enduring mysteries about how biogenetic and environmental factors interact to influence developmental pathways" (p. 13).

Shonkoff and colleagues (2009) published an updated summary of research linking the processes of neural development, development of physiological control mechanisms, and the environment in which a child is raised. Given that the nerve pathways in the brain, in response to messages contained in the infant's genes, are finalizing their development during the early part of life, Shonkoff raised an intriguing yet crucially important question. Can the physical, psychological, and social environment in which the infant is raised after birth impact the way in which the child's genetic information is translated into physiologic and neural functioning? If so, are these environmental effects on gene functioning transitory or permanent? Shonkoff refers to this process as "biological embedding," and refers to the interaction between genes and environment as involving "epigenetic pathways" (p. 2254). Epigenetic changes affect the way a gene is expressed physiologically without affecting the underlying gene structure or nucleotide sequence. They are becoming an increasingly important component of research on human diseases (Feinberg 2018).

In their conclusion regarding the epigenetic influences on neural development, Shonkoff and colleagues offer the following perspective:

> This model is based on mounting evidence that the origins of many adult diseases can be found among adversities in the early years of life that establish biological "memories" that weaken physiological systems and produce latent vulnerabilities to problems that emerge well into the later adult years. . . . Beginning as early as the first weeks after conception and continuing into early infancy, the immature "organism" "reads" key characteristics of its environment and prepares to adapt to an external world that can vary dramatically in its levels of safety, sufficiency, and peril. When early experiences prepare a developing child for conditions involving a high level of stress or instability, the body's systems retain that initial programming and put the stress response system on a short-fuse and high-alert status. (p. 2257)

I would like to focus particular attention on the final sentence of the above. Shonkoff seems to be saying that early childhood experiences can impact a child's stress response system in ways that affect response to stress not only in childhood but also in adulthood. Berg and colleagues (2017) found that allostatic load and associated adverse health outcomes in adults were greatest among those who had experienced high levels of stress as children. Conversely, Slopen et al. (2017) found a significant association between positive experiences during childhood, such as emotionally supportive parents and a supportive school environment, and lower rates of cardiovascular disease as adults.

Recall from our discussions of allostatic load in Chapters 4 and 6 that the hypothalamus within the brain senses the level of stress in the environment, and conveys messages to the adrenal gland and other parts of the stress response system to react accordingly. A chronically elevated stress response, or allostatic load, can have serious consequences for the cardiovascular and other systems. An exaggerated allostatic load associated with the stress of socioeconomic disadvantage or perceived racial discrimination appears to be a major contributor to the health disparities we have been discussing.

What would be the consequences of a young child developing an overly active allostatic response system—either by lowering the threshold of stress to which the body will respond, or increasing magnitude of the stress response for a given level of stress? This type of "biological embedding" of an exaggerated stress response, if it persists throughout childhood and adulthood, could be a major contributor to the types of adult health disparities we have been studying.

McEwen (2012) has described the consequences of these types of early childhood interactions. He describes how the social environment in which a child is raised can "get under the skin" to affect later physiological and behavioral responses. "The brain is the central organ of stress and adaptation. The social environment as well as the physical environment have powerful effects on the body and the brain through the neuroendocrine, autonomic, and immune systems. Two important processes are evident: The first process is the biological embedding of early experiences . . . that determines operating ranges of physiological systems for the effects of later experiences, and the second process is the cumulative wear and tear of the physical and social environment on the brain and body acting through the neuroendocrine, autonomic, metabolic, and immune systems" (p. 17180).

Halfon's perspective on the importance of adopting a life course perspective in addressing inequalities in health is consistent with those of McEwen and Shonkoff. He describes the ways in which the impacts of social deprivation during sensitive periods of a child's development can extend the impact of that deprivation so as to involve long-term changes in biological and behavioral functioning. Halfon (2012) suggests "that the patterns of morbidity that are established in childhood largely hold steady throughout the rest of the lifespan, presaging higher rates of morbidity, disability, and chronic disease in adults" (p. 672).

Barr (2017) has reviewed the research into how toxic levels of stress in childhood can contribute to early development of cardiovascular disease (CVD). In Chapter 4 I described the process by which chronic elevation of allostatic load can contribute to cellular injury in the lining of the arterial circulation system. The principal mechanism is through elevated levels of the stress hormone cortisol triggering inflammation in the inner layers of arteries and arterioles. As discussed in Chapter 6, Thurston and Matthews (2009) have identified thickening and stiffening of the arteries of 18-year-olds raised in highly stressful circumstances. This type of damage to the arteries is a major risk factor for the development of high blood pressure and other types of CVD. While the actual arterial injury is not clinically apparent until age 18, the chronic elevation of blood cortisol levels that contributed to the injury has been detected in children as young as 3–4 who have grown up in a highly stressful environment, leading Barr to conclude that "independent of subsequent behavioral patterns, children experiencing high levels of adversity during childhood may be on a road to early CVD . . ." (p. 1420).

In a technical report issued by the American Academy of Pediatrics as background for their 2012 policy statement described above, Shonkoff and Garner (2012) come to a similar conclusion: "Beginning prenatally, continuing through infancy, and extending into childhood and beyond, development is driven by an ongoing, inextricable interaction between biology (as defined by genetic predispositions) and ecology (as defined by the social and physical environment) . . . [which] can affect lifelong behavior, development, and health" (p. e234).

Once a toxic childhood environment gets under a child's skin, the consequences can be substantial. Are these changes, though, lifelong and irreversible? If they were irreversible, there would seem to be little point in pediatricians and other health providers developing clinical and policy interventions to counteract them. Braveman and Barclay (2009) emphasize the importance of adopting a "Life Course Perspective" in evaluating the causes and potential solutions to health disparities that originate in childhood. Such a perspective focuses on the early childhood experience, looking at how that experience subsequently affects adolescent behavior and eventually adult health.

Wise (2009) reviews the research in support of adopting a Life Course Perspective such as that described by Braveman and Barclay. He acknowledges both the complexity and the importance of early genetic and environmental interactions, but stresses that the ability of the child's neurological and physiologic systems to respond to changing environmental circumstances does not stop in early childhood. Rather, that capacity to change continues into adolescence and, albeit at a somewhat slower rate, into adulthood. Questioning those who adopt a strict, deterministic approach to the early life course, Wise emphasizes that "the emerging science of the life course in no way suggests that the impact of early exposures is any less amenable to intervention than are the impacts of any other influences on human health. . . . Rather, these observations suggest a developmental reality that is far more dynamic and dependent on the provision of efficacious services than is usually implied by life-course representations" (p. S208).

Rutter (2012) supports Wise's perspective on the amenability of early, adverse epigenetic impacts on neurological and physiological functioning to targeted intervention. Referring to the body's "neuroplasticity"—its capacity to be molded during certain critical periods by environmental forces both positive and negative—he underscores that "despite some early claims on the fixity of such periods, it is now evident that they are not immutable; that plasticity extends into adult life, although it diminishes with increasing age; and that intervention can alter plasticity" (p. 17150).

The 2012 policy statement by the American Academy of Pediatrics that encouraged those who study child development to adopt an "ecobiodevelopmental" approach to child development also offered explicit recommendations for pediatricians and other pediatric health providers. When it comes to reducing or reversing the childhood impacts of toxic stress, "the profession of pediatrics plays an important role in designing, implementing, evaluating, refining, and advocating for a new generation of protective interventions. Pediatric providers are uniquely qualified and placed to assist in translating recent advances in developmental science into effective interventions for the home, the clinic, and the community" (p. e226).

Mischel's Marshmallow Experiment and the Predictive Ability of Childhood Behaviors

The above discussion describes the ways that early childhood experiences can affect brain and physiological functioning in children, and as a consequence their patterns of behavior. Among preschoolers, children growing up in low-income families, having experienced the social and psychological stresses associated with low-income communities, are at a greater risk of displaying problematic behaviors at an early age (Brown et al. 2012). These types of behaviors are associated with later problems in school and in other contexts.

Is it only problematic children whose behaviors are associated with future measures of health and well-being? Will seemingly well-behaved preschool children show signs of differential behaviors that also are associated with future well-being?

In the 1960s, psychologist Walter Mischel and his colleagues (1988) began a study of preschool-aged children at the Bing Preschool—a high-quality preschool, open to children from diverse backgrounds, operated in association with Stanford University's Department of Psychology. Bing includes among its classrooms a room referred to by the children there as "The Game Room." (The author's child spent time in The Game Room, enjoying it thoroughly, while he was a student at Bing in the early 2000s.) The Game Room is often equipped with a variety of toys and other apparatus of intense interest to preschoolers, as well as with a one-way window that allows experiments to observe children at play. Parents give informed consent for their children to participate in experimental activities in The Game Room.

Mischel invited children who were about four years old into The Game Room one at a time. Each child was given the following proposition: As a reward for playing alone in The Game Room, with the toys and other paraphernalia there, the child was shown a plate with two marshmallows on it. All the child had to do was play until the teacher/researcher returned (usually about 15 minutes), and the child would be given the reward.

The child was also told that if they did not want to wait for the teacher to return to get the reward, they could simply push a button in the play area, and the teacher would return right away. If the child chose to push the button, there would still be a reward, however the reward would be one marshmallow, rather than the two that were available for waiting. How would the child respond? Would they wait, or would they push the button?

Some children waited the full 15 minutes, and enjoyed the full reward. Others chose the smaller reward earned by not having to endure the stress of waiting. When each child received the selected reward, the experiment was over, and the child returned to the regular classroom.

Mischel then kept track of the children as they grew into adolescence. By contacting the families, he learned that, as adolescents, the children who didn't ring the bell (that is, they were able to wait 15 minutes for the larger reward) were:

- more academically and socially competent
- more verbally fluent
- more rational, attentive, and able to plan ahead
- more able to deal with frustration and stress

As four-year-olds, these children already had differing time perspectives that offered them differing levels of rewards associated with their differing responses to the opportunity to wait for a greater reward, as compared to accepting a smaller reward without the stress of waiting. Their time perspective as four-year-olds was associated with their personality characteristics and level of academic success as adolescents.

Did the children who chose to wait have different patterns of brain connections and different levels of stress response than those who chose not to wait? Alternatively, were their different responses associated with learned behaviors that were independent of underlying brain circuitry? While Mischel was not able to answer these questions explicitly, his results nevertheless point out the principle emphasized by the researchers cited above, that the social environment into which the child is born and in which it is raised can affect brain functioning and physiologic stress responses, potentially in ways that will persist into adolescence and adulthood.

Boyce and colleagues (2012) evaluated a diverse group of kindergarten children in Berkeley, California—across the San Francisco Bay from the Bing School. They observed several cohorts of children in the classroom, evaluating the children's behavior in the learning environment, observations of their interactions with their peers, and their family SES background. Based on information provided by the teacher, classroom behavior was categorized as adaptive or maladaptive based on factors such as how well they paid attention, how well they interacted with other children, and how well they did academically. Social interaction with peers was categorized as dominant or subordinate based on direct observation by the researchers. Boyce found that children from higher and lower SES backgrounds were equally likely to be in either a dominant or a subordinate position in their peer interactions. However lower SES children were more likely to show maladaptive pattern behavior. Growing up in a lower SES environment appears to increase the risk a child will, as early as the beginning of kindergarten, demonstrate behaviors that will likely impede that child's subsequent educational attainment.

Bogart and colleagues (2013) evaluated the behavior of a racially and ethnically diverse group of fifth-grade students from schools in Alabama, California, and Texas. They looked at behaviors such as aggression toward other children (both physical and nonphysical), retaliatory behavior, and school delinquency. They first compared the behaviors of students from different racial or ethnic groups, and then evaluated the extent to which these differences were reduced when family SES was taken into account. They found striking racial/ethnic differences, with both black and Latino students more likely to display these problematic behaviors in school. When they took into account parents' SES, these racial/ethnic differences nearly went away. After further controlling for students' experiences of racial discrimination, the racial/ethnic behavioral differences were no longer apparent.

Ross and Mirowsky (2011) describe a model in which low levels of parental education will put a child at increased risk of developing behavioral patterns that not only impede the child's early educational success, but will also increase the child's risk of developing unhealthy lifestyles and health-related behaviors. "Because education develops competence on many levels, it gives people the ability and motivation to shape and control their lives. High levels of education increase sense of personal control; the belief that one can master, control, or effectively alter the environment. In contrast, the poorly educated may not possess the resources necessary to achieve their goals, which produces a sense of powerlessness, fatalism, and helplessness" (p. 592). They found that children of parents with low levels of education who themselves had low levels of education were, when they were adults, the most likely to have unhealthy behaviors (for example, smoking, diet, alcohol, exercise) and worse health status.

Shonkoff (2012, p. 17302) links these early patterns of maladaptive educational and health-related behavior to the neurological and physiological impacts of early childhood stress. "At the time of school entry, children differ in how well they are able to focus and shift their attention, manage their feelings, control their impulses, follow rules and directions, and adapt to a variety of other demands." He links these differences in what he calls "executive function" to the "multiple developmental impediments that limit the ability of children with normal cognitive potential to benefit from available learning opportunities. These include emotional problems associated with fear and anxiety, maladaptive social adjustment, disruptive behaviors, impairments in executive functioning, and a range of other difficulties." Shonkoff attributes these outcomes to the epigenetic impact of stress in the early childhood experience.

The Center on the Developing Child at Harvard University (2011) published an informative paper describing the importance of executive function in early child development. They suggest that "Having executive function in the brain is like having an air traffic control system at a busy airport to manage the arrivals and departures of dozens of planes on multiple runways" (p. 1). They describe the typical pattern by which young children develop executive function, with the most rapid development taking place between ages 3 and 6. Fortunately, most children entering kindergarten at age 5–6 have developed a sufficient level of executive function to be able to control their emotional impulses and focus on the process of learning and of getting along with other people (both the teachers and their fellow students).

What if a child entering kindergarten has experienced delay in the development of executive function as a consequence of growing up in a high-stress environment? Kate Taylor, a writer for the *New York Times*, describes such a child (Taylor 2015). When the girl entered kindergarten at a private, charter school in Brooklyn, "She racked up demerits for not following directions or not keeping her hands folded in her lap. Sometimes, after being chastised, she threw tantrums. She was repeatedly suspended for screaming, throwing pencils, running away from school staff members or refusing to go to another classroom for a timeout."

In a paper I wrote intended for schoolteachers and administrators (Barr 2018), I explain how executive function in young children is dependent on the development of certain nerve connections within the developing child's brain. Just as elevated levels of cortisol adversely impact blood vessels, they also adversely impact the formation of nerve connections. The 6-year-old girl described by Taylor had not yet fully developed her "air traffic control system"—her full executive function capacity. As I emphasize for teachers, this child is not brain-damaged. Rather, she had experienced a delay in her neural capacity for executive function. Unfortunately, being treated by her teacher as a troublemaker who didn't belong in kindergarten, the child was at risk of internalizing this concept of herself and as a result reduced her sense of her own self-efficacy, defined by psychologist Albert Bandura (1997) as "beliefs in one's capabilities to organize and execute the courses of action required to produce given attainments" (p. 3).

Without this sense of her own capacity to succeed in school, the girl was likely to have been at increased risk of dropping out of high school, as described in a report by the American Public Health Association (APHA) (APHA 2018). As described in the APHA report, "high school graduation is the social determinant that most strongly predicts long-term health. Students who do not graduate high school on time are less likely to attain higher education, practice health-promoting behaviors, earn living wages or access social capital" (p. 2). The APHA also emphasizes the role of delayed neural development of the brain in contributing to this risk. "The result is that chronic stress can negatively impact development of the prefrontal cortex—the part of the brain that controls some of our most sophisticated intellectual functions as well as emotional and cognitive regulation" (p. 4).

In the Mischel marshmallow experiment, did the children who chose to wait have different patterns of brain connections and different levels of executive function and stress response than those who chose not to wait? We cannot answer this specific question, but we can say with some certainty that, as early as the preschool years, children show differential patterns of behavior in response to stressful circumstances and in the context of self-control, and that these differential responses have been repeatedly linked both to subsequent educational attainment and subsequent health-related behaviors. Many if not most of these early childhood differences can be linked to the experience of having grown up in a lower SES context. From what we have learned in earlier chapters, we know that reduced educational attainment and worse health-related behaviors can have lifelong adverse consequences on adult health status.

In an editorial published in a special edition of the *American Journal of Public Health* focused on "Child Maltreatment: Breaking the Intergenerational Link," Merrick and Guinn (2018) summarize the findings of a series of articles included in the journal. "Research on intergenerational continuity of violence and adversity finds that individuals who experience abuse, neglect, or other forms of childhood adversity are more likely than are nonexposed individuals to have children who go on to have similar adverse childhood experiences" (p. 1117). The child who experiences toxic levels of stress in early childhood may unconsciously and unwillingly pass those experiences on to their own children.

Disparities in Childhood Asthma

The above discussion provides strong evidence that the "toxicity" of the social and economic environment into which a child is born and in which a child grows up can trigger fundamental changes in the brain and associated stress response mechanisms, which in turn can affect early child behavior, the quality of a child's social interactions, and the level of education a child is able to attain. All of these factors will influence health status as an adult.

There is a second group of illnesses that has shown a similar pattern of epigenetic inheritance based on the quality of a child's environment. These are respiratory allergies, in particular asthma. The prevalence of asthma has been steadily increasing for several decades, with rates higher in developed countries than in developing countries (Ho 2010). The United States has seen a steady increase in the prevalence of asthma over the period 2001–16, with the highest rates among poor children and black children (CDC 2018).

Asthma is an illness in which the cells lining the airways respond to the presence of certain foreign substances by swelling, producing increased amounts of thick mucus, and by spasm of the muscles lining the airways, with consequent narrowing of the airways and difficulty breathing. This response is brought on by an interaction between certain foreign substances and an immune protein in the body, immune globulin E, referred to by the abbreviation IgE. IgE is analogous to the protective protein immune globulin G (IgG) antibodies produced in response to certain viruses and other types of infections. While the stimulation of IgG is protective for the body, the stimulation of IgE can be harmful. It is the interaction of IgE with foreign substances recognized as toxic that triggers a cellular cascade leading to the symptoms of asthma. The most common types of substances that trigger this response are certain types of air pollution, certain household irritants, and tobacco smoke.

Fortunately, most people, while bothered by air pollution and other irritants, will not develop an asthma attack in response. In order for the irritant to trigger an asthma attack, the affected individual must have "imprinted" a sensitivity to it in the body's IgE memory. In a manner analogous to the imprinting of increased allostatic response to stress, the imprinting of an allergic reaction to certain foreign substances takes place in two critical time periods: during fetal development in the uterus, and in early childhood development (Durham and colleagues 2011).

North and Ellis (2011) have reviewed research on the role of epigenetics in allergic diseases such as asthma. "There is increasing evidence pointing to the influence of prenatal and early life exposures on the development of allergic disease. A growing body of literature supports the theory that transient environmental pressures can have permanent effects on gene regulation and expression through epigenetic mechanisms" (p. 35). The process of sensitization to asthma involves two steps. First, an individual's IgE encounters a foreign substance and imprints the chemistry of that substance in its memory. Second, an individual encounters that substance again, at a later time. Having previously imprinted the substance as foreign, the IgE triggers an allergic response, often involving the airways.

Not everyone will develop these allergic responses on repeated exposure to a foreign substance. Certain individuals are born with an increased risk of developing asthma and other forms of allergic symptoms. These individuals are born with a condition referred to as "atopy." Atopic individuals are at substantially increased risk of developing asthma and other forms of allergy through this IgE imprinting process. It is not necessary to have inherited atopy as a child in order to develop asthma; however, a substantial majority of those with asthma are also atopic.

An interesting aspect of the condition atopy is that it is possible to develop it without having inherited it, and once having developed it, to then pass it on to one's children and grandchildren. Atopy seems to involve epigenetic changes in the chemical coating of the DNA molecule that are transmissible across generations, without there being any change in the underlying genetic structure (Kuriakose and Miller 2010).

There are clear racial and ethnic disparities in the prevalence and severity of asthma among children in the United States. In 2016 the highest prevalence rates were among black children (15.7 percent) and Puerto Rican Hispanic children (12.9 percent), as compared to 7.1 percent among white children (CDC 2018). There are also racial/ethnic differences in the severity of asthma among those children who have asthma and where they went for care for their asthma. In 2016 5.2 percent of black children and 5.6 percent of Hispanic children with asthma received treatment in the emergency room as their usual source of care for their condition, as compared to 1.8 percent of white children.

Lozano and colleagues (1995) addressed the question of racial differences in asthma in a study of children with asthma from low-income families in the Seattle-Tacoma area of Washington State. All of these children were on Medicaid, all had access to the same health care facilities, and all had approximately the same rate of well-child visits to the doctor (although the black children had fewer office visits specifically for management of their asthma). Nevertheless, the black children were significantly more likely to need emergency room treatment or hospitalization for their asthma.

The authors acknowledged that "the dichotomous definitions of race used in this study obscure the complexity of the meaning of African American ethnicity." They suggested that in order to understand why black children with asthma are so much sicker than white children of comparable SES who also have asthma, we will need to undertake further research "to discern which institutional, cultural/behavioral, and societal characteristics mediate the influence of African American race on the use of health services" (p. 473).

Rosenstreich and colleagues (1997) also studied the frequency of asthma treatment in a sample of 476 children from eight inner-city areas in the United States. All lived in poor or low-income neighborhoods, and all had asthma. Given the inner-city origins of these children, very few were white—78 percent of the children were black and 16 percent were Hispanic. Thus, we are not able to make meaningful black/white racial comparisons from this study.

The purpose of this study was not to assess the influence of race on asthma, but rather the impact of allergy to the components of common household dust. The authors were interested in three dust components in particular: cat dander, dust mites, and cockroaches. The authors first performed standard skin testing among the children to determine the extent to which they were allergic to these three allergens. They then visited the homes of the children and vacuumed up all the dust in the child's bedroom. They analyzed the dust in a laboratory for the presence of the same three antigens. The authors then divided the children into four groups for each of the three allergens they studied:

Group 1: children with no allergy to a specific antigen and low levels of the antigen in their bedroom dust

Group 2: children with no allergy to a specific antigen and high levels of the antigen in their bedroom dust

Group 3: children with allergy to a specific antigen and low levels of the antigen in their bedroom dust

Group 4: children with allergy to a specific antigen and high levels of the antigen in their bedroom dust

For each of the three antigens studied, they compared the rate of hospitalization among these four groups. For dust mites and cat dander, the children with allergy and high bedroom exposure to the allergen were no more likely to be hospitalized for their asthma than the children in the other three groups. However, the children with allergy to cockroaches and high levels of cockroaches in their bedroom were between two and four times more likely to end up in the hospital than children in the other three groups. The combination of allergy to cockroaches and the presence of cockroaches in a child's bedroom was also associated with more severe wheezing, more unscheduled medical visits, and more frequent changes in the caregiver's plans to get treatment for the child with asthma.

The Rosenstreich study was of mostly black inner-city children from low-income families. The Lozano study was of black and white children in one large metropolitan area, also from low-income families. The Rosenstreich study did not compare asthma severity by race; the Lozano study did not compare asthma severity by the frequency of cockroaches in the child's bedroom. One has to wonder, though, if we were able to go back to the homes of the children from Seattle-Tacoma in the

Lozano study, whether we would find more cockroaches in the bedrooms of the black children than the white children?

Gaffin and Phipatanakul (2009) studied household factors that contribute to the rising asthma prevalence in the United States. They cite elevated levels of IgE among six-month-old children as predictive of asthma during childhood, and identify a series of factors commonly found inside homes that place a child at this increased risk of developing asthma. Principal among these risk factors are dust mites, furred pets, cockroaches, mold, and rodents, with cockroaches one of the worst. The authors note that "inner city children sensitized and exposed to cockroaches suffer the highest morbidity" (p. 130). It seems clear that children growing up in the most run-down neighborhoods, which are often the most racially segregated neighborhoods, grow up in lower quality housing with concomitant increased exposure to the very factors most likely to trigger asthma in children.

Another factor that may contribute to the added severity of the black children in the Lozano study is the nature of racial residential segregation in the Seattle area. Recall from our discussion in Chapter 6 of contributors to racial disparities in lung cancer, that blacks living in racially segregated communities consistently experience higher rates of air pollution. Abel and White (2011) studied patterns of air pollution in the Seattle area for the period 1990–2007, and identified two closely linked results: (a) the worst sources of air pollution were concentrated in one area of south central Seattle, and (b) minority residents were concentrated in the most polluted areas. In 1990, the period in which Lozano gathered his data about childhood asthma severity, seven of the Seattle's 10 worst air polluters were located in the same neighborhoods where minority populations were concentrated.

Inner-city, low-income neighborhoods are often segregated by race or ethnicity. If the characteristics of the neighborhoods of black children and white children were to differ systematically and in ways that could be tied directly to asthma severity, we might be able to explain why a racial difference in asthma severity persists after taking into account SES.

Meng and colleagues (2006) addressed this issue in a study of asthma severity among children with asthma. Rather than exposure to home allergens as a risk factor for asthma morbidity, they looked at exposure to air pollution resulting from vehicular traffic in a child's neighborhood of residence. They divided the density of the neighborhood traffic into three categories—low, medium, and high—and then analyzed differences in the severity of asthma symptoms among these categories. Not surprisingly they found a clear association between traffic density and asthma. Using the annual frequency of hospitalization or visits to the emergency room for the treatment of asthma as a measure of severity, they found this frequency to be:

- 8 percent for children living in low traffic density neighborhoods
- 17 percent for children living in medium traffic density neighborhoods
- 22 percent for children living in high traffic density neighborhoods

They then looked to see if there was an association between the family income of these children and their traffic exposure. As illustrated in Figure 7.2, they found a clear association, with exposure to traffic density falling as family income rises.

Children living below the poverty line are more than twice as likely as children at or above three times the poverty line to be exposed to high traffic density in their neighborhood. The researchers then looked to see if there was an association between the child's race/ethnicity and the exposure to traffic density. These results are also shown in Figure 7.2 and demonstrate a clear racial difference, with black children nearly twice as likely to experience heavy traffic density as white children.

California has had a problem for many years with air pollution related to heavy traffic volume and other associated factors. Southern California has had a particularly severe problem with air pollution and its impact on children with asthma. Fortunately, Southern California has taken a number of steps to reduce the level of air pollution. As reported by Berhane and colleagues (2016), decreases in air pollution levels between 1993 and 2013 were associated with significant decreases in asthma

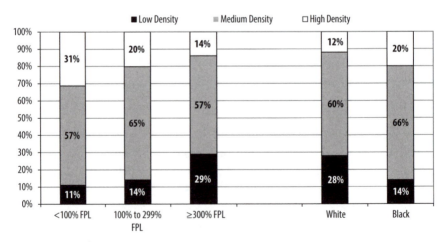

Figure 7.2. Traffic density of residential neighborhood for children with asthma in California, by family income and race. Family income measured as percentage of federal poverty level (FPL). *Source*: Adapted from Meng et al. 2006.

severity among children. The largest decreases in air pollution were in those communities with the highest pollution levels at the start of the study.

It should also be noted that exposure to secondhand tobacco smoke is a significant risk factor for developing asthma. Given the higher rates of smoking among adults with low levels of education and income, low-income children are at increased risk of exposure to secondhand smoke in the home environment. Kum-Nji and colleagues (2012) studied low-income children coming for treatment (not necessarily asthma related) in an inner-city pediatric clinic, and found that 60 percent of the children were exposed to secondhand smoke at home. Among the children exposed to smoke, 69 percent had a mother who smoked.

Holtby and colleagues (2011) found that nearly one million children in California were exposed to secondhand smoke, with black children substantially more likely than other racial/ethnic groups to be exposed. Tobacco smoke, indoor allergens, and air pollution all affect low-income children, and especially low-income black children, disproportionately.

Williams and colleagues (2009) have reviewed the range of factors contributing to disparities in childhood asthma. They note that "illness and social adversity tend to cluster in the same people and places, so that individuals and areas that are at risk for 1 adverse condition tend to be at risk for multiple social ills" (p. S174). That adversity clusters by income, and it often clusters by race. Given the history of residential racial segregation in our country, black children are often the ones most adversely affected. As concluded by Williams, for asthma as well as other conditions, "residential segregation is a central determinant of black/white disparities in SES at the individual, household, and neighborhood levels and, thus, is a fundamental cause of racial disparities in health in the United States" (p. S177).

Confronting Pollution in the Water Children Drink: The Case of Flint, Michigan

We should recall that air pollution is not the only form of pollution children in racially segregated communities experience. In 2014 children in Flint, Michigan, began to be exposed to toxic levels of lead in their drinking water, due to a change in the city's water source. Dr. Mona Hanna-Attisha and her colleagues at a hospital in Flint measured the levels of lead in children's blood both before and after the change in the city's water source (Hanna-Attisha et al. 2016). They reported that "incidence of elevated blood lead levels increased from 2.4% to 4.9% after water source change, and neighborhoods with the highest water lead levels experienced a 6.6% increase" (p. 283). Neighborhoods that were both poor and predominantly black showed the highest blood lead levels. A study by Sadler, LaChance, and Hanna-Attisha (2017) found that "children living in older homes in neighborhoods of generally poorer housing condition have been disproportionately affected by higher rates and greater increases in pediatric [blood lead levels] during this water lead-leaching event" (p. 766).

In an interview conducted by Bridget Kuehn (2016), Dr. Hanna-Attisha described the chronic challenges the children in Flint have faced: "Our population was already rattled with toxic stresses. We have a 40% poverty rate, high rates of unemployment, high rates of violence, and high rates of single parents. We have no grocery stores in Flint. The people in Flint have a 20-year lower life expectancy than people in a neighboring suburb. We were already struggling with every barrier to our children's success. Then we gave them lead. This is added toxic stress to the toxic stresses we already had" (p. 968).

David Bellinger, a Professor of Environmental Health at Harvard, has accurately described the challenges poor, minority children typically face: "The burden of childhood lead poisoning has always weighed most heavily on populations that are politically and economically disenfranchised . . . . Were Flint more affluent, it's unlikely that the contamination would have continued for 18 months after citizens first voiced complaints about water quality" (Bellinger 2016, p. 1102).

Disparities in Childhood Obesity

Obesity is a major public health concern in the United States. Obesity-related illnesses such as heart disease and kidney disease are a principal contributor to SES and racial/ethnic disparities in life expectancy and level of disability. Accordingly, there has been growing national attention on ways to reduce obesity at all ages.

Obesity among children is a central concern in this national effort. Obesity as a child is highly predictive of obesity as an adult, with obese children more likely to develop high blood pressure, high cholesterol, and diabetes as adults (CDC 2013). In addition, the earlier obesity occurs, the earlier related illnesses begin to occur. A growing number of adolescents in the United States is developing Type II diabetes, an illness previously referred to as "adult onset diabetes" since it rarely occurred in children. Among black and American Indian children between the ages of 10 and 19, Type II diabetes occurs substantially more often than Type I diabetes—formerly referred to as "child onset diabetes" (CDC 2017).

The term "obese" is intended to be used in a purely descriptive sense, without normative or value judgments attached to it. The ratio of one's weight (measured in kilograms) to the square of one's height (measured in meters), referred to as the Body Mass Index (BMI), is used to describe obesity. Using federal standards (US Department of Health and Human Services, National Institutes of Health 2019), an adult with a BMI between 18.5–24.9 is considered to be of a normal weight; those with a BMI of 25–29.9 are described as overweight; and those with a BMI of 30 or greater are described as obese. These divisions between BMI categories were established based on changes in the relative risk of illness.

Children are categorized on a somewhat different basis, using where a child is on a BMI-for-age growth chart using a percentile ranking (with separate charts for girls and boys) (CDC 2013). Child weight is classified based on the following percentile categories:

- Underweight   less than the 5th percentile
- Healthy weight   5th percentile to less than the 85th percentile
- Overweight   85th percentile to less than the 95th percentile
- Obese   equal to or greater than the 95th percentile

As discussed below, substantially more than 5 percent of children in the United States are obese, which seems inconsistent with defining obese as having a BMI that is at or above the 95th percentile. Principles of mathematics would suggest that no more than 5 percent of children can be at or above the 95th percentile. This seeming inconsistency is because the distribution of childhood BMI in the 1980s, a period when far fewer children were obese, was used to establish these categories (Ebbeling and Ludwig 2008). Thus, if we state that "10 percent of a certain group of children are obese," what we are actually saying is that 10 percent of today's children have a BMI that is equal to or greater than the 95th percentile of BMIs for a child in the 1980s of the same gender and age.

In the period 1976–80, using this definition of obesity, 5.5 percent of children in the United States were obese, ranging from 5.0 percent for children aged 2–5 and aged 12–19 to 6.5 percent for children aged 6–11. By 2004 the rate of childhood obesity in the United States was 17.1 percent, with rates of 13.9 for ages 2–5, 18.8 for ages 6–11, and 17.4 for ages 12–19 (Ogden and Carroll 2010). While obesity rates leveled off somewhat between 2004 and 2010, by 2016 the overall rate of childhood obesity was 18.5 percent, with rates of 13.9 for ages 2–5, 18.4 for ages 6–11, and 20.6 for ages 12–19 (Hales et al. 2017).

Geserick and colleagues (2018) analyzed the pattern of BMI change over time in more than 50,000 children in Germany from birth through age 15–18. They found that the greatest risk of developing childhood obesity occurred between two and six years of age. It was in these preschool years when the most rapid increase in BMI

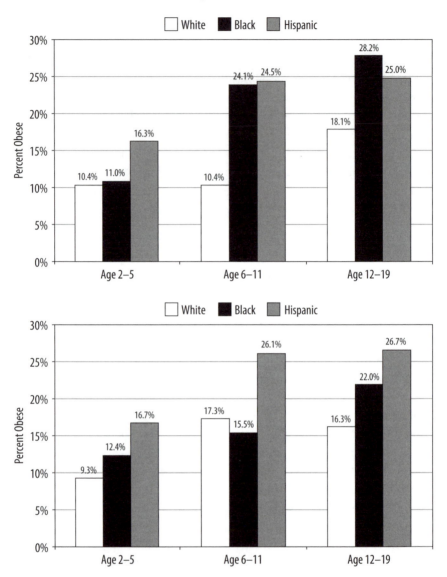

Figure 7.3. Rates of obesity among girls (*top*) and boys (*bottom*) in the United States, 2016. *Source:* Based on Ogden and colleagues 2018.

percentile occurred among those children who were obese at age 15–18. Of those children who were obese by age three, 90 percent remained obese as adolescents.

If we look at obesity rates by gender and by race/ethnicity, we see some striking differences (Ogden et al. 2018) (Figure 7.3). Depending on which age group we look at, in 2016 the rate of obesity for black girls was between 1.1–2.39 times

Table 7.1. Obesity Rates and Risk Factors for Obesity among Adolescents (Age 12–17) in California in 2005 by Household Income as a Percentage of Federal Poverty Line

	< 100% FPL	100–199% FPL	200–299% FPL	≥ 300% FPL
Obesity rate	21%	20%	16%	8%
Did not get at least 60 minutes of physical activity on any day in past week	18%	16%	14%	13%
Drank soda in the previous day	71%	67%	67%	55%
Ate fast food in the previous day	49%	49%	46%	37%
Mean number of fast-food outlets within ½ mile of home	5.5	4.6	3.4	2.5

Source: Hastert and colleagues 2008.

greater than the rate for white girls, while the rate for Hispanic girls was between 1.4–2.4 times greater than the rate for white girls. Among boys, the black rate was 0.9–1.3 times the white rate, while the Hispanic rate was 1.5–1.8 times the white rate. It is interesting to note that the highest rates were found in black girls and Hispanic boys.

Disparities in rates of obesity do not only exist among racial/ethnic groups. Childhood obesity also affects children in low-income families disproportionately, independent of race/ethnicity. Hastert and colleagues (2008) looked at obesity rates in 2005 among adolescents aged 12–17 in California, based on household income as a percent of the federal poverty line (FPL). As shown in Table 7.1, they found the obesity rates to be consistently higher in lower income families. When they also looked at known risk factors for adolescent obesity, they also found consistent income related gradients, with lower income adolescents less likely to have regular exercise and more likely to have recently consumed soda or fast food.

As suggested by Michelle Obama's *Let's Move* program, introduced in 2009 to reduce childhood obesity nationally, low levels of regular exercise are a major risk factor for obesity. Kimm and colleagues (2002) followed the exercise patterns of 1,213 black girls and 1,166 white girls from the age of 9 through the age of 19. They surveyed the girls on a regular basis about their exercise patterns, and calculated how many times per week each girl expended one metabolic equivalent (MET) of energy in exercise. At age 9–10, the median energy expenditure for white girls was 30.8 MET-times per week, and that of black girls was 27.3 MET-times per week. Between age 9–10 and age 15–16 there was a dramatic drop-off in energy expenditure for both groups of girls. The drop-off was substantially greater, however, for the black girls than for the white girls. By age 15–16, the median energy expenditure for white girls had fallen to 10.3 MET-times per week. It remained at about this level through age 18–19. From age 15–16 through age 18–19, the median expenditure for black girls was zero.

The authors then evaluated the association between parental education and income and the observed decline in physical activity during adolescence. For white girls, there was an inverse association between parental education and decline in activity only during the preadolescent years. For black girls, there was also an inverse association between parental education and decline in activity, but it was only evident during the later adolescent years.

Franzini and colleagues (2009) followed 650 fifth-grade children in Birmingham, Los Angeles, and Houston for the months of May to September, measuring their levels of physical activity, while also measuring the quality of the social environment and the physical environment of the neighborhood in which they lived. Consistent with Kimm's study, they found that black and Hispanic children had lower levels of exercise than white children, after controlling for parents' education. They found a strong association between the social environment and the children's exercise level. In a follow-up study (Franzini et al. 2010), the researchers walked through the several blocks surrounding each child's home, recording various aspects of the residential environment. They found that, compared to higher income neighborhoods, "characteristics of the physical environment favorable to outdoor physical activity are less prevalent in poorer neighborhoods: the physical environment is less safe, less comfortable, and less pleasurable for outdoor physical activity" (p. 272). While income was a stronger predictor of the social environment of the neighborhood, high levels of minority race among residents, either black or Hispanic, continued to be associated with a worse social environment after controlling for income. The adverse impact of residential racial segregation over and above its association with a low-income environment appears to extend to the risk of child and adolescent obesity (Kimbro and Denney 2013).

Beyond the nature of the physical environment in low-income and minority communities, the food environment to which children are exposed also has an important role in affecting obesity rates. Recall from Table 7.1 that, compared to their higher income peers, lower-income adolescents in California were also more likely recently to have consumed both soda and fast food. They also had many more fast-food outlets within one-half mile of their home. A federal study reported that a lack of venues such as supermarkets to purchase healthy foods, coupled with greater access to fast-food restaurants and convenience stores, creates a substantial risk of adolescent obesity due to increased consumption of soda and fast foods with high fat and calorie content (CDC 2011). Babey and colleagues (2011) studied food environment near homes and schools in California, calculating the ratio of unhealthy food outlets (for example, fast-food restaurants, convenience stores, liquor stores) to healthy food outlets (for example, grocery stores, produce vendors) within a half mile of children's schools and one mile of children's schools (two miles in rural areas). For all of California they found this ratio to average 7.9. They then compared the consumption of fast foods and sodas by adolescents, based on this ratio in their home and school neighborhood. They found that adolescents exposed to a higher ratio of unhealthy to healthy food sources consumed significantly more sodas and fast foods than those in lower-ratio neighborhoods. In a similar study of preadolescent children living in New Haven, Connecticut, Carroll-Scott and colleagues (2013) found that students living within a 5-minute walk of a fast-food outlet had higher BMI and less healthy eating habits.

Often referred to as "food deserts," areas with a predominance of unhealthy food sources are typically found in low-income and minority communities. In their study of the food environment of adolescents, Hastert and colleagues (2008) found that "adolescents with household incomes below the poverty line have an average of 5.5 fast food outlets and convenience stores within one-half mile of home, more than twice as many as teens with household incomes of at least 300% FPL" (p. 2). D'Angelo and colleagues (2016) found that 50 percent of public schools with a majority of Hispanic students had a fast-food restaurant within about 2,500 feet, while 21 percent of public schools with a majority of white students had a fast-food source so close. The predominance of food deserts in low-income and minority neighborhoods provides yet one more example of the harmful health effects associated with residential racial segregation.

There is another important aspect of child and adolescent obesity that we should consider. Perceptions of child obesity may vary by culture. In my research about perceived cultural barriers to health care, we conducted focus group sessions with ethnically homogeneous, low-income patients (Barr and Wanat 2005). One focus group included Pacific Islander patients, such as those from Tonga and Samoa. In asking these patients to described cultural barriers they perceived in the care process, the participants emphasized their resistance to and resentment of physicians consistently bringing up the issue of obesity. They perceived this as negative stereotyping of their ethnic group, and expressed little concern about their children's body image.

Creighton and colleagues (2012) studied 1,610 families in Los Angeles County, looking at the association of patterns of food consumption for first- and second-generation Mexican immigrants. They found second-generation immigrants to be at a substantially higher risk for obesity, in close association with their increased propensity to consume sweetened drinks and fast foods.

Garcia (2004) describes his experiences in a health clinic serving a largely Mexican immigrant community in California.

> "No come nada," the Mexican mother of a two-year-old boy said to me at morning clinic, pointing to her toddler, who at thirty-eight pounds is far above the normal weight for his age. "He hasn't eaten anything in three days." . . . Deciphering the code of Mexican culture in present-day California, I think the mother means that the child doesn't eat as much as Mama would like him to—that he doesn't eat as much as he did when he was a hungry, rapidly growing, normal infant. (p. 215)

Parents who perceive a heavier child as a healthier child may not respond positively to health providers characterizing their child as "obese" and urging them to change how they feed the child. Some suggest that especially for some Mexican American boys and African American girls, a large body is not always considered undesirable.

Hager and colleagues (2012) interviewed 304 low-income mothers of children between 12 and 32 months of age. They asked the mothers to look at a series of silhouette images of toddlers of varying BMI percentiles who were of a similar age as their own child. The images ranged, at increments of 16 percentile points, from a toddler at the 1st percentile of the BMI distribution (that is, an underweight toddler) to a toddler at the 96th percentile. They then asked the mother, "Which picture looks most like your child?" They then asked the mothers, "Which picture do you want your child to look like?"

Two-thirds of the mothers were at or below the poverty line; 73 percent were unmarried; 81 percent had no education beyond high school. Seventy-one percent of the mothers were black, 22 percent were white, and 2 percent were Hispanic. Fifty percent of the mothers were obese themselves.

Seventy percent of the mothers selected an image that was inaccurate, defined as being two images (32 percentile points) or more different from their own child's actual BMI percentile, based on measurement by the researchers. Among mothers of overweight toddlers (that is, BMI percentile ≥85), 94 percent were inaccurate in their assessment, all of whom selected an image two steps or more smaller than their child's actual size. Mothers who themselves were overweight or obese were more likely than normal weight mothers to perceive their child as smaller than they actually were. The accuracy of the mother's perception did not differ based on the mother's race or SES. The mother's satisfaction with their toddler's actual body size was highest among mothers of overweight children. Parental perceptions of how a "healthy" child should look seem to vary based on personal and cultural beliefs held by the mother.

Addressing the Causes of Childhood Health Disparities

We have seen that, in a manner similar to health disparities among adults, dispari-ties among children fall largely along SES and racial/ethnic lines. Children born into a low-income home and community environment experience substantially greater levels of stress than those in higher income communities. These toxic levels of stress can "get under the child's skin," causing biochemical and neurological changes in the child's response to stress and to environmental toxins. These changes can influence how the child's genetic inheritance is expressed, both physiologically and behaviorally. The adverse effects of economic disadvantage are often exacer-bated by the effects of residential segregation, both economic segregation and ra-cial segregation. Black and other minority families are disproportionately concen-trated in neighborhoods with higher levels of air pollution, higher levels of household allergens, and higher concentration of "food deserts"—areas with large numbers of fast-food outlets and few healthy food outlets.

It is essential that we appreciate the profound effects the stress of inequality can have on the development of children. It is equally essential that we avoid approach-ing the physiologic and behavioral responses children develop in response to stress as a *fait accompli*. The same scientific evidence that has documented the "imprint-ing" of toxic stress on children's neural and hormonal systems has also reinforced the ongoing plasticity of those same systems. As underscored above by Wise (2009) and Rutter (2012), well-designed interventions that target children, adolescents, and young adults have the potential to reverse many of the harmful effects of early ex-periences of inequality. These interventions include those that increase educa-tional opportunity, improve access to health care, and enhance children's percep-tions of their own self-efficacy. In order to be effective in the long term, efforts at reducing child health disparities must focus particular attention on reducing the impact of the inequality and social injustice that are the root causes of most of these disparities.

CHAPTER EIGHT

All Things Being Equal, Does Race/Ethnicity Affect How Physicians Treat Patients?

The discussion in Chapter 6 explored the various ways that race and SES interact to affect health status. We found that, after taking into account differences in SES, blacks and other minorities continue to have worse health status than whites for a broad range of conditions. I attributed part of this difference to the physiological effects over time of the stress associated with being in a minority racial/ethnic group. I also attributed part of the difference to the neighborhood effects of decreased social capital that accompany continued residential racial segregation across a range of SES. However, I left unexamined the possible contribution of racial differences in access to medical care. This chapter explores this issue in more depth.

Clearly, racial/ethnic differences in SES will be associated with racial/ethnic differences in access to medical care. For more than a century, the United States has approached medical care as a market commodity. In the words of economist Uwe Reinhardt, "Americans have . . . decided to treat health care as essentially a private consumer good of which the poor might be guaranteed a basic package, but which is otherwise to be distributed more and more on the basis of ability to pay" (Reinhardt and Relman 1986, p. 23). While the Affordable Care Act is intended to make health care more broadly available to those without access to affordable health insurance, the hesitance of many states to expand Medicaid eligibility has meant that low-income and poor individuals still have had to go without access to affordable care. Because many racial/ethnic minority groups, especially blacks and Hispanics, have substantially lower SES on average than whites and Asians, we would expect those same groups to have less ability either to obtain health insurance or to pay for care directly. However, access to care is not only an issue of ability to pay.

Zuvekas and Taliaferro (2003) undertook a comprehensive review of various factors that affect access to medical care for different racial/ethnic groups. While the availability of health insurance was an important contributing factor, it alone did not fully explain observed differences. For both blacks and Hispanics, the authors were able to identify two other contributing factors:

1. characteristics of the individual that do not directly pertain to SES, including factors such as age, sex, family size, and employment
2. health care system capacity, which includes the number of available physicians and the characteristics of local hospitals, and the availability of other types of local health care facilities

The authors found that, even when they took into account these factors as well as access to health insurance, there remained substantial gaps in the rates at which different types of health care services are used by different racial/ethnic groups. The authors concluded that "much of existing disparities remains to be explained, presenting a challenge to policies to eliminate them" (p. 139). These conclusions were echoed by Kirby and colleagues (2006), who analyzed data gathered in 2000–01 by the federal government about access to health care. They summarized their findings in the following way: "Consistent with earlier studies, we find insurance status and socioeconomic differences explain a significant part of the disparities. Additionally, neighborhood racial and ethnic composition account for a large portion of disparities in access, and language differences help explain observed disparities in the use-based access measure. However, much of the differences between racial and ethnic groups remain unexplained" (p. I-64).

While much of the focus on disparities in access to care is on black/white differences, differences also exist for other racial/ethnic groups. Andrews and Elixhauser (2000) reviewed the barriers to access faced by Hispanics. Roubideaux and colleagues (2004) reviewed the obstacles faced by American Indians and Alaskan Natives. Both studies identified barriers similar to those identified by Zuvekas and Taliaferro. A comprehensive review by the Agency for Healthcare Research and Quality of the US Department of Health and Human Services (2003) and a report prepared jointly by Brown and colleagues of the UCLA Center for Health Policy Research and the Kaiser Family Foundation (2000) came to similar conclusions. For a variety of reasons, blacks, Hispanics, and American Indians have had less access to needed medical care than whites and Asians, and only a part of this difference can be explained by differences in SES.

Residential Segregation and Access to Medical Care

In Chapter 6 we discussed the ways racially based residential segregation is associated with worse health outcomes through increased stress and greater exposure to environmental toxins. Racially based segregation is also associated with lower access to medical care, and to lower quality of the care that is available. Gaskin and colleagues (2012) examined the association between residential segregation and access to primary care physicians in metropolitan areas. They found that African Americans and Hispanics were substantially more likely than whites or Asians to live in an area with a documented shortage of primary care physicians. For African Americans, as the level of segregation increased, the odds of being a primary care shortage area increased. Wong and colleagues (2017) studied access to care for men living in Philadelphia who had been diagnosed with localized prostate cancer, and confirmed that black patients experienced significantly longer travel times in order to see a physician for follow-up monitoring and care.

Even when primary care physicians were available to those living in highly segregated residential areas, those physicians had lower incomes and worked with constrained financial resources, with resultant decreases in the quality of the coordination of care, the ability to spend adequate time with patients, and the ability to obtain specialty care when needed (Reschovsky and O'Malley 2008). Among older patients covered by Medicare, when patients are able to see a physician, black patients are more likely to receive care identified as having low value in affecting outcomes (Schpero et al. 2017).

Beyond its impacts on access to primary care, residential segregation has also been shown to be associated with impaired access to high quality hospital care. Hasnain-Wynia and colleagues (2007) examined the records of 320,000 patients who received care from one of 123 different hospitals, assessing the quality of care received based on 13 established measures of clinical quality. They found that minority patients (defined as black, Hispanic, or Asian) experienced lower quality of care while in the hospital than nonminority patients, and that hospitals that served a larger proportion of minority patients tended to be lower quality than those seeing more nonminority patients.

Joynt and colleagues (2011) look at the quality of hospital care received by elderly black and white patients on Medicare who received treatment for one of three serious conditions: heart attack, congestive heart failure, or pneumonia. As their measure of quality they used the frequency with which patients needed to be readmitted within 30 days of discharge for treatment of the same problem. They found that black patients were more likely to be readmitted than white patients, and that being treated in a hospital serving mostly minority patients (rather than the patient's race) was the principal factor explaining the quality disparity.

Jha and colleagues (2011) reported a similar study, in which they ranked hospitals according to scales of clinical quality and cost. They "found that the 'worst' hospitals . . . care for double the proportion . . . of elderly black patients as the 'best' hospitals" (p. 1904). They also found that elderly Hispanic patients and patients on Medicaid were more likely to be found in the "worst" hospitals than in the "best."

The quality of surgery available at hospitals also varies by the racial and ethnic composition of the patients using the hospital. Dimick and colleagues (2013) found that black patients needing surgery were more likely than white patients to receive care at a low-quality hospital and that "Racial segregation was also a factor, with black patients in the most segregated areas 41–96 percent more likely than white patients to undergo surgery at low-quality hospitals" (p. 1046). Using the frequency with which a hospital performed a specific surgical procedure as a measure of quality, Liu and colleagues (2006) found that black and Hispanic patients were less likely than white patients to receive care at high-volume hospitals. Similarly, Lucas and colleagues (2006) studied surgical mortality rates among Medicare patients nationally, concluding that "Black patients have higher operative mortality risks across a wide range of surgical procedures, in large part because of higher mortality rates at the hospitals they attend" (p. 281).

In a study of hospital death rates among infants born at very low birth weight (VLBW) (that is, less than 1,500 g), Morales and colleagues (2005) found that the risk-adjusted chance of death for VLBW infants was higher in minority-serving hospitals. This association was the same whether the infant was white or black. Profit and colleagues (2017) came to similar conclusions in their study of more than 18,000 VLBW infants cared for in one of the 134 neonatal intensive care units (NICU) in California. They found that the quality of care for black and Hispanic infants as compared to white infants varied within NICUs, with even larger disparities found between NICUs.

Racial disparities in the quality of hospital care parallel the racial disparities that exist in the quality of nursing home care. In a national study of nursing homes certified by the federal government, Smith and colleagues (2007) identified the following associations:

- Black nursing home patients are concentrated in a relatively small number of nursing homes. Two-thirds of black residents are in just 10 percent of all homes.
- There is a strong inverse association between the percentage of black residents in a nursing home, and the quality of care in that home. The more racially segregated the patients in the home, the lower the quality of care provided in that home.
- There is a strong association between the level of racial segregation among patients in a nursing home and the level of racial segregation of the metropolitan area in which the home is located.

Other studies of the association between the level of segregation in a nursing home and the quality of care in the home have confirmed these findings, with the consequence that black nursing home residents are more likely to develop pressure ulcers (Li and colleagues 2011; Bergstrom and Horn 2011) and less likely to receive flu vaccine (Cai and colleagues 2011).

While there are consistent racial disparities in the quality of care received in nursing homes, there do not appear to be substantial racial disparities in the quality of end-of-life care. Sharma and colleagues (2017) gathered data collected between 2011 and 2015 as part of a large national study of aging. Based on interviews with family members or others who assisted patients who had died, most of the deaths occurred in the patient's home. While not all respondents were satisfied with the quality of the care provided during the patient's last month of life, there were no racial disparities in the overall quality of the care received. Kutney-Lee and colleagues (2017) reported the results of a survey of more than 50,000 family members of patients who had died in a Veterans Affairs hospital nationally. While the family of black veterans who had died were somewhat less likely than those of white veterans to report excellent overall care for their family member while in the hospital, there were no racial disparities in the receipt of palliative care or hospice care for their family member.

In summary, for black Americans, where a person lives seems to be associated with access to primary care, the quality of available hospital care, and the quality of available nursing home care.

Racial/Ethnic Disparities in the Treatment of Heart Disease

To understand other ways in which racial/ethnic differences in access to care come about, we need to look at data from a study by Gornick and colleagues (1996). While the study is from the 1990s, its conclusions are still instructive. The authors looked at detailed data collected by the federal government about annual rates of use in 1993 of a wide range of medical care services by those age 65 or older who were covered by Medicare. They were able to obtain data from more than 26 million subjects and were able to sort these subjects into approximate income quartiles. To do this, they used the median household income from the 1990 census for all households in the same zip code as the subject. Previous research has established that the median income of the zip code of residence is a good proxy for an individual's actual income. People by and large tend to live in neighborhoods in which the other residents have similar income levels.

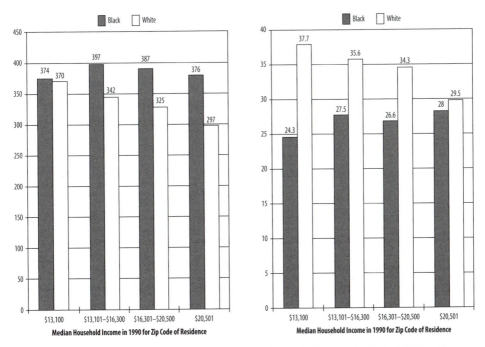

Figure 8.1. *Left*: Hospital discharges in 1993, by race and household income for 1990. *Right*: Hospital discharges in 1993 for treatment of ischemic heart disease, by race and household income for 1990. Rates for both figures are per 1,000 Medicare beneficiaries per year. *Source*: Based on Gornick et al. 1996.

Once they had the data broken down by income quartile, they then compared utilization rates between black and white subjects. Figure 8.1 displays graphically data on two different measures of health care utilization.

The graph on the left shows the rate at which blacks and whites were discharged from the hospital, not differentiating the problem for which the subjects were in the hospital. It can be seen that, in the lowest income quartile, whites and blacks were hospitalized at about the same rate. However, as income increases, the gap between the black rate and the white rate widens. The black rate stays approximately the same across income levels, while the white rate falls consistently. This finding—that at most income levels blacks tend to be sicker than whites—is consistent with my discussion in previous chapters.

The graph on the right side of the figure shows the rates at which subjects were discharged from the hospital after treatment for one specific disease: ischemic heart disease (IHD). IHD is due to clogging of the arteries that feed the heart, typically caused by chronically elevated cholesterol levels. The clogging of these vessels leads to an inadequate blood supply to the heart muscle, with inadequate delivery of oxygen to the heart tissue (ischemia). The blockage in the arteries can lead either to severe pains in the chest triggered when the heart is under an increased work load such as exercise (referred to as angina) or to permanent damage to the heart tissue from lack of oxygen (a heart attack).

IHD is a disease that affects whites more so than blacks, reflected by the black/white differences in discharge rates for the treatment of IHD, shown in the graph on the right of Figure 8.1. The widest gap is for the lowest income quartile, with the white rate more than 50 percent higher than the black rate. As incomes rise, we see different patterns for whites and blacks: as white incomes rise, the rate of IHD goes down; as black incomes rise, the rate of IHD goes up. Within the top income quartiles, the rate of treatment for IHD is about the same for the two groups.

These data simply state the rate at which blacks and whites were hospitalized for the treatment of IHD. They do not say anything about what went on in the hospital. After undergoing cardiac catheterization to identify where and how severe the blockage of the arteries to the heart is, there are two principal treatments for patients with IHD to unclog the clogged arteries:

1. Angioplasty, a procedure by which a thin balloon attached to a wire is threaded through the aorta and into the clogged artery. When the balloon is inflated, it compresses the material clogging the artery, thus opening the artery back up to blood flow.
2. Coronary artery bypass graft (referred to by its acronym, CABG, pronounced just like the leafy vegetable), by which a surgeon cuts out a small piece of a vein from the patient's lower leg and grafts it into the clogged artery in such a way that it bypasses the clog.

Once a Medicare beneficiary is admitted to the hospital, they face only a single charge that covers all the care necessary to treat their illness. The entire remainder of the bill, often amounting to tens of thousands of dollars, is paid by Medicare. Thus, for Medicare beneficiaries admitted to the hospital, income and ability to pay should not affect the treatment given in the hospital. However, despite the leveling of the SES field by the Medicare system, the patterns of care received by blacks and whites with IHD were strikingly different (Figure 8.2).

The graph on the left side of Figure 8.2 compares the rate at which blacks and whites with IHD were treated with angioplasty; the graph on the right compares the rate at which the two groups were treated with CABG. The mean rate of angioplasty across income groups for whites was more than twice the mean rate for blacks. The mean rate of CABG across income groups for whites was 2.5 times the mean rate for blacks. In addition, the income gradient we saw for the rate of

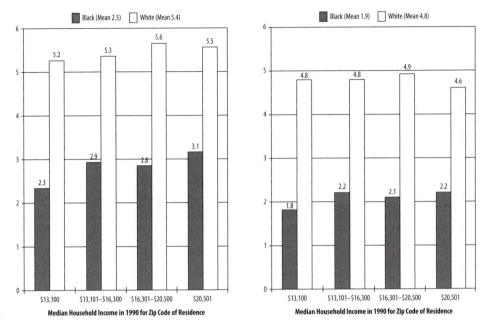

Figure 8.2. *Left*: Angioplasty procedures 1993 for treatment of ischemic heart disease, by race and household income for 1990. *Right*: Coronary artery bypass graft procedures 1993 for treatment of ischemic heart disease, by race and household income for 1990. Rates for both figures are per 1,000 Medicare beneficiaries per year. *Source*: Based on Gornick et al. 1996.

hospitalization for IHD is no longer there for either procedure. At all levels of income, the gap between the rate at which the procedure was used in white and black patients is approximately the same. For some reason, blacks hospitalized for the same disease and covered by the same insurance received substantially lower rates of these potentially lifesaving procedures.

In a society that has prohibited racial discrimination both by law and by the dictates of our Constitution, we would like to be able to presume that all individuals, regardless of their race/ethnicity, will receive the same treatment if they:

- have the same disease
- have the same type of health insurance
- are treated by the same doctors in the same hospitals

The study by Gornick and colleagues (1996) looked at patients with the same disease and the same insurance (Medicare). However, it was unable to determine the extent to which blacks and whites were treated by the same doctors or in the same hospitals. As described above, there are often systematic differences between black and white patients in the doctors and hospitals from which they receive treatment. Many of the hospitals used more often by blacks had less advanced technology available for care (Groeneveld et al. 2005). Bach and colleagues (2004) identified clear patterns of difference in the training and location of the physicians treating black and white Medicare patients. Those physicians who treated a disproportionate share of blacks often had less training and less access to important clinical resources.

What, though, if we are able to equalize all three aspects of care: nature of the disease, type of insurance, and source of treatment? Will racial disparities persist in the type of care received? A seminal study by Peterson and colleagues (1994) conducted in the system of hospitals operated by the US Department of Veterans Affairs (VA) was able to address this issue specifically. The VA operates a series of hospitals and clinics throughout the country, many affiliated with academic medical centers. Veterans discharged from military service under honorable circumstances are eligible for care in the VA system. For those veterans whose income falls below certain levels, that care is free. Once a veteran has established eligibility, they can go to any VA facility for care.

Peterson and colleagues were able to obtain data on more than 33,000 veterans who were discharged from one of the 158 hospitals operated by the VA after treatment for a heart attack. The authors asked two questions:

1. Did black and white veterans with a heart attack (caused by a blocked artery to the heart) get cardiac catheterization at the same rate?
2. Once diagnosed with cardiac catheterization, did black and white veterans receive treatment to unblock the artery at the same rate?

For both analyses, the authors took into account a number of factors other than the veteran's race that might affect the answers to these questions, such as age and co-existing medical conditions, as well as the type of treatment facilities available in the hospital to which the veteran came for care. In order to avoid differences based on sex, they looked only at the care provided to male veterans. Their results are shown in Table 8.1.

Before adjusting for individual patient characteristics and the characteristics of the hospital, we can see that blacks received a different level of care than whites. Blacks were significantly less likely than whites to have undergone cardiac catheterization, a necessary diagnostic step before either angioplasty or CABG can be performed. Among those patients who had undergone cardiac catheterization, blacks were significantly less likely to have received either angioplasty or CABG within 90 days of their discharge from the hospital. When the authors used statistical techniques to control for patient and hospital characteristics, these differences persisted,

Table 8.1. Treatment of Patients with an Acute Heart Attack at a Veterans Affairs Hospital, by Race of the Patient

	Black	White
Number of patients	4,522	29,119
Received cardiac catheterization	33.7%	36.9%*
Received CABG surgery	5.1%	9.6%*
Received angioplasty	4.2%	6.2%*
Received either CABG surgery or angioplasty	9.0%	15.3%*

Source: Peterson et al. 1994.
*$p < 0.0001$

Table 8.2. Survival of Patients with an Acute Heart Attack Treated at a Veterans Affairs Hospital, by Race of the Patient

	Proportion Still Alive	
Time after Heart Attack	Black	White
30 days	85.2%	82.7%*
One year	71.4%	69.2%**
Two years	64.2%	63.0%

Source: Peterson et al. 1994.
*$p < 0.0001$ **$p < 0.002$

albeit at a somewhat reduced level. Despite having the same disease, the same method of paying for care, and being treated in the same hospitals by the same doctors, black veterans with a heart attack were less likely than white veterans to receive the most advanced care available at that time for the treatment of heart attacks.

Peterson and colleagues followed this analysis with a second one, addressing the question of whether the increased rate at which white veterans received these procedures was associated with an increased rate of survival after the heart attack. They followed the veterans in the study for two years, measuring how many were still alive at 90 days, one year, and two years. As shown in Table 8.2, the results were striking. Despite their increased treatment with these advanced procedures, white veterans were no more likely to survive two years after their heart attack. In fact, at 90 days and at one year after the heart attack, the survival rate among black veterans was actually higher than that for white veterans.

One important aspect of the study of the VA system by Peterson and colleagues limited the extent to which the results could be generalized to our health care system more broadly: the VA system may have patterns of care that differ systematically in some way from the care more generally available. To address this issue, Peterson undertook a similar study in a very different setting (Peterson et al. 1997).

They went to the Duke University Medical Center—one of the leading academic medical centers in the country—and obtained the records of 11,127 whites and 1,275 blacks treated at that facility for IHD. All the patients had narrowing of the coronary arteries (the arteries to the heart muscle) documented on cardiac catheterization; all were covered by health insurance. The authors addressed the following question: "whether racial differences in the use of coronary angioplasty and bypass surgery were evident among patients with documented coronary disease" (p. 480).

The authors did not find a significant difference in the percentage of blacks and whites receiving angioplasty within 60 days of their cardiac catheterization (29 percent compared to 30 percent). They did find a significant difference in the rate of CABG surgery, with 26 percent of blacks and 37 percent of whites receiving this treatment.

The authors then addressed a second question: "whether differences in clinical history, severity of disease, anginal symptoms, coexisting illness, or access to care in cardiac subspecialties accounted for the difference in treatment" (p. 480). To address this question, they stratified the subjects according to the following measures of the severity of their disease: number of coronary arteries affected by a blockage (there are three principal coronary arteries), the severity of the anginal chest pain the patient was experiencing (mild versus severe), and the extent to which one of the interventions was expected to prolong the patient's life (< 2 months, 2 months to 1 year, >1 year). In each case they found that the more severe the disease, the wider the gap between whites and blacks in their access to treatment.

In the five years following their diagnosis of IHD, 27 percent of the blacks died and 20 percent of the whites died. About half of the blacks' excess risk of death was because they had on average more severe disease than white patients. When the authors used statistical adjustment to compare blacks and whites with the same severity of disease who had received the same treatment, they found no significant black/white difference in the likelihood of death. If blacks had received the same levels of treatment as whites, they would still have had a higher likelihood of dying within five years, due to the greater severity of their cardiac disease on average. If blacks had received the same levels of treatment as whites with the same level of disease, there would have been no racial difference in their chance of death. The racial difference in five-year mortality that remained after adjusting for disease severity was apparently due to under-treatment of black patients.

Subsequent research has shown that the findings of the two studies of Peterson and colleagues are more widespread than the specific systems of care they studied. Among the studies looking at racial differences in care for IHD was one by Canto and colleagues (2000), which looked at the records of 26,575 Medicare beneficiaries found to be appropriate for revascularization under nationally recognized standards. These authors found that "blacks, regardless of sex, are significantly less likely than whites to receive this potentially lifesaving therapy" (p. 1094).

From these studies, it seems clear that there was a consistent disparity in access to revascularization treatments for blacks with IHD, and that these differences could not be explained by the availability of health insurance or other factors related to SES. While documenting this disparity, these studies did not identify the reason for the disparity. When a black person with the same severity of heart disease and the same type of insurance as a white person does not receive revascularization therapy, while the white person does receive it, there are two possible explanations:

1. A physician recommended the treatment to both patients, and the black patient declined the recommended treatment.
2. A physician recommended the treatment to the white patient but did not recommend it to the black patient.

To understand the cause of the documented disparity in access to revascularization therapy, it was crucial to differentiate between these two explanations. If the first were the principal source, efforts to reduce the disparity should focus on educating blacks to be sure they understand the therapeutic benefits of the therapy. If the second explanation were accurate, efforts should focus instead on making physicians aware of the discriminatory outcomes of their care.

Hannan and colleagues (1999) undertook a study to differentiate between these two alternative causes. They were able to review the records of 1,261 patients in New York State who had recently undergone cardiac catheterization. The patients included in the study were 42 percent female and 58 percent male; they were 54 percent white, 25 percent black, and 21 percent Hispanic. Based on an independent review of the results of the catheterization, each patient had been identified as "appropriate" for CABG surgery according to criteria previously developed by the RAND corporation. Among those who were deemed appropriate for surgery, the researchers also identified a subgroup for whom CABG surgery was considered "appropriate and necessary" according to the RAND guidelines.

The patients were followed for three months to determine whether they actually underwent CABG surgery. The researchers found blacks and Hispanics were significantly less likely than whites to undergo the procedure. These results are shown in Table 8.3. These differences remained statistically significant after adjusting for individual characteristics such as age, gender, type of insurance, and extent of the disease.

The researchers were then able to contact the physician who had treated 241 of the patients in the study. All of them had been deemed appropriate for CABG by

Table 8.3. Percentage of Subjects for Whom CABG Surgery Was "Appropriate" or "Appropriate and Necessary" Who Underwent CABG Surgery within Three Months of Angiography

	Percentage of Those Appropriate for CABG Who Received CABG	Percentage of Those Necessary for CABG Who Received CABG
White	57	63
Black	45	49
Hispanic	46	57

Source: Hannan et al. 1999.
Note: Differences statistically significant, $p < 0.001$

Table 8.4. Percentage of Physicians Who Reported That They Did Not Recommend CABG Surgery, by Patient's Sex and Race/Ethnicity

	Percentage of Physicians Who Reported That They Did Not Recommend CABG Surgery	Sample Size
Male patients		
White	85	53
Black	95	41
Hispanic	87	45
Female patients		
White	92	38
Black	88	32
Hispanic	97	32
Total	90	241

Source: Hannan et al. 1999.
Note: All subjects were deemed "appropriate" for CABG surgery by study reviewers. Differences not statistically significant: chi square $= 4.32$, $p = 0.504$.

the study reviewers, but none had received it. They specifically asked these physicians (92 percent of whom were cardiologists) if they had recommended CABG surgery to the patient, breaking down the physicians' responses by the race/ethnicity and sex of the patient. These results are shown in Table 8.4.

For the 241 patients who did not receive CABG within three months of their diagnosis, all of whom were found to be appropriate for the procedure by independent reviewers using a nationally recognized scale of appropriateness, 9 out of 10 did not have the procedure because their physician did not recommend it to them. While the percentages differ somewhat by the race/ethnicity and sex of the patient (these differences were not found to be statistically significant), it seems clear that in the vast majority of patients, regardless of race/ethnicity, if they did not receive a revascularization procedure it was because their physician did not recommend it to them. In only a small group of patients—about 1 in 10—the physician recommended the procedure but the patient did not follow the physician's recommendation.

The findings of Hannan and colleagues were supported by a study of patients at a large VA hospital (Gordon et al. 2004). These researchers reviewed the records of 113 patients whose physician had recommended that they undergo angioplasty based on the results of cardiac catheterization, and 45 patients whose physician had recommended that they undergo CABG surgery. None of the 113 patients declined angioplasty; 2 of the 45 recommended for CABG declined treatment, leading the authors to conclude that "patient decisions to decline recommended invasive cardiac procedures were infrequent and may explain only a small fraction of racial disparities in the use of invasive cardiac procedures" (p. 962).

If we extrapolate these findings to the two studies by Peterson and colleagues, it seems clear that the principal contributor to different rates of revascularization procedures in patients with similar types of disease and similar insurance was physician reluctance to recommend the procedure to some who might otherwise be appropriate for the procedure. The racial/ethnic group that was principally affected by this pattern of reluctance was blacks with heart disease. Physician reluctance appears to be an important factor in perpetuating racial disparities in access to advanced care for heart disease.

These and other studies had such profound implications for the care of cardiac disease that the American College of Cardiology and the Association of Black Cardiologists, in collaboration with the Kaiser Family Foundation, undertook a comprehensive review of the available literature addressing the issue of racial/ethnic disparities in cardiac care, issuing their report in 2002 (Lillie-Blanton et al. 2002). The reviewers were able to identify 81 different studies that had been published between 1991 and 2001. From their analysis of these studies, the reviewers reported (p. 1) that the majority of the peer-reviewed studies investigating racial/ethnic differences in cardiac care

- are methodologically rigorous
- compare African Americans to whites
- find a racial/ethnic minority group less likely than whites to receive the procedure or treatment under study

The reviewers then assessed the methodological strength of the studies, conducting a separate, more in-depth analysis of the 44 studies (54 percent) found to be methodologically strong. From these studies the reviewers concluded (p. 1) that

- there is credible evidence that African Americans are less likely than whites to receive diagnostic procedures, revascularization procedures, and thrombolytic therapy
- racial/ethnic differences in care remain after adjustment for clinical and socioeconomic factors

It seems that the racial/ethnic disparity in cardiac care identified by Peterson and colleagues is widespread, and its presence is well supported by extensive scientific literature. The best evidence to date suggests that the root of the disparities lies in physician behavior, and not in patient refusal of recommended procedures. The implications of this finding are discussed in more depth in the following chapter.

Vaccarino and colleagues (2005) looked at data on the treatment of nearly 600,000 individuals who had sustained a heart attack between 1994 and 2002 to see if they could identify evidence that the extensive research and discussion of racial/ethnic disparities in cardiac care that occurred during that time had resulted in any decrease in that disparity. They concluded that, despite more than a decade of research, "rates of reperfusion therapy, coronary angiography, and in-hospital death after myocardial infarction . . . vary according to race and sex, with no evidence that the differences have narrowed in recent years" (p. 671).

Race/Ethnicity and the Treatment of Cancer

Lung cancer continues to be a major cause of death in the United States, especially for those in lower SES groups for which the rate of smoking remains high. In 2015 the age-adjusted death rate from lung cancer per 100,000 population was 49.9 for white men and 59.1 for black men. For white women it was 34.9; for black women it was 30.8 (CDC 2018).

Part of the reason that black men continue to die from lung cancer disproportionately is poor access to medical care, with the result that the cancer is often diagnosed when it is at a later stage of development. Late-stage lung cancer carries with it an extremely poor prognosis. However, Blackstock and colleagues (2006), in a review of the records of 995 patients with a particularly invasive form of lung cancer that had already spread, found that so long as they received equivalent therapy for their disease, "the outcome for African American patients was the same as that observed for non–African American patients" (p. 407).

If lung cancer is identified when it is still in an early stage, having not yet spread to the lymph tissue or other organs in the body, the prognosis can be improved dramatically with aggressive care, usually involving the surgical excision of the tumor. Bach and colleagues (1999) looked specifically at the treatment and survival of nearly 11,000 patients treated between 1985 and 1993, all of whom were on Medicare and all with this early form of lung cancer. They found that five years after their diagnosis, 34 percent of the whites were still alive while only 26 percent of the blacks were alive.

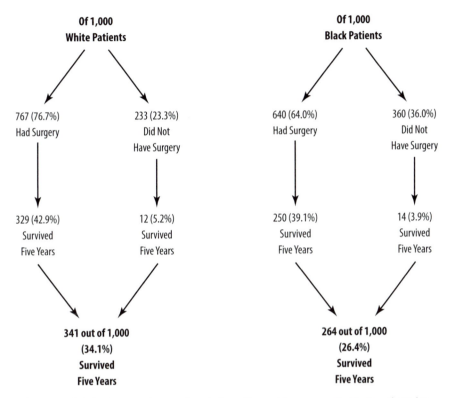

Figure 8.3. Relation between the rate of surgical resection and five-year survival for hypothetical cohorts of a thousand black and a thousand white Medicare beneficiaries age 65 or older with early-stage lung cancer. *Source*: Based on Bach et al. 1999.

Previous data had shown that patients with this form of cancer who receive surgery to resect their tumor have a 40 percent chance of surviving for five years after their diagnosis. Those who do not have surgery have less than a 5 percent chance of surviving five years. The researchers looked further at the data to see which patients had received surgery for their disease and which patients had been treated without surgery. They found clear differences in the pattern of treatment for blacks and whites (Figure 8.3).

Of the whites in the study, 76.7 percent had surgery for their disease. Of the blacks, 64 percent had surgery. Based on the marked differences in five-year survival—41.2 percent for those with surgery and 4.4 percent for those with no surgery—it was the lower rate of surgery among black lung cancer patients that was principally responsible for the black/white difference in survival. If the same percentage of blacks had undergone surgery as whites, their estimated survival rate would have been 30.8 percent.

Lathan and colleagues (2006) undertook a study similar to that of Bach. They were able to obtain data from a tumor registry of 21,219 patients who had been diagnosed with early-stage lung cancer. The authors asked two questions:

1. Which of these patients underwent further invasive testing (often involving procedures with some danger) to get confirmation that the tumor had not spread?
2. Of those who had undergone the procedure to confirm that the tumor was still localized, how many had surgery to remove the tumor?

As with the Bach study, these authors found that the overall survival of blacks was less than that of whites, and that the rates of both invasive testing and surgery were lower in blacks than in whites. For those who had surgery, there was no black/white difference in survival. These authors did explore the reasons for the lower rate of surgery among blacks, and found two explanations:

1. The doctors were less likely to recommend surgery in black patients (67.0 percent) than in comparable white patients (71.4 percent).
2. Once surgery was recommended, slightly more black patients (3.4 percent) refused surgery than white patients (2.0 percent).

Looking at factors that influence patients' decisions regarding surgical treatment of lung cancer, Margolis and colleagues (2003) had become aware that patients at a VA hospital at which the authors work frequently expressed a belief (not supported by scientific evidence) that exposing a cancerous tumor to air during surgery would increase the chances that the tumor would spread to other parts of the body. Concerned that such an inaccurate belief may prevent patients from agreeing to lung cancer surgery with a proven potential benefit, the authors administered a survey questionnaire to 626 patients coming to the clinic for treatment of lung cancer or other lung ailments. Thirty-eight percent indicated that they believed exposing a lung tumor to air during surgery would increase the chances that it would spread. Ten percent indicated that this belief would be a reason to oppose surgery if their doctor recommended it to them. Black subjects were significantly more likely than white subjects to believe the risk of spread due to air exposure (61 percent versus 29 percent), and were more likely to indicate that they would oppose surgery based on this belief (19 percent versus 5 percent). The authors cautioned that they were measuring attitudes and not actual decisions in the face of a diagnosis of lung cancer. Nevertheless, they indicated that an irrational fear of tumor spread caused by surgery, coupled with a lower level of trust in the medical care system, may be an important factor explaining at least part of the reduced rate of surgery among blacks with early-stage lung cancer.

Following up on the issues raised by Margolis, James and colleagues (2011) explored further the issue of patient perceptions of the risk of causing spread of a cancerous tumor by exposing it to air during surgery. They conducted focus group discussions and interviews with 42 mostly black patients recruited from a primary care clinic in the Midwest that served mostly low-income patients. Subjects were age 45 or older and did not have cancer at the time of the interview. Many of the study subjects agreed with the concept that exposing a tumor to air could cause it to spread and as a consequence worsen the outcomes of treatment.

Cykert and Phifer (2003) used decision theoretic modeling to address the issue of who refuses recommended surgery for lung cancer, and why. Under this type of modeling subjects (not actual patients, but rather subjects who are asked to imagine that they had lung cancer) are asked a series of questions about which of two alternative states they would prefer. An example might be, "Would you rather have surgery for lung cancer with an x percent chance of living five years or treat the lung cancer without surgery with a y percent chance of living two years?" The terms x and y are quoted as actual percentages. For subsequent questions, these percentages are altered to determine if the subject will change their answer in response. From this type of research, it was possible to estimate how often subjects would refuse surgery, and how different people weigh the dangers of surgery with the risk of living with lung cancer without surgery. They found that black subjects had a somewhat more positive view of living with lung cancer without surgery, but that this difference in views did not seem to have a substantial impact on the likelihood that subjects would actually refuse surgery if offered. These researchers also identified an association between trust in the medical care system and an expressed willingness to undergo surgery.

Cykert and colleagues (2010) followed up on these issues by surveying 386 patients who had been recently diagnosed with early-stage lung cancer. Before a treatment plan had been determined, the researchers asked the patients about their attitudes toward cancer, their trust in the medical care system, their level of communication with their provider, and their coexisting medical conditions. They found that 66 percent of white patients and 55 percent of black patients had undergone surgery within four months of their initial diagnosis. Consistent with the data cited above, patients who believed that exposure to air during surgery could cause the tumor to spread were less likely to undergo surgery, and black patients were more likely to hold this view. Other factors were also associated with lower rates of surgery. These included reporting worse patient-provider communication, lacking a regular source of care, age, and coexisting medical conditions. When all these factors were included in the analysis, the authors reported that they did not find a higher rate of surgical refusal by race. "Paradoxically, we found that black patients with higher trust scores received cancer surgery less often, suggesting that physicians' surgical recommendations may have been framed in less favorable terms. . . . Implicit bias, negative perceptions of communication, and lack of a primary care physician likely create obstacles to health equity that are too difficult to overcome without systematic solutions" (p. 2374).

In 2006 the *Journal of Clinical Oncology* published a special issue that focused on racial disparities in the treatment of lung cancer. In it Dr. Otis Brawley, of the Winship Cancer Institute at Emory University, was asked to submit an editorial. Summarizing the findings of the research in that issue and previous research, he stated that the scientific data "demonstrate that there are significant differences in treatments offered to patients with early stage . . . lung cancer" (p. 332). He went on to broaden his discussion of racial disparities in care, acknowledging that "blacks are at a greater risk to receive less than optimal treatment for a number of cancers" (p. 333).

As in the early studies of cardiac revascularization, it has been difficult to determine how much of the black/white difference in the rate of surgery for lung cancer was because blacks refused recommended treatment at a higher rate, or because the doctors recommended surgery less often to blacks than to whites. However, differing levels of trust in the medical care system and in the recommendations of physicians seem to play an important role.

While lung cancer is the leading cause of death due to cancer in the United States for both men and women, breast cancer is the second leading cause of cancer death for women. While death rates from breast cancer declined substantially in the 1990s with the widespread use of mammography screening, black/white racial disparities have persisted. While black women and white women in the United States are equally likely to develop breast cancer, black women are more likely to die from breast cancer. In 2015 the death rate from breast cancer per 100,000 white women was 19.8, while the death rate per 100,000 black women was 27.6 (US Department of Health and Human Services 2018 [see Ref. 6]).

For much of the 1990s, black women had lower rates of mammography, with higher rates of having late-stage cancer at the time of diagnosis. The survival rate of late-stage breast cancer, in which the tumor has spread beyond the breast, is substantially lower than early-stage cancer, with the tumor confined to the breast. By the late 1990s, however, mammography rates among black and white women had largely equalized. Despite comparable rates of mammography, black women continue to be more likely to have their cancer diagnosed at a later stage, with consequent higher death rates (Chatterjee et al. 2013). While tumor biology may play a role, delays in treatment and lower quality of the treatment available to black women contribute to the continuing disparity in death rates (Fedewa et al. 2011). Part of the disparity in treatment quality is due to the hospital in which a woman receives treatment, with black women more likely to receive treatment in lower-quality hospitals (Freedman et al. 2013). Molina and colleagues (2015) were also able to determine that women screened for breast cancer at lower-quality hospitals experienced delay in diagnosis, which may place them at increased risk of the cancer having spread.

Race/Ethnicity and the Treatment of Pain

There is a medical condition in which it seems counterintuitive to believe that individuals would refuse treatment when offered: the treatment of pain that results from a serious injury. Dr. Knox Todd was an emergency physician on the medical staff of the UCLA Emergency Center. In this capacity he often treated injuries that were very painful. One of the most consistently painful of these injuries is a fracture of a long bone in either the arm or the leg. Todd and colleagues (1993) reported their study of the ways in which a person's ethnicity was associated with the treatment they received for the pain of an isolated long-bone fracture. By studying long-bone fractures in patients without other serious injuries, they were able to evaluate the way emergency physicians treated what was essentially a constant level of pain across patients.

They looked at the treatment given to all patients between the ages of 15 and 55 coming to their emergency room over a two-year period for the treatment of an isolated long-bone fracture. Given the community served by their emergency room, these individuals were either Hispanic (31 patients) or white (108 patients). Fifty-six different physicians were involved in the care of these patients. They found that, in the face of this very painful injury

- 17 of the 31 Hispanics (55 percent) received no medication for pain during their treatment
- 28 of the 108 whites (26 percent) received no medication for pain during their treatment

Despite having a serious injury that by its very nature is associated with high levels of pain, the Hispanics were twice as likely as the whites to receive no pain medication while in the emergency room.

Critics of this study suggested that different ethnic groups may respond to and express pain differently. If Hispanics were more stoic in the face of their injury, expressing fewer symptoms of pain to their physician, this might explain why the doctors administered less pain medication. The authors of the study acknowledged that "it is certainly true that not all patients with similar injuries experience (or express) the same degree of pain." However, they expressed their opinion that "we do not believe it likely that the degree of pain evoked by the separate injuries [of the two ethnic groups] is likely to explain the difference in analgesic use" (p. 1538).

Based to a certain extent on the attention given to his earlier publication, Todd moved to a faculty position with the Emory University School of Medicine, in Atlanta, Georgia. There he was able essentially to repeat his earlier study, this time examining persons coming to the emergency room of a large, inner-city community hospital in Atlanta that was affiliated with Emory (Todd et al. 2000). He evaluated the medical records of 217 individuals coming to the emergency room over a 40-month period for treatment of an isolated long-bone fracture. Given the racial makeup of Atlanta, these included 127 blacks and 90 whites. They found that

- 54 of the 127 blacks (43 percent) received no medication for pain during their treatment
- 23 of the 90 whites (26 percent) received no medication for pain during their treatment

As with the earlier study in Los Angeles involving whites and Hispanics, in this study the blacks were nearly twice as likely to receive no pain medication while in the emergency room. With this study, the authors were keenly aware of the importance of documenting the extent to which the patients expressed painful symptoms. By thoroughly reviewing the medical records of these patients, they found that 54 percent of the blacks and 59 percent of the whites had a notation in their medical record that they had expressed painful symptoms. The nearly twofold difference in withholding pain medication in blacks and whites was because the doctor did not order the medication, not because the patient did not want the medication.

Building on the work of Todd and his colleagues in Los Angeles and Atlanta, Tamayo-Sarver and colleagues (2003) reported their study of a nationally representative sample of individuals discharged from an emergency room for treatment of one of the following conditions:

- an isolated fracture of a long bone (753)
- a back injury (1,311)
- a migraine headache (606)

They limited their study to patients who were either white, black, or Hispanic.

While the pain associated with a fracture of a long bone is more consistent across patients, the pain associated with a back injury or a migraine headache is more subjective, depending on the nature of the patient and the severity of the problem. Back injuries can range from a relatively minor muscle sprain to the more severe pain associated with ruptured disc and pinched nerve. To a large extent, it is up to the physician to assess how severe the pain from these two conditions is, based on a combination of the doctor's exam and their interpretation of the patient's expression of symptoms.

In treating these types of symptoms, the physician will have two choices: first, whether to treat the patient with pain medication, and second, whether to use an opioid or nonopioid medication. Nonopioids include medications such as ibuprofen or Tylenol. Opioids include medications such as codeine or hydrocodone. As a rule, opioids provide significantly more pain relief than nonopioids, but carry a higher potential for abuse.

The researchers first looked to see if any pain medication was given to the individuals in their study with these conditions. There was no significant racial/ethnic difference in the rate at which patients with a long-bone fracture received at least some pain medication. For back pain and migraine headache, whites were the most likely to receive a medication for pain, and blacks were the least likely to receive such a medication. The authors then looked at only those patients who received the more effective opioid type of medication. They evaluated the likelihood a black or Hispanic would receive an opioid medication, using as a baseline comparison the rate at which whites received an opioid. These results are shown in Figure 8.4.

There is a clear pattern of blacks receiving an opioid medication less often than whites. These differences were statistically significant for the treatment of back pain and migraine headache, but did not reach statistical significance for the treatment of a long-bone fracture. Largely due to sample size, the Hispanic rate of opioid treatment did not reach statistical significance for any of the three specific conditions. When the authors looked at all Hispanics as compared to all whites, the Hispanics were significantly less likely to receive an opioid medication.

The authors of the study speculated why emergency room doctors were less likely to use the more effective opioid medication in blacks and Hispanics, particularly in those conditions for which the physician's assessment of the level of pain experienced by the patient is more subjective. They suggested that differences in patient assertiveness, impaired communication between physician and patient, perceptions of social distance between physician and patient, and differences in the physician's perception of the patient all may have contributed to the observed differences.

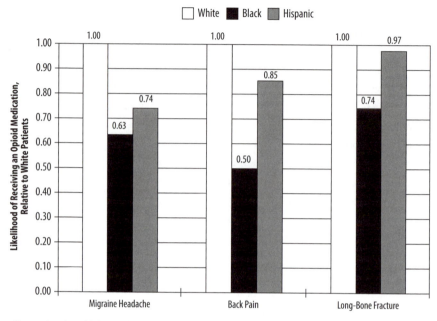

Figure 8.4. Racial/ethnic differences in the likelihood of receiving an opioid pain medication as part of treatment in an emergency room. White is the reference group. *Source*: Based on Tamayo-Sarver et al. 2003.

Singhal and colleagues (2016) report that "emergency physicians might rely on subjective cues such as race-ethnicity, often unknowingly, when prescribing opioids for pain-related complaints, especially for conditions that are often associated with drug-seeking behavior" (p. 1). They examined a large database of emergency department visits, selecting patients treated for one of five specific conditions that often involve pain medication: toothache, back pain, abdominal pain, long-bone fracture, or kidney stones. The authors suggest that, in the experience of emergency physicians, the first three conditions are often associated with drug-seeking behavior, while the latter two are not. They found that black patients were less likely than white patients to receive treatment with an opioid medication for back pain or abdominal pain, with no racial difference for the other causes. The authors suggest that "These disparities may reflect inherent biases that health care providers hold unknowingly, leading to differential treatment of patients based on their race" (p. 11).

Shah and colleagues (2015) looked specifically at the treatment of more than 67,000 patients nationally who received emergency department treatment for acute abdominal pain during the period 2006–10. While patients who complained of mild abdominal pain experienced no racial disparity in receiving pain medication, among those with either moderate or severe pain, blacks and Hispanics were significantly less likely to receive a narcotic medication while in the emergency room. They also found these disparities to be greatest in those hospitals that treat the largest numbers of minority patients.

In an editorial accompanying the second study by Todd and colleagues, Marcus Martin, an emergency physician at the University of Virginia, discussed his years of experience in emergency rooms in a variety of settings: "I have witnessed the tendency, particularly among trainees, to withhold pain medication from those who visit the emergency department frequently because of fears of substance abuse. I have also witnessed the influence of the nursing staff on trainees regarding the withholding of pain medication" (2000, p. 78). Taylor and colleagues (2008) published a commentary on the issue of effective pain treatment, confirming that "many patients and physicians hold unsubstantiated fears that addiction will result from opioid use during appropriate pain management" (p. 89), but emphasizing that data show that this belief is greatly exaggerated, especially in the case of severe pain.

Goldfrank and Knopp also responded editorially to the second Todd study: "We believe that Todd et al. have identified a crucial problem not only for emergency medicine but also for the house of medicine. There is a growing body of evidence that minority patients are not receiving timely and appropriate medical care when compared with non-minority groups. . . . If we cannot assure each and every patient that he or she will receive comparable high-quality care, we have abdicated our moral authority" (2000, p. 79).

Concern that patients coming to the emergency room with subjective complaints of pain may be drug abusers seeking a prescription for an opioid may have increased in light of the growing national opioid epidemic. By the end of 2017 nearly 15,000 people died from overdoses of prescription medications containing opioids such as codeine, hydrocodone, or oxycodone. Nearly 30,000 people died from injecting synthetic opioids such as fentanyl (CDC 2018). Recalling from our discussion in Chapter 4 regarding "deaths of despair," the recent increase in deaths due to the overdose of prescription opioids occurred largely among middle-aged whites with low levels of education, many living in rural areas, while deaths due to fentanyl overdose have had the greatest impact on low-income, urban communities of color. It seems apparent that blacks and Hispanics who come to the emergency room have been at risk for being treated based on their race or ethnicity in addition to the nature of their illness or injury. This risk may have increased in the context of the opioid epidemic. It has become most important for physicians and other providers of emergency room care to be aware of and to learn to avoid the types of biased treatment of pain documented in earlier research. I reexamine this issue in the following chapter when I address ways in which racial/ethnic stereotypes can be invoked by physicians, often inappropriately and unknowingly, in making clinical decisions.

Race/Ethnicity and the Treatment of Kidney Failure

In chronic medical conditions such as hypertension and diabetes, the kidneys can sustain permanent damage over a period of years. In other conditions, the kidneys can be damaged more acutely. When the kidneys stop working properly, the only ways to keep a person alive are either to administer kidney dialysis or to transplant a kidney from another person into the person whose kidneys have failed. Whatever the cause, these conditions are referred to collectively as end-stage renal disease (ESRD).

In 2015 more than 700,000 people in the US suffered from ESRD (CDC 2018). Due largely to disproportionate rates of diabetes and high blood pressure, in 2015 African Americans were nearly four times more likely to develop ESRD than whites. Fortunately, Congress adopted a policy several decades ago making any patient with ESRD automatically eligible for Medicare, thus removing most financial barriers to receiving adequate treatment for ESRD.

Most people who develop ESRD will be treated with kidney dialysis, typically performed several times a week at a dialysis center. Those undergoing dialysis are able to lead relatively normal lives, although they must make room in their schedule for dialysis visits. Receiving a surgically transplanted kidney frees the person from the limits of dialysis, often leading to a substantially higher quality of life. People with transplanted kidneys can travel freely, play many sports, and enjoy essentially normal personal and professional lives.

As early as 1991, a comprehensive review of the literature on the treatment of ESRD came to three conclusions: "First, in the United States end-stage renal disease is more common in racial minorities than in whites. Second, fewer blacks than whites undergo kidney transplantation. Third, the rate of survival of renal allografts is lower among blacks than whites" (Kasiske et al. 1991, p. 306). They were not able to identify the source of this lower rate of graft survival in blacks, but speculated that it may be a combination of biologic and SES-related factors.

Recognizing this disparity in access to kidney transplantation for blacks, Alexander and Sehgal (1998) undertook a prospective study of 7,125 patients who developed kidney failure requiring the initiation of kidney dialysis. They identified four steps that all patients go through in the process of moving from kidney dialysis to kidney transplantation.

Step 1: Medical evaluation to determine if the patient is both medically suitable for and possibly interested in receiving a kidney transplant.

Step 2: Once a patient has been found to be medically suitable for a transplant, determine if the patient is definitely interested in obtaining a transplant.

Step 3: For those patients found to be medically suitable and definitely interested, a thorough workup, involving a series of tests and evaluations, must be completed before the patient is eligible to receive a transplant.

Step 4: Once the patient has completed the required workup, the patient's name is then placed on a regional list of patients awaiting transplant. Patients to undergo a transplant are subsequently selected from this list based on established criteria that are largely independent of the patient's race/ethnicity.

Using multivariate statistical analysis to take into account such factors as age, gender, income, underlying medical condition, and years of dialysis treatment, the authors found that:

Step 1: Blacks and whites were equally likely to be medically suitable and possibly interested.

Step 2: Blacks were less likely than whites to express a definite interest in obtaining a transplant.

Step 3: For those patients who were medically suitable and who had expressed a definite interest in obtaining a transplant, blacks were less likely than whites to have the pretransplant workup completed during the four-year study period.

Step 4: For those patients who had completed the pretransplant workup, blacks were less likely than whites to have their name placed on the transplant waiting list.

From these results, it seems that the disparity in access to kidney transplantation is due to a combination of factors, including hesitance to undergo the procedure on the part of blacks and reluctance on the part of the physician to refer blacks.

The relative contribution of patient preferences or physician reluctance was explored in a study by Ayanian and colleagues (1999). They conducted interviews with 1,392 patients at a point approximately 10 months after they had begun kidney dialysis, asking them specifically about their preferences regarding dialysis versus transplantation. Their study sample was approximately evenly split between blacks and whites, and between men and women. They found that blacks were less likely to want a transplant: 76 percent of black women and 81 percent of black men wanted a transplant, while 79 percent of white women and 86 percent of white men wanted

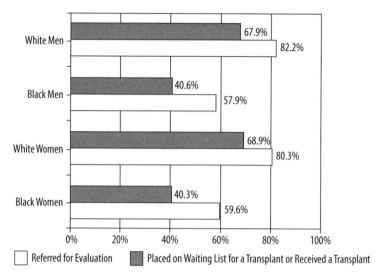

Figure 8.5. Racial and gender differences in referral for pretransplant evaluation and placement on a transplant waiting list / receiving a transplant. *Source*: Based on Ayanian et al. 1999.

a transplant. On further questioning blacks were also found to be less certain of this preference.

The authors were then able to follow the subjects for between three and four years to determine which patients were actually referred for the pretransplant workup and which were placed on the transplant waiting list. Using multivariate statistical methodology, they were able to control for both social and demographic factors and for the patient's previously expressed interest in obtaining a transplant. They were thus able to compare the outcomes of blacks and whites with the same level of interest in receiving a transplant and similar medical and SES backgrounds. These results are shown in Figure 8.5.

Epstein, Ayanian, and colleagues (2000) explored in more depth the process by which patients are selected for transplantation. They first used a panel of independent experts to review the available literature on the treatment of ESRD, and based on that review to define the clinical criteria by which someone with ESRD could be determined to be either "appropriate" or "inappropriate" for a transplant. Using these criteria, they then reviewed the records of 1,518 patients between the ages of 18 and 54, selected at random from the list of all those receiving dialysis in a five-state area. They reviewed who actually was referred for a pretransplant evaluation, who was placed on a waiting list, and who actually received a kidney transplant. Their results are shown in Table 8.5, broken down by whether the patient was deemed appropriate or inappropriate for a transplant based on the independent review.

Table 8.5. Racial Differences in the Treatment of Kidney Failure, Sorted by Appropriateness for Kidney Transplantation

	Appropriate for Transplant (percent)	Inappropriate for Transplant (percent)
Referred for pretransplant evaluation		
Black	90.1	38.4
White	98.0	57.8
Placed on transplant waiting list		
Black	71.0	17.4
White	86.7	30.9
Received kidney transplant		
Black	16.9	2.2
White	52.0	10.3

Source: Epstein et al. 2000.
Note: Differences statistically significant, $p < 0.01$

Not surprisingly, blacks who were medically appropriate for a transplant were less likely than whites to undergo each of these three steps. What is somewhat surprising from this study is the extent to which individuals who, based on an independent chart review were medically inappropriate for a kidney transplant, were nonetheless referred for evaluation, placed on the waiting list, and actually underwent a transplant. Of those thought to be inappropriate for a transplant who received a transplant, more than 80 percent were white. It seems that the disparity in access to kidney transplantation has two aspects to it.

1. Blacks who are medically appropriate for a transplant are less likely to undergo the steps that are preparatory for a transplant and to receive a transplant.
2. Whites who are medically inappropriate for a transplant are nonetheless referred for evaluation and receive a transplant at disproportionately high rates.

In their discussion of these findings, the authors commented: "Our results suggest that lower rates of renal transplantation among black patients in part reflect racial differences in clinical characteristics that make fewer blacks clinically appropriate candidates for transplantation. However, blacks also appear to receive fewer transplants, regardless of the clinical indications, a pattern that results in the relative underuse of transplantation among blacks who are appropriate candidates for transplantation and the relative overuse among whites who are inappropriate candidates" (p. 1542).

Research has shown that blacks with ESRD have substantially lower access to kidney transplantation, even after taking into account medical appropriateness and personal preferences. The system of treating ESRD and the physicians within that system appear to be less aggressive in moving blacks toward transplantation than whites. Recall that in the review by Kasiske and colleagues (1991), once a kidney was transplanted into a black patient, the rate at which that kidney survived and continued to function was lower in blacks than it was in whites. Young and Gaston (2000) reviewed the scientific literature exploring the causes of this racial disparity in allograft survival. They conclude that there are two general explanations for this outcome:

1. If the blood type and distribution of tissue antigens are sufficiently different between the donor of a kidney and the recipient of a kidney, these differences increase the likelihood that the recipient's immune system will attack the transplanted kidney, thus shortening its survival. There are enough differences in the blood types and tissue antigens of whites and blacks that whites tend to be a better match when a kidney becomes available. As the vast majority of donated kidneys come from whites, the result is that a donated kidney is more likely to go to a white patient than to a black patient.

2. Even when tissue antigens are matched closely, blacks continue to experience shorter survival times of a transplanted kidney. Possible explanations for this finding include a higher prevalence and increased severity of hypertension in blacks with kidney disease. (Hypertension itself can damage kidney tissue. See the discussion of the detrimental effects of allostatic load in Chapter 4.)

Young and Gaston point out that the system of allocating kidneys based on similarities in tissue antigens originated in the 1980s. As many of the newer drugs that suppress immune response to transplants had not yet been developed, it was much more important at that time to get the closest tissue match as possible. Accordingly, it became common practice to pass over a black patient and allocate a donated kidney to a white patient. However, with newer drugs available, the authors concluded that "in light of the increasing recognition of nonimmunologic factors . . . on long term survival, it may be time to formulate a new approach to organ allocation" (p. 1549).

The United Network for Organ Sharing (UNOS) is the nonprofit organization that maintains the national registry for the allocation of deceased donor kidneys for transplantation (United Network for Organ Sharing 2018). Based on the extensive and consistent data that the lower rate of kidney transplantation among black patients as compared to white patients was largely due to delays in referring patients to be placed on the transplant waiting list, UNOS made a fundamental change in the system by which deceased donor kidneys were allocated for transplantation

(Melanson et al. 2017). Previously, priority for allocation of a donated kidney was based on the time a patient had been on the waiting list. As the time it took to refer a black patient for placement on the list was significantly longer than for a white patient, in 2014 UNOS began measuring waiting time based on the date on which a patient first started kidney dialysis. By September 2016 the rate of kidney transplantation among black and Hispanic patients had increased significantly. While blacks and Hispanics continue to spend longer times in the process of being evaluated for and referred to the waiting list, under the new policy disparities in access to transplantation among blacks, Hispanics, and whites had been eliminated.

The success in eliminating racial and ethnic disparities in access to kidney transplantation pertains to access to deceased donor transplantation. Beginning in the 1990s there has been a substantial increase in the number of kidney transplantations that were done transplanting a kidney from a live donor rather than a deceased donor. Long-term success of a transplanted kidney is greater when the kidney is from a live donor rather than a deceased donor. Kidneys donated by a live donor are allocated according to a combination of tissue matching and time on the waiting list. By 2015 nearly one-third of transplanted kidneys were from live donors (United States Renal Data System 2017). Purnell and colleagues (2018) evaluated the changes between 1995 and 2014 in the rates of differing racial and ethnic groups receiving a live donor kidney transplantation. The authors reported that "between 1995 and 2014, disparities in the receipt of live donor kidney transplantation increased from 1995–1999 to 2010–2014" (p. 49).

Among patients eligible for kidney transplantation in 2014, 11.4 percent of white patients, 2.9 percent of black patients, and 5.9 percent of Hispanic patients received a kidney from a live donor. In an editorial written in response to these data, Jay and Cigarroa (2018) conclude that "Despite improvements in disparities related to access to the waiting list and deceased donor kidney transplantation rates among black and Hispanic patients, large disparities in live donor kidney transplantation rates remain" (p. 26).

Race/Ethnicity and the Treatment of Mental Illness

In 1999 Dr. David Satcher, the US Surgeon General, released the first Surgeon General's Report ever to focus on mental health (US Department of Health and Human Services 1999). In 2001 Dr. Satcher released a supplement to that report titled *Mental Health: Culture, Race, and Ethnicity* (US Department of Health and Human Services 2001). The report found overall rates of mental illness in blacks and whites to be similar, however, "Carefully gathered evidence indicates that African Americans are diagnosed accurately less often than white Americans when they are suffering from depression and seen in primary care, or when they are seen for psychiatric evaluation in an emergency room" (p. 66).

Schizophrenia is a major mental illness that is associated with potentially lifelong consequences and substantially worse prognosis when compared to what are referred to as "affective disorders" such as depression. After reviewing extensive evidence regarding how mental illness is diagnosed and treated, the report identified major racial disparities. "For many years, clinicians and researchers observed a pattern whereby African Americans in treatment presented higher than expected rates of diagnosed schizophrenia and lower rates of diagnosed affective disorders. When structured procedures were used for assessment, or when retrospective assessments were made via chart review, the disparities between African Americans and whites failed to emerge. One explanation for the findings is clinician bias: Clinicians are predisposed to judge African Americans as schizophrenic, but not as suffering from an affective disorder" (pp. 66–67).

One study cited by the report reviewed care provided to patients with mental illness in emergency rooms. It found that in treating mental illness, the ER physicians (who were mostly white) spent less time with their black patients, and were more likely to prescribe antipsychotic medicines (for treatment of conditions such as schizophrenia) to the black patients (Segal et al. 1996). A more recent study looked at care provided to patients in psychiatrists' offices. It found that psychiatrists spent less time with their black patients than with comparable white patients (Olfson et al. 2009).

Akincigil and colleagues (2012) compared rates of diagnosis and treatment of depression in more than 33,000 Medicare patients nationally. Again consistent with the original finding of the Surgeon General's Report, they found that black patients as well as Hispanic patients were less likely than white patients to be diagnosed and treated for depression. These findings are of increased significance in the context of the increased severity of depressive symptoms often found in blacks who experience depression. Hankerson and colleagues (2015) report that, while African Americans have lower prevalence of experiencing a major depressive disorder, "African Americans have depressive episodes that are more disabling, more persistent, and more resistant to treatment relative to their White counterparts" (p. 21). Accordingly, undertreatment of depression may have substantial adverse impacts on the lives of blacks who do experience mental illness.

Perhaps not surprisingly, when asked about their experience obtaining treatment for a mental health condition, both blacks and Hispanics were significantly more likely than whites to report perceived discrimination on the part of the mental health provider (Mays et al. 2017). Those who do experience discrimination in the care process are less likely to continue with treatment for their mental health condition.

While I have focused mainly on the black/white differences identified in the Surgeon General's Report from 2001, I would like to emphasize that other racial and ethnic minority groups were also found to have disparate patterns of diagnosis and treatment of mental illness. For example, among Hispanics being treated for mental illness, bilingual patients were evaluated differently when interviewed in English as opposed to Spanish. Similarly, a critical issue raised in the report was whether Asian Americans will manifest symptoms of mental illness in a manner that is similar to those in Western societies, or whether ethnic and cultural factors may lead to Asians having different ways of expressing the symptoms of mental illness.

Reviewing the Patterns of Racial Disparity in Access to Care

I have looked at research on the patterns and possible causes of racial disparities in access to care across a range of illnesses. I have looked at the treatment of ischemic heart disease, cancer, severe pain associated with traumatic injuries, treatment of kidney failure, and treatment of mental illness. I have found consistent patterns of care, with blacks and Hispanics having less frequent access than whites to optimal medical treatment. I could have looked at other conditions and found the same pattern, such as access to replacement knee joints for seniors with severe arthritis (Skinner et al. 2003; Cisternas et al. 2009), access to routine flu shots for seniors (Schneider et al. 2001), or access to HPV vaccine for adolescents (Ylitalo and colleagues 2013).

Part of the explanation for these disparities may have to do with racial/ethnic differences in preferences for treatment or trust in the system. In each of the conditions I have looked at, I have found even larger disparities that seem to originate in the decisions physicians make about which treatments to apply in which patients. By the end of the 1990s, the issue of racial/ethnic disparities in access to care was a major national policy issue.

The National Academy of Sciences advises the federal government on scientific issues affecting national policy. As one of the principal agencies of the academy, the National Academy of Medicine (formerly the Institute of Medicine [IOM]) advises the government on the application of medical science to health policy. In 1999 Congress requested that the IOM undertake a thorough review and analysis of the scientific evidence that dealt with racial/ethnic disparities in care. Specifically, Congress asked the IOM to

- assess the extent of racial and ethnic differences in health care that are not otherwise attributable to known factors such as access to care (for example, ability to pay or insurance coverage)
- evaluate potential sources of racial and ethnic disparities in health care, including the role of bias, discrimination, and stereotyping at the individual (provider and patient), institutional, and health system levels
- provide recommendations regarding interventions to eliminate health care disparities (Smedley et al. 2003, p. 3)

To do this, the IOM convened a committee of nationally respected scientists and experts. This committee looked at more than 100 published scientific studies addressing the quality of medical care provided to different racial/ethnic groups. In most of these studies, the analysis was able to control for factors such as SES, access to health insurance, coexisting illnesses, and demographic factors such as age and gender.

In 2003 the IOM published a report describing their findings titled *Unequal Treatment: Confronting Racial and Ethnic Disparities in Healthcare* (Smedley et al. 2003). In a summary of the report, the committee stated what was perhaps their principal finding: "The study committee was struck by the consistency of research findings: even among the better-controlled studies, the vast majority indicated that minorities are less likely than whites to receive needed services, including clinically necessary procedures" (Institute of Medicine 2002, p. 2).

The committee reviewed studies in a wide range of conditions, including cardiovascular disease, cancer, cerebrovascular disease (for example, stroke), kidney transplantation, HIV/AIDS, asthma, diabetes, pain relief, rehabilitation, maternal and child health, children's health, mental health, and more. They separated the root causes of the disparities they found into three general categories: barriers to care within the health system, patient-level factors such as mistrust and personal preferences, and provider-level factors such as the effects of prejudice and bias under conditions of uncertainty.

It was clear to the IOM committee that racial/ethnic disparities in care were a national problem that required a change in national policies to address them. The committee recommended that the federal government support the systematic gathering of data on patterns of care so as to monitor the levels of racial/ethnic disparities that exist, and to support and conduct further research on issues surrounding the reduction or elimination of those disparities. As part of this initiative, the US

Department of Health and Human Services amended the goals of its *Healthy People 2020* initiative (a national initiative to set goals for the improvement of the health of the American people) to include "achieve health equity, eliminate disparities, and improve the health of all groups" (CDC 2018). In 2011 the government expanded this effort with the publication of its *Action Plan to Reduce Racial and Ethnic Disparities* (US Department of Health and Human Services 2011). An explicit goal of the Action Plan was to achieve "a nation free of disparities in health and health care" (p. 11).

In addition to the *Unequal Treatment* report and the change to the *Healthy People 2020* goals, Congress also directed the US Agency for Healthcare Research and Quality (AHRQ) to prepare a yearly *Health Disparities* report. The first report was issued in 2003, and faced immediate controversy. Within a month of its publication, news reports circulated suggesting that the report drafted by AHRQ had been rewritten so as to play down the persistence of race as a factor in care, dismiss the possibility of physician prejudice as a contributing factor, and minimize the adverse health impacts of disparities in access to care (Geiger 2004). The controversy surrounding the alleged interjection of politics into what was intended as a scientific document triggered a congressional investigation (US Congress 2004) and a series of commentaries in the *New England Journal of Medicine* (Bloche 2004; Steinbrook 2004). In response to the controversy, Dr. Carolyn Clancy, director of AHRQ, made both the original draft of the report and the final published version publicly available (Clancy 2003). Following the initial controversy, subsequent annual disparities reports have been well received. One of the most controversial aspects of the 2003 *Health Disparities* report was its assertion that racial bias on the part of physicians was not a serious issue. The earlier IOM report had come to quite a different conclusion, finding that "bias, stereotyping, prejudice, and clinical uncertainty on the part of healthcare providers may contribute to racial and ethnic disparities in healthcare" (Smedley et al. 2003, p. 12).

The 2016 *Health Disparities* report concluded that "Overall, some disparities were getting smaller from 2000 through 2014–2015, but disparities persist, especially for poor and uninsured populations in all priority areas: While 20% of measures show disparities getting smaller for Blacks and Hispanics, most disparities have not changed significantly for any racial and ethnic groups . . ." (US Agency for Healthcare Research and Quality 2018). The issue of racial bias on the part of physicians and other health care providers, raised in this chapter as one of the possible contributors to observed disparities, remains highly controversial. I address it in some depth in the following chapter.

CHAPTER NINE

Why Does Race/Ethnicity Affect the Way Physicians Treat Patients?

In the previous chapter I looked at the way patients in certain racial/ethnic groups—primarily blacks—receive a different level of treatment for a wide range of illnesses and conditions. These differences are due in part to factors pertaining to the patient, factors such as personal preferences about treatment options and trust in physicians' recommendations. Even after taking into account these patient-level factors, blacks and other minority racial/ethnic groups continue to receive less care and care that is of lower quality than whites. They receive *Unequal Treatment*—the title of the report addressing these issues by the Institute of Medicine of the National Academy of Sciences (IOM). In the opening words of that report, "Racial and ethnic minorities tend to receive a lower quality of healthcare than non-minorities, even when access-related factors, such as patients' insurance status and income, are controlled. The sources of these disparities are complex, are rooted in historic and contemporary inequities, and involve many participants at several levels, including health systems, their administrative and bureaucratic processes, utilization managers, health professionals, and patients" (2003, p. 1).

In the middle of the twentieth century, overt racial discrimination was the norm in many parts of the United States. Blacks were not permitted in many hospitals and clinics meant for whites (Thomson 1997). Black doctors, fully licensed and certified, were not permitted to join the staff of white hospitals. The discrimination was conscious, and it was intended. Fortunately, a series of civil rights laws passed in the 1960s, backed up by targeted lawsuits, made this type of racial discrimination in medical care illegal (Reynolds 1997).

It is understandable that some people reacted defensively when the experts involved in creating the IOM report stated that "bias, stereotyping, prejudice, and clinical uncertainty on the part of healthcare providers may contribute to racial and ethnic disparities in healthcare" (Smedley et al. 2003, p. 12). Since the publication of the IOM report, there has been continuing debate as to whether doctors and other health care providers allow racial/ethnic bias or prejudice to affect their treatment decisions.

Even before the IOM report was published, the issue of physician bias was hotly debated. One example of this debate was a panel discussion convened at a joint meeting of the American Heart Association and the American College of Cardiology (2001). The purpose of the panel was to discuss the causes of the observed disparities in the treatment of cardiovascular disease, such as those discussed in the previous chapter. One of the panelists was Dr. Elizabeth Ofili, chief of cardiology and a professor at Morehouse School of Medicine. In reviewing the research on the treatment of heart disease, she concluded, "What America has to deal with, obviously, is the legacy of race and racism. And one of the reasons that we've always had difficulty discussing that topic is that none of us thought that providers, when they go into a relationship with a patient, necessarily are racist in their interactions. But, as all of us have looked at the record and the track of publications, we know that there are obviously differences. . . . So we must honestly begin to look at those issues, while not necessarily racism, perhaps something related to that" (p. 4).

Jerome Kassirer, editor of the *New England Journal of Medicine*—the journal in which many of the important studies about racial disparities in care have been published—responded to Ofili's remarks: "Inadequate health education, differences in preferences for invasive management, and a delivery system that is unfriendly to certain cultures. That isn't necessarily prejudice, it simply defines the kinds of delivery systems that provide care. . . . There are all kinds of potential alternative explanations rather than racism as an explanation" (pp. 7–8).

Dr. Sally Satel, a psychiatrist and frequent political commentator, responded to Ofili's comments by saying, "Is racial bias one of the reasons for disparities? Possibly. It's certainly a hypothesis that people can entertain; but thus far, virtually every study that has been held up as an example of bias, I have found unconvincing" (p. 13).

These excerpts provide a good summary of the principal arguments heard as part of the debate on the role of racial/ethnic bias on the part of physicians and other providers. These arguments can be summarized in the following manner:

Argument 1: Because of the legacy of racism in this country, it is important to consider racism and other forms of racial bias as sources of disparities of care when other explanations are inadequate.

Argument 2: There are many other possible explanations for the disparities that have little to do with racism.

Argument 3: It is difficult to believe that physicians are racist, regardless of what the studies suggest.

The Study of Racial Bias among Physicians

In the 1980s—20 years after the enactment of civil rights laws making racial discrimination in medical care illegal—there were continuing patterns of racial differences in care. The Council on Ethical and Judicial Affairs of the American Medical Association (1990) undertook a comprehensive study of this issue. In it they found that "recent studies have suggested that even when blacks gain access to the health care system, they are less likely than whites to receive certain surgical or other therapies. . . . Whether the disparities in treatment decisions are caused by differences in income and education, sociocultural factors, or failures by the medical profession, they are unjustifiable and must be eliminated" (p. 2344). After reviewing the evidence available at that time and considering possible causes, the report concluded that "disparities in treatment decisions may reflect the existence of subconscious bias. This is a serious and troubling problem. Despite the progress in the past 25 years, racial prejudice has not been eliminated in this country. The health care system, like all other elements of society, has not fully eradicated this prejudice" (p. 2346).

Responding to the admonition from the American Medical Association to identify the causes of continuing racial disparities in care, and to published reports such as those of Peterson and colleagues discussed in the previous chapter, Schulman and colleagues (1999) undertook what was to become a highly controversial study of the way physicians use a patient's race in making clinical decisions about the treatment of heart disease. Their intent was to have physicians review the medical records of blacks and whites with the same level of heart disease, and then indicate what treatment they would recommend if the patient were in their practice. In order to do this they videotaped an interview with eight different patients, each complaining of chest pain. Each patient was shown in a physician's examining room, dressed only in a skimpy examining gown. They then showed the videotapes to a series of physicians who had never seen the patients before and asked for the physicians' recommendation.

The patients in the videos, however, were not true patients. They were professional actors, each reading a script. The scripts had been created in consultation with a group of cardiologists. The scripts read by the actors were of two types: one conveying information suggesting that the patient had a relatively low risk for heart disease based on their previous medical background, and one suggesting that the patient's risk was relatively high. Similarly, the script read by the actors describing their current symptoms sometimes was written to suggest a low probability of the chest pain being caused by heart disease, and sometimes was written to suggest that the pain probably was coming from the heart. Finally, after responding to a series of questions, the physicians were then shown the results of a test that, if abnormal, is indicative of probable heart disease. Thus, the researchers were able to compare physicians' responses to patients with exactly the same type of disease who differed only in their race.

To take into account other factors that might influence the physicians' decisions, the researchers selected the patients so that they also differed by age and sex. Of the eight actors, there were

- four blacks and four whites
- four men and four women
- four patients who stated their age to be 55, and four patients who stated their age to be 70

Thus, there was one actor or actress for each of the eight possible combinations of race, sex, and age. However, the words read by the actors and actresses were the same, varying only in their description of their pain and their medical background, as described above.

To recruit practicing physicians to participate as subjects in the study, the researchers contacted those who had registered to attend either the 1996 annual meeting of the American Academy of Family Practice or the 1997 annual meeting of the American College of Physicians, requesting their participation while attending the meeting. By selecting these two professional organizations, the researchers were able to have physicians whose practices were principally in primary care rather than cardiology. They were able to recruit 720 physicians; each viewed a single videotaped interview and responded to questions about the patient shown on the tape. The researchers then compared the average of the responses across all subjects. There were a total of 144 tapes, each with a unique set of patient and examination circumstances. Each of the tapes was viewed by five separate subjects. The subjects were unaware that the purpose of the study was to assess their response to the race of the patient.

The first part of the study asked the physician-subjects to estimate how likely it was, in their opinion, that the patient had clinically significant heart disease. Across the various levels of disease represented on the tapes, there was not a significant difference for blacks and whites. There were differences across age and sex, with the physicians estimating that women were less likely than men and the younger subjects were less likely than the older subjects to have significant heart disease. Thus, the physicians responded appropriately to the differing descriptions on the tapes about the nature of the pain and the patient's medical background, correctly identifying those patients intended to convey more serious disease on the tapes.

Table 9.1. Odds Ratio of Referral for Cardiac Catheterization According to the Race, Sex, and Age of the Patient

	Mean Rate of Referral (percent)	Odds Ratio for Referral
Race of patient		
White	90.6	—
Black	84.7	0.6*
Sex of patient		
Male	90.6	—
Female	84.7	0.6*
Age of patient		
55 years	89.7	—
70 years	85.6	0.7**

Source: Schulman et al. 1999.
Note: The odds ratio compares the odds of the indicated category receiving a referral to the odds of the comparison category.
*$p = 0.02$ **$p = 0.09$

The final step in the study was to show the physicians the results of a cardiac stress test that was suggestive of heart disease. The subjects were then asked whether they would, or would not, recommend that this patient undergo cardiac catheterization—the first step in the diagnosis and ultimate treatment of ischemic heart disease. To analyze these results, the researchers used multivariate statistical analysis to take into account the various differences in the attributes of the patients on the tapes. These results are shown in Table 9.1.

In a multivariate analysis that compares the relative frequencies of two possible outcomes (in this case, to refer or not to refer), the statistic used to make the comparison is referred to as the "odds ratio." For those who are not familiar with this statistic, it is calculated in two steps (Blalock 1979):

Step 1: Calculate the ratio within each comparison group of those who did demonstrate the outcome under study and those who did not. For the comparison by race, for blacks the ratio is 84.7 percent / 15.3 percent = 5.54; for whites the ratio is 90.6 percent / 9.4 percent = 9.64.

Step 2: Divide the ratio for black patients by the ratio for white patients. In this case, this "odds ratio" is calculated as 5.54/9.64 = 0.6.

It should be noted that an odds ratio of 0.6 does not imply that blacks were referred for catheterization only 60 percent as often as whites. In fact, they were referred 93.5 percent as often, which is 84.7 percent / 90.6 percent. This is referred to as the "risk ratio" and is a statistic that compares the likelihood of a specific outcome for one group as compared to another.

In addition to reporting these outcomes, the researchers looked for what is referred to as an "interaction effect," looking to see if the physicians who were the subjects of this study responded to the race of the patient differently for males and females. They did find this to be the case. Again using multivariate analysis, there was no evidence that physicians responded to black males any differently than to white males or white females. However, they did consistently recommend significantly less often that black females be referred for catheterization. When this difference, found only in black females, was averaged across all black patients, male and female, the resulting rate of referral for blacks as a group independent of the sex of the patient was significantly lower than the rate for whites as a group.

Does this finding—that the physicians referred black *women* less often than the other groups—provide evidence of racial prejudice on the part of the physician? Here is how the authors interpreted their findings: "Our finding that the race and sex of the patient influence the recommendations of physicians independently of other factors may suggest bias on the part of the physicians. However, our study could not assess the form of bias. Bias may represent overt prejudice on the part of physicians or, more likely, could be the result of subconscious perceptions rather than deliberate actions or thoughts. Subconscious bias occurs when a patient's membership in a target group automatically activates a cultural stereotype in the physician's memory regardless of the level of prejudice the physician has" (p. 624).

The problem, of course, is that only black women were referred less often. The race of the patient in combination with her gender led the physicians to refer the black women less often. Did this in itself constitute race bias, or gender bias, or neither, or both? This was the controversy that rapidly surrounded the Schulman study. Helft and colleagues (1999) pointed out this problem in a letter to the editor published a few months after the original study. Adding further to the controversy, the news media often misrepresented the meaning of the odds ratio, reporting that blacks were 60 percent as likely as whites to be referred.

The confusion and controversy generated by the Schulman study prompted the *New England Journal of Medicine* to publish an article explaining the appropriate use of odds ratios, risk ratios, and the implications of the female/black interaction effect (Schwartz et al. 1999). The issue of whether the Schulman study provides evidence of race bias on the part of the physicians who were the subjects of the study continues to be controversial, with responses falling generally into the three categories of argument described above.

Rathore and colleagues (2000) used the original tapes from the Schulman study to carry the analysis of this issue one step further. They used only two of the tapes from the original study, one showing the 55-year-old black female and one showing the 55-year-old white male. All other aspects of the content of the tapes were identical. Rather than showing the tapes to practicing physicians, they showed them to 164 medical students in their first or second year of medical school. (Students at this stage of their medical education typically have had no training in the formal diagnosis and treatment of heart disease.) They then asked the students to estimate how healthy the patient was based on their need for glasses, their need to use a wheelchair, and how likely it was that they suffered from angina pain. (Note that the tapes contain no information specific to the need for glasses or a wheelchair.) Overall, the medical students saw no difference in the needs of the two patients for glasses or the use of a wheelchair. However, the students were significantly more likely to attribute the white male patient's symptoms to angina than those of the black female. As discussed by the authors, "If patient race or sex influences physician recommendations about treatment, then our study indicates that these biases may be present at the earliest stages of medical training. . . . Thus, differences in diagnosis and health state rating may derive from preformed ideas brought to medical training. These biases may not be conscious but may still influence clinical decisions" (p. 564).

As with the original Schulman study, these results suggest that an unconscious form of bias, affecting their perceptions of blacks and women, may affect the reasoning and decisions of both medical students with little clinical training and physicians with substantial clinical experience.

Perceptions of Racial Bias in Care among the Public and among Physicians

In the months following the controversy generated by the publication of the Schulman study, the Kaiser Family Foundation, a nonprofit health policy research center, conducted a national survey of public perceptions about the ways in which race and ethnicity affect medical care (Kaiser Family Foundation 1999). Among the questions they asked in the survey were several about the quality of medical care for blacks and whites. When asked how the quality of care received by blacks compared to that received by whites, white respondents gave the following answers:

- 23 percent indicated that they believe blacks receive lower-quality care
- 67 percent indicated that blacks and whites receive the same level of care

For black respondents, the percentages were essentially reversed:

- 64 percent said that blacks receive lower-quality care
- 27 percent said they receive the same level of quality care

The surveyors then asked respondents whether they believed the following state-ment to be true or false: "African Americans with heart disease are just as likely as whites who have heart disease to get specialized medical procedures and surgery." Thirty-three percent of white respondents thought this statement was false; 56 percent of black respondents thought it was false. A subsequent question asked, "How often do you think our health care system treats people unfairly based on their race / ethnic background?" Forty-six percent of whites, 56 percent of blacks, and 51 percent of Latinos responding to the survey indicated that they think this happens either very often or somewhat often. It seems to be a common perception among diverse groups in the United States that blacks get less care and lower-quality care than whites, for reasons based on race rather than economic factors such as health insurance. While whites are less likely to hold this belief, a substantial seg-ment of white respondents reported this view for each of these three questions.

The Kaiser Family Foundation (2002) subsequently conducted a survey of a na-tionally representative sample of practicing physicians about their perceptions of these same issues. Of the 2,608 physicians who responded, 69 percent indicated that they thought the health care system "never" or "rarely" treats people unfairly because of their race; 29 percent indicated that this occurred "often" or "somewhat often." Sixty-five percent of physicians found the statement to be false that African Amer-icans with heart disease are treated the same as whites with heart disease.

Both in the public at large and among practicing physicians, there seemed to be a fairly broad awareness of the differences in medical care access and quality faced by blacks. While the physicians seemed more aware of the specific barriers faced by blacks with heart disease, they saw less unfair treatment in the health care system more generally, compared to respondents from the general public.

Finding a broad general awareness among practicing physicians of the racial dis-parities in the treatment of heart disease does not tell us what physicians perceive as the cause of those disparities. Lurie and colleagues (2005) surveyed 344 cardi-ologists specifically about their understanding of the sources of the observed racial differences in the treatment of heart disease. They asked the cardiologists several of the same questions used in the earlier Kaiser Family Foundation survey of pub-lic attitudes.

1. What were the principal factors that contribute to racial disparities?

Sixty-nine percent of physicians viewed health insurance as a principal source of disparities; 47 percent viewed educational differences among patients as a source of disparities; 34 percent believed that the patient's race/ethnicity was a source of dis-parities in treatment.

2. How strong is the evidence that blacks with heart disease are less likely than whites with heart disease to get specialized medical procedures and surgery?

More than 60 percent of the cardiologists rated the strength of this evidence as "strong" or "very strong."

3. In what health care settings is it likely that patients receive different levels of care based on their race/ethnicity?

Thirty-four percent of respondents felt that disparities in care occurred in the health care system in general; 12 percent indicated that these disparities occurred in the hospital or clinic in which they worked; 5 percent felt that these disparities occurred among their own patients.

These cardiologists seemed to be saying that they believed the research documenting racial disparities in the care of heart disease, but did not perceive racial disparities to exist in the context of their own practice. To them, the disparities existed largely because of social and economic factors, principal among them SES and access to health insurance. Consistent with argument 2 described above, these doctors interpret the evidence as not indicative of racial bias on the part of physicians but rather indicative of factors unrelated to bias. Consistent with argument 3 above, a substantial minority of the physicians in this study simply didn't believe that racial disparities existed, despite what the evidence said.

There are voices within the medical profession, however, that interpret the growing body of evidence as indicative of racial bias within the medical profession. H. Jack Geiger, a longtime civil rights activist and leading academic physician, argued, "The alternative explanation is racism—that is, racially discriminatory rationing by physicians and health care institutions. We do not yet know enough to make that charge definitively. Furthermore, if racism is involved it is unlikely to be overt or even conscious. As Escarce and colleagues have noted, 'Race . . . may influence physicians' clinical decisions in ways that physicians do not even recognize but that are not justified by medical need'" (1996, p. 816).

Is Racism on the Part of Physicians a Source of Racial Disparities in Care?

It is understandable that this question is one to which people often react defensively. However, it is a question that must be addressed directly if we are to understand the processes by which blacks and other minorities seem consistently, across diseases and across time, to receive a lesser level of care than comparable whites.

To illustrate this point, let me describe an incident I experienced earlier in my medical career.

I was on duty in a busy urgent care center when I pulled the next chart off the rack and called the patient into the examination room. Accompanied by his wife, he limped into the room with the aid of a cane. The patient was worried about the pain in his knee. He was 67, a retired federal worker who had played perhaps too hard during his college sports days. He had had arthroscopic surgery two years earlier to remove torn cartilage, but was once again getting pain, swelling, and occasional locking of his knee. The knee problem was affecting both his very active life and his part-time work as a local radio show host. He had consulted his regular doctor about his knee and had gone to physical therapy as prescribed. The pain elicited by therapy had prompted the therapist to urge him to go back to a physician for reassessment. His regular doctor had been too busy to see him that day, so the patient found himself in my examining room.

Clearly, the knee was not normal. I could feel fluid in the joint, the knee was stiff, and when I tried to move it there was a popping noise and the patient winced in pain. I got x-rays, which showed narrowing of the joint space and degenerative changes. My assessment was that there was a combination of degenerative and internal structural problems that might or might not be amenable to further arthroscopic procedures. I wanted to refer the patient to an orthopedist after first obtaining an MRI.

Out of professional courtesy, I phoned the patient's regular doctor before taking these steps. Yes, the doctor said, there might be structural problems amenable to surgery, but there was something about the patient I should know. The business office at the doctor's practice had recently referred the patient to a collection agency for nonpayment of earlier bills. It appeared that he was cashing the checks he received from Medicare and taking the money for his own personal use, without paying the doctor's bills. Rather than running up a bill for the MRI and the orthopedic consultation and risk being cheated out of more money, the doctor advised me, I should prescribe ibuprofen for several weeks and have the patient return to see his regular doctor at a later date.

I was startled to hear this, coming as it did, from one of the senior physicians in our community. I was being asked to choose economics over clinical judgment. There seemed only one thing to do: I shared my dilemma with the patient and his wife.

He was simultaneously shocked and embarrassed. Yes, he said, there had been a problem with a late bill. The reason for the delay had been his confusion in working his way through the Medicare system, a new phenomenon for him. He had carefully sent every bill he received to Medicare. As each check came back from Medicare, he made a note of the check and sent a supplemental claim on to his private insurance carrier, as he had been instructed. As soon as the payment came in from the private company, it was his intent to endorse all the checks over to his doctor. The only problem was, this process took so long that before he received the checks from the private insurer he got an overdue notice from the collection agency. He had immediately taken his entire file down to the doctor's business office and spent more than two hours going over each charge with the clerk. He was embarrassed that he had not realized he was expected to send in the Medicare checks as soon as he had gotten them, without waiting for the supplemental checks from the private company. A quick call to the business office confirmed this information. As far as they were concerned, there was no problem with this patient's account.

I was able to obtain an MRI within a few days. It confirmed extensive degenerative changes and demonstrated three separate structural problems that might be helped by arthroscopic surgery, including a loose body in the joint (perhaps the cause of the locking the patient had been experiencing). The patient consulted an orthopedist shortly thereafter.

Why had my colleague told me that this man was cashing the Medicare checks without any evidence that this was actually the case? More important, why did my colleague confuse the patient's unfamiliarity with the Medicare system with dishonesty? Finally, on what basis had he recommended that I withhold potentially helpful diagnostic steps? Was it because the patient was black? If the patient had instead been a retired white entrepreneur, would the internist have assumed that a delay in submitting the Medicare checks indicated malfeasance sufficient to warrant the withholding of care?

Was my colleague a racist?

I learned what a racist is in 1963. I had grown up in a largely white, middle-class neighborhood in Berkeley, California. While there certainly were racial tensions at Berkeley High School, the issues of racism and civil rights seemed distant to us. Then I saw images on television of what racism does when it is given political power. Theophilus Eugene "Bull" Connor was a high school dropout who at the age of 66 had risen to the position of police commissioner in Birmingham, Alabama. In April and May 1963, the Rev. Martin Luther King Jr. led a series of nonviolent marches and demonstrations to protest continued racial segregation in Birmingham. On May 23 a group of more than 1,000 children, ranging in age from 6 to 18 years, began a march from a park in Birmingham toward the downtown area. Bull Connor instructed the firefighters under his command to turn high-power fire hoses on the child demonstrators. Images of these children being hit with the blast of the fire hoses, some of which are shown in Figure 9.1, were carried on nationwide TV, including the TV in my living room.

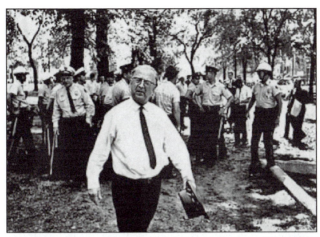

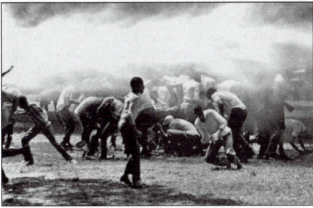

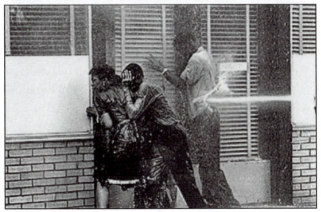

Figure 9.1. Bull Connor and his response to the Children's Civil Rights March, Birmingham, Alabama, 1963. *Source*: Photos © Charles Moore, used by permission.

As described in social studies courses offered to high school students in Alabama, "televised reports of police dogs lunging at African-American citizens and people being washed down the streets by water from powerful fire hoses dramatized the plight of African-Americans in segregated areas. The events in Birmingham helped mobilize the administration of President John Kennedy to begin efforts leading to the most far-reaching civil rights legislation in history, the Civil Rights Act of 1964. The name 'Bull' Connor thus came to symbolize hard-line Southern racism" (Nunnelley 2006).

As a high school student in Berkeley in 1963, I learned what a racist is. Bull Connor was a racist.

Was my physician-colleague a racist?

If I answer "yes" to this question, I seem to be saying that my colleague was no different from Bull Connor. My colleague likely saw the same TV images of Birmingham that I did. These images became an indelible part of our history and our culture. No, my colleague was not a racist, not in the way that Bull Connor was a racist. As described by Bradby (2010), "Physicians who contribute to cultural discordance with Black patients are not 19th century–style racists and doubtless know that racism is wrong. The health-damaging effects of 21st century subtle racism differ dramatically from the operation of 19th century institutionalized segregationist racism" (p. 11).

In his contribution to the book *Anatomy of Racism*, Kwame Anthony Appiah distinguishes what he refers to as "extrinsic racism" from other forms of racial prejudice. He states that "extrinsic racists make moral distinctions between members of different races because they believe that racial essence entails certain morally relevant qualities. The basis for the extrinsic racist's discrimination between people is their belief that members of different races differ in respects that *warrant* the differential treatment" (1990, p. 5).

I have no evidence that, nor do I find it credible that, my colleague practices medicine under the belief that patients who are black warrant differential treatment because of their race. Nor does he believe that there are distinctions between blacks and whites that entail morally relevant qualities.

What, then, led my colleague to attribute our patient's tardy payment of bills to an intent to steal the checks coming from Medicare, rather than to a confusion about the proper sequencing of insurance checks? I believe the most likely explanation for my colleague's misattribution was his inappropriate invocation of a racial stereotype, probably without his conscious awareness that he was doing so.

Racial Stereotypes as a Source of Racial Bias

A stereotype, according to the *Oxford English Dictionary*, is "a preconceived and oversimplified idea of the characteristics that typify a person." It can also be an attitude derived from such a preconception. Stereotypes pervade American culture. Consider the cab driver traveling down a one-way street in Manhattan. Ahead he sees two young men flagging him down. Both appear to be stylishly dressed. One is on each side of the street. The potential fare on the right is white; the fare on the left is black. Which does he pick up? The cabby can easily rationalize that he is safer picking up the white customer. After all, the statistical chances of a black customer robbing him are higher than the chances of a white customer robbing him—even though the chances are overwhelming that neither will rob him. The cabby maintains a negative stereotype of black customers, and often acts on it. As a result, black men in search of a cab on the streets of New York have found it harder to get a cab to stop than white customers.

Danny Glover, a well-known black actor, had just such an experience. Despite his fame, he continued to have difficulty getting a cab to stop for him on the streets of Manhattan. He noticed repeatedly that cabs would pass him by, only to pick up a white customer farther down the block. He filed a complaint with the New York City Taxi and Limousine Commission, which sent out decoys to test Glover's assertion that cab drivers systematically passed by black customers to pick up a white customer. In response, the City of New York changed the law. They determined that all those in New York City share equally in the right to public transportation. Now, cab drivers who discriminate based on the race of the customer are subject to losing their license to operate a cab. Between 1997, when the program was established, and 2006 the rate of noncompliance was cut by two-thirds. The *New York Times* reported a story of a cab driver who was fined several thousand dollars for refusing to pick up a black woman and her daughter on a street in Manhattan, then stopping to pick up two white women farther down the block (Mueller 2015).

Calvin Sims (2006), a *New York Times* correspondent, described his successful experience hailing a cab in Manhattan, a success he attributed to making illegal the use of racial stereotypes in selecting cab customers. "Last weekend, I did a remarkable thing. I hailed a cab. It was late, around 2 a.m. and I had just finished dinner with friends in SoHo. I was alone, and raised my hand, looking for an available yellow cab. As if by magic, one drove by, stopped and I stepped in. That may not sound like anything extraordinary, but it was the first time I can remember getting a cab to carry me uptown that late at night without having to hide in the shadows while white friends procured one for me."

Can we draw a direct analogy between the thought processes of a cab driver in New York and physicians' decisions that contribute to racial disparities in care? When we do, we see that the thought processes are often the same, invoking the same type of racial bias, and with the same results. Recalling the data discussed in the previous chapter about kidney transplantation, consider the kidney specialist who monitors the dialysis treatment of patients with kidney failure. He knows that there are not enough donated kidneys to make a kidney transplant available to all who need it. He needs to choose which patient to send to the transplant surgeon to be placed on the waiting list for a kidney. Money is not an issue, as all patients with permanent kidney failure have their medical care paid for by the federal Medicare program. With the advances in posttransplant care, racial matching of donor and recipient is much less of an issue.

To successfully maintain a transplanted kidney, a patient must follow a complex regimen of antirejection drugs. People with lower levels of education often have a harder time keeping up with complex treatment protocols. Blacks have, on average, lower levels of educational attainment than whites. Based on this stereotype—that blacks will do more poorly than whites because of their lower levels of education— might a kidney specialist favor whites over blacks when deciding which patient to recommend for transplantation?

This reasoning, of course, is not justifiable. It's not the average level of education that's important, it is each patient's actual level of education. In addition, there is a strong moral argument to suggest that those from lower socioeconomic backgrounds deserve the best of care independent of how far they got in school. Might, though, physicians such as my colleague make inappropriate associations such as these, based on their holding a view that certain stereotypic characteristics apply to patients who are black?

This is the question addressed by van Ryn and Burke (2000) in the context of treating heart disease. They studied a stratified random sample of 618 patients who had recently undergone cardiac catheterization as the initial stage of their evaluation for possible heart disease. Each patient had recently seen a physician in follow-up consultation to discuss the results of the test. Of the 193 physicians involved, 88 percent were cardiologists. The researchers administered a survey to the patients to gather data about their demographic characteristics, their current emotional status, their work and social support characteristics, and their general attitudes about the medical care process. The patients in the study were 57 percent white and 43 percent black; 53 percent were male and 47 percent female. The average age was 65 years, with ages ranging from 28 to 92 years. The average educational level was 12 years of schooling, with patients ranging from 8 years to more than 17 years of education.

Table 9.2. Differences in Physicians' Perceptions of Patients Undergoing Cardiac Catheterization, Based on the Race of the Patient

	White (percent)	Black (percent)
"Not at all likely" to abuse alcohol or other drugs	79	67
"Not at all likely" to fail to comply with medical advice	57	42
"Very" to "extremely likely" to participate in cardiac rehabilitation	47	34
"Very" to "extremely likely" to strongly desire a very physically active lifestyle	26	14
"Very" intelligent (versus unintelligent)	26	13
"Very" to "somewhat" educated (versus uneducated)	41	31
"Very" pleasant	53	27
"Very" rational	37	20

Source: van Ryn and Burke 2000.
Note: All comparisons remain statistically significant ($p \leq 0.05$) after controlling for actual demographic circumstances.

The researchers administered a separate survey to the physicians, conducted within two weeks of the patient's follow-up encounter. They asked the physicians for their perceptions of the patient from a number of perspectives, some pertaining to how well the patient would follow physicians' directions and be an active participant in a rehabilitation program if they were to receive a cardiac revascularization procedure (angioplasty or CABG surgery). Of the physicians, 84 percent were white, 1 percent were black, 3 percent were Hispanic, and 11 percent were Asian, with 1 percent "other" races or ethnicities.

The researchers then compared the physicians' attitudes toward and descriptions of the patients, first simply comparing physicians' responses for whites to their responses for blacks. They then used multivariate analysis to see if the differences in physicians' perceptions of their white and black patients were still significant after controlling for the patients' SES, demographics, and other individual variables. They found consistent differences in physicians' perceptions of and attitudes toward their white and black patients (Table 9.2). Most of these perceptual differences had direct relevance to the clinical decision of whether to recommend that the patient undergo a revascularization procedure.

As compared to their white patients, the physicians perceived their black patients as less intelligent, less well educated, and less likely to have the personal characteristics most conducive to a successful rehabilitation from a cardiac procedure, *even when the patients' actual levels of education, income, and personal desire to participate in rehabilitation were identical to that of white patients.* In their summary of their findings, the authors stated, "Black patients [with coronary artery disease] were more likely to be seen as at risk for noncompliance with cardiac rehabilitation, substance abuse, and having inadequate social support. In addition, physicians rated Black patients as less intelligent than White patients, even when patient sex, age, income and education were controlled. Physicians also report less affiliative feelings toward Black patients. . . . Physicians' understanding of epidemiologic evidence regarding population-based likelihoods may function as stereotypes, and be applied to assessments and perceptions of individuals regardless of actual individual characteristics" (pp. 821–22).

Van Ryn and colleagues (2006) then looked at a subset of patients from the original study, all of whom were appropriate for CABG surgery based on an independent review of the patient's medical record. They looked to see for which patients the physician had recommended surgery, based on the physician's response to the original survey. Using multivariate analysis they were able to determine which characteristics—either those reported by the patient or the attitudes of the physician expressed about the patient—were associated with an increased likelihood of a recommendation for surgery.

The researchers did their analysis in two steps. They first asked if the patient's race was associated with a recommendation for surgery. They found that physicians recommended surgery less often in black men as compared to white men. There were no significant differences in the rate at which physicians recommended surgery for black or white women. They then looked only at the male patients, including in the analysis the physicians' responses about their impressions of the patient they had seen (Table 9.2). They found that, after taking into account physicians' perceptions of the patient's level of education and the patient's desire for a physically active lifestyle, there was no longer a racial difference in the likelihood of recommending surgery. These results suggest that the physicians use a two-stage process in their reasoning:

1. Compared to their white patients, they perceive their black patients to be less well educated and to be less likely to desire a physically active lifestyle, even when the patients are identical in these regards.
2. Independent of the patient's race, they are less likely to recommend surgery in patients whom they perceive to be less educated and less likely to desire a physically active lifestyle.

From these studies, it seems apparent that physicians tend to attach certain stereotypic characteristics to members of certain racial or ethnic groups—in this case, black. Whether or not the patient is poorly educated, a physician may assume that a black patient is less well educated than a comparable white patient, based on the average difference in educational attainment between population groups. Recalling the studies of pain relief in the emergency room context discussed in the previous chapter, whether or not a specific emergency room patient has a tendency to abuse narcotic drugs, an emergency room physician may assume that they have such a tendency based on the higher observed prevalence of narcotic abuse among the population of black or Hispanic patients in the context of a busy, inner-city emergency room. And finally, whether or not a patient is actually diverting Medicare checks to their own benefit, a physician may assume that they are based on the higher crime rate observed among the black population as compared to the white population.

Having to act in the face of uncertainty, particularly when time is an added constraint, is the situation in which unconscious racial stereotypes are most likely to exert their effects. As a *New York Times* article on racial stereotyping reported (Goode 2002a), "unconscious biases . . . can shape behavior, even when people do not consciously endorse such biases. Studies suggest that those hidden stereotypes or attitudes are often activated in situations where people are forced to respond quickly and automatically."

When a child is brought to the emergency room with a broken arm or leg or with a fractured skull, one thing the ER physicians must do, both ethically and legally, is ask themselves, "Are this child's injuries the result of child abuse?" If the physician believes that child abuse may have occurred, they are then obligated by law to report this concern to the local child protection agency. Lane and colleagues (2002) reviewed the medical records of 388 children younger than three years who had been seen at an urban children's hospital for treatment of one of these injuries. They wanted to see if the race of the child was independently associated with the likelihood that the treating physician submitted a report of suspected child abuse.

Before looking at whether a report was submitted, they first had a group of pediatric experts review the medical record and evaluate the likelihood, based on the information in the record, that the child's injuries were the result of abuse. They grouped the records into three levels of likelihood: likely due to an accident and not abuse; cause of injury indeterminate; likely due to abuse. They then compared rates of referral for suspected abuse by race/ethnicity, and by likelihood of abuse.

Of the 388 children in the study, 196 (51 percent) were minority (black or Hispanic) and 192 (49 percent) were white. Based on the review of the medical record, 54 of the minority children (28 percent) and 24 of the white children (12 percent) had injuries that were likely due to child abuse—a minority/white ratio of 2.3:1. When the researchers then looked at which children were reported as likely to be victims of abuse, they found that 101 of the minority children (53 percent) and 43 of the white children (23 percent) had reports filed—also a minority/white ratio of 2.3:1. On the surface, it would seem that the greater rate of referral of minority children reflected the greater likelihood that minority children are the victims of abuse.

A closer look, however, raises concerns over stereotype bias on the part of the physicians treating these children. The researchers then looked at the children judged likely to have accidental injuries and not abuse. Of the minority children, 108 (55 percent) were judged likely to have accidental injuries, while 145 of the white children (76 percent) were likely to have had accidental injuries. Despite the likelihood that the injuries were accidental, physicians were substantially more likely to refer minority children in this group than they were white children. Among those children with probable accidental injuries who were covered by private insurance (18 percent of minority and 73 percent of white children), researchers found that 15 percent of minority children and 7 percent of white children were referred for suspected abuse—a minority/white ratio of 2.1:1. Among children with accidental injuries covered by Medicaid insurance (82 percent of minority and 27 percent of white children), 32 percent of minority children and 18 percent of white children were referred—a minority/white ratio of 1.8:1. This compares to a minority/white referral rate of 1.1:1 for children found likely to have been the victims of abuse.

Under the pressure of treating injured children, often in an emergency room context, it appears that physicians were using the following reasoning:

1. Minority children are more likely to be the victim of child abuse than white children.
2. This injured child is minority.
3. Therefore it is more likely that this child's injuries are the result of child abuse than if the child had been white, and I will accordingly use a lower threshold of suspicion to report this family to Child Protective Services.

The physicians applied this reasoning, even when the available clinical information indicated that the likely cause of the injury was accidental. As a result, many more of the minority children seen at this hospital for treatment of their injuries had reports of suspected abuse submitted, regardless of the likely nature of the injury. These results parallel a study by Ellsworth and colleagues (2010) evaluating the likelihood that infants born to black mothers would be screened for having been exposed *in utero* to drugs of abuse. The authors found that, in a manner similar to the study of suspected child abuse, "Infants born to black mothers were more likely than those born to white mothers to have screening performed whether they met [established] screening criteria or did not" (p. e1379).

Puumala and colleagues (2016) surveyed 154 ED physicians who worked at hospitals in the upper Midwest that had a large number of American Indian children as patients. They administered a survey that assessed a physician's level of explicit bias against American Indian children. They found that those physicians who reported seeing larger numbers of American Indian children had, on average, higher levels of explicit bias against these children. Given the important role the emergency department plays in providing care for many American Indian children, the authors voiced concern that "given the unique, time-stressed environment of EDs, providers may have increased reliance on classification and cognitive short-cuts leading to greater use of stereotypes" (p. 562).

The practice of medicine often involves making clinical judgments and treatment decisions under conditions of tremendous uncertainty. Knowing what to do when you do not have all the facts is the basis of "the art of medicine." When to recommend a kidney transplant, when to recommend a cardiac revascularization procedure, when to administer pain medication, when to recommend that a patient with a sore knee see an orthopedist are all examples of medical judgment under conditions of uncertainty. Each represents a condition under which unconscious racial or ethnic stereotypes may influence the decision of a physician, even one who abhors and disavows the type of explicit racism exemplified by Bull Connor.

Referred to as "stereotype bias," this type of reasoning has been recognized for some time by social psychologists as distinct from the type of explicit racism described above by Appiah. Research by Devine (1989) suggests that negative racial stereotypes are "automatically activated in the presence of a member . . . of the stereotyped group. However, conscious racism and unconscious stereotype bias, are conceptually distinct cognitive structures" (p. 5). Fiske (1998) reviewed the social psychology literature on stereotype bias. She found that the use of racial stereotypes is an unconscious process that is often used to assist in decision making under situations of uncertainty or inadequate data. It is based on cultural norms learned early in the process of psychological development. "People learn cultural stereotypes early, before they can critically evaluate the validity of these (predominantly negative) stereotypes. Through repeated encounters in a variety of contexts, the stereotypes become automatically activated" (p. 360).

Thus, a person who has consciously disavowed the racist belief "that members of different races differ in respects that *warrant* the differential treatment" (Appiah 1990, p. 5) may nonetheless invoke unconscious negative stereotypes of black patients under certain circumstances. This appears to be the process invoked by my colleague in his recommendation about the patient with the sore knee, by the physicians in the studies by van Ryn and colleagues, and in other research discussed above. While these physicians discriminated against their black patients based on unconscious stereotypes, they are not racists in the way that Bull Connor was a racist.

Unconscious Aversion as a Form of Racial Bias

Another form of racial bias may affect physicians, even though it exerts its effects unconsciously, as illustrated in the following narrative of a physician-patient encounter. The patient, a colleague of mine, is a nationally known scholar. A number of years ago he was disappointed to learn that his primary care physician, from whom he had received only the best of care for more than a decade, was planning to retire.

"Oh, and before I forget," his doctor told him, "I realize that I never arranged for you to see a skin specialist about that rash on your legs that never seems to get better. I've set you up to see one of the best dermatologists in town. He can see you next week." The doctor's office had contacted the dermatologist's office to request that they squeeze the patient, a senior professor at the university, into the dermatologist's busy schedule. For such a distinguished individual, they were only too happy to oblige.

When he arrived at the dermatologist's office, my colleague was given a clipboard and asked to complete the requisite paperwork—name, insurance carrier, employer, occupation, and the like. He was then shown into the examination room. The dermatologist soon opened the exam room door, the clipboard and recently completed forms in his hand. "Professor _____?" he called out, and then stepped fully into the room. As my colleague reports, when the dermatologist realized the black man sitting in the room was the professor, his jaw dropped. The doctor spent a hasty few minutes in the room with the patient, holding tightly to the clipboard the entire time. He rarely established eye contact with the patient and did not come physically close to him. He never touched the patient's skin, even to shake hands.

The *Oxford English Dictionary* defines an *aversion* as "a mental attitude of opposition or repugnance; a fixed, habitual dislike; an antipathy." It seems clear that, as described by my colleague, the dermatologist had an aversion to black patients. It was most likely not a conscious attitude; rather, it was an unintended and probably unconscious reaction to seeing that a black man was the distinguished professor he had agreed to see.

Dovidio and Gaertner (1998) reviewed an extensive research literature that documents what they refer to as aversive bias toward blacks and other minorities. They are careful to distinguish aversive bias from explicit racism of the type described above by Appiah. They see explicit racism as a conscious attitude that is expressed openly, while aversive bias "represents a subtle, often unintentional, form of bias that characterizes many white Americans who possess strong egalitarian values and who believe that they are not prejudiced" (p. 5). Rather than the open hostility toward blacks felt by explicit racists, aversive bias often involves "discomfort, uneasiness, disgust, and sometimes fear."

It seems apparent that the dermatologist my colleague saw exhibited aversive bias. No doubt he would ardently deny any conscious feeling of prejudice toward blacks— he would likely have asserted that he was "color-blind" in treating his patients. However, his behavior, as described by my colleague, is nearly identical to that cited by the IOM report on *Unequal Treatment*: "Socially conditioned implicit prejudice may be manifested in healthcare providers' nonverbal behaviors reflecting anxiety (for example, increased rate of blinking), aversion (for example, reduced eye contact) or avoidance (for example, more closed postures) when interacting with minority rather than white patients" (Smedley et al. 2003, p. 162).

As described by Dovidio and Gaertner (1998), the social psychology research literature suggests that those who exhibit aversive bias "frequently assert that they are color-blind; if they do not see race, then it follows that no one can accuse them of being racist. Finally, their negative feelings will get expressed, but in subtle, rationalizable ways that may ultimately disadvantage minorities or unfairly benefit the majority group" (p. 7).

Appiah (1990), in his discussion of conscious and unconscious forms of racial bias, acknowledges that unconscious, aversive bias may be qualitatively different than conscious, extrinsic racism: "To the extent that their prejudices are really not subject to any kind of rational control, we may wonder whether it is right to treat such people as morally responsible for the acts their racial prejudice motivates, or morally reprehensible for holding the views to which their prejudice leads them" (p. 9).

For many in the United States, it was easy to see Bull Connor as morally responsible and morally reprehensible for holding his views and acting on them, to the substantial detriment of the black children marching peacefully in Birmingham in 1963. It is much more difficult to see the dermatologist as morally reprehensible.

When a person is suddenly startled, they typically will blink their eyes. The more startling the stimulus, the stronger the eye-blink will be. This is not a conscious reaction—it reflects an unconscious reaction to an external stimulus. Using electronic sensors attached to the skin around the eyes, Phelps and colleagues (2000) were able to measure the strength with which research subjects blinked their eyes in response to certain images shown on a computer screen. They showed a group of research subjects a random series of black and white faces. The subjects tended to blink more strongly when they were shown a black face than when they were shown a white face. They did not do so consciously; their response was unintended and unconscious. They then studied brain images of the subjects obtained from an

MRI machine while they were being shown the series of faces. The subjects' brains tended to show activation in different areas of the amygdala (a region of the brain involved in emotional learning and evaluation) when shown a white face rather than a black face. The researchers interpreted these findings as suggesting that subjects go through different unconscious evaluative processes in response to white and black faces. These unconscious emotional reactions reflect previous social learning and not conscious attitudes.

If I unconsciously blink harder when I see a black face than I do when I see a white face, will I also have a more negative implicit response to the black face? Greenwald and colleagues (1998) developed an Implicit Association Test (IAT) that shows subjects two sets of words and sees how quickly they can identify the similarity or difference in the concepts represented by the words. Subjects responded more quickly when the words were similar ("flower" and "pleasant") than if the words represented disparate concepts ("insect" and "pleasant").

Researchers have adapted the IAT as an online test of associations between facial images and words (Project Implicit). Available online, subjects are shown simultaneously a word and a picture of a face, and are asked to indicate as quickly as possible if the word has positive or negative connotations. The face is changed at random from that of a white person to that of a black person. Studies of more than 1 million online subjects have found that white subjects in the United States consistently take a longer time to identify a word as having positive connotations when it is paired with a black face than when it is paired with a white face. Conversely, they are quicker to identify a word with negative connotations when it is paired with a black face than with a white face (Nosek et al. 2007). Subjects who demonstrate these implicit associations of white+good and black+bad will usually state that they have no personal race bias. Black subjects typically do not show this implicit association.

Many physicians have taken the IAT, and have demonstrated the same pattern of implicit associations as the general public: white physicians demonstrate the association, while black physicians do not (Sabin and colleagues 2009). One study looked at the IAT responses of 210 primary care physicians in Denver, Colorado, and demonstrated the pattern of implicit association for both black and Hispanic faces (Blair and colleagues 2013). A study of 211 first year medical students at Johns Hopkins University (Haider et al. 2011) found an implicit negative association with black faces demonstrated by white and Asian medical students, but not by black or Hispanic students. Interestingly, when the students repeated the test with faces representing upper class and lower class individuals, they found a similar pattern of response. In an editorial response to this study, van Ryn and Saha (2011) suggested that "Implicit attitudes may contribute to unequal care by influencing not only physicians' assessments and clinical decision making but also the way they interact with patients. Implicit attitudes affect verbal communication and nonverbal behaviors, such as rates of blinking, eye contact, and indicators of friendliness, even among people with egalitarian explicit attitudes" (p. 996).

Dovidio (2001) described 50 years of research documenting the presence and power of unconscious racial bias in large segments of our population. Through the experience of growing up and living in our racially divided society, individuals may unconsciously come to associate certain negative characteristics with members of a minority race or ethnicity. The person who acts based on these internalized associations is often unaware that another person's race may have influenced their decision. While most people openly endorse fair and equal treatment of all racial groups and disavow overt racism, they nonetheless harbor some type of negative feelings or association toward blacks or other minorities. As Dovidio describes it, this type of unconscious, unintended bias is "embedded fundamentally in people's group identities and in a society's institutions and its culture" (p. 830).

Lawrence (1987) reviewed the legal implications of racial discrimination that is rooted in unconscious bias: "Americans share a common historical and cultural heritage in which racism has played and still plays a dominant role. Because of this shared experience, we also inevitably share many ideas, attitudes, and beliefs that attach significance to an individual's race and induce negative feelings and opinions about non-whites. . . . We do not recognize the ways in which our cultural experience has influenced our beliefs about race or the occasions on which those beliefs affect our actions" (p. 322).

Because of the unconscious nature of certain types of racial bias rooted in the cultural history of the society in which we grew up, it is difficult to attach the legal concept of conscious intent to these biases, even when their outcomes are clearly discriminatory.

Racial Bias in Police Responses to Civilians: Black Lives Do Matter

In their review of two decades of research into experiences of racial discrimination and health status, Lewis and colleagues (2015) found "consistent associations between exposure to discrimination and a wide range of . . . diagnosed mental disorders as well as objective physical health outcomes" (p. 407). They also reported "that across studies, higher-SES African Americans consistently report more discrimination than do their lower-SES counterparts" (p. 420).

A team of researchers from National Public Radio, the Robert Wood Johnson Foundation, and Harvard T. H. Chan School of Public Health has published a series of reports of surveys of a nationally representative sample of adults from a range of racial and ethnic backgrounds. In their report on the experiences of African Americans (National Public Radio et al. 2017), they found that "African Americans report extensive experiences of discrimination, across a range of situations" (p. 1). The three most common contexts in which African Americans reported experiencing discrimination were being paid equally at work, applying to jobs, and interacting with the police. A central finding of the study was that 60 percent of survey respondents reported that they or a family member had been unfairly stopped or unfairly treated by the police because they are black. They also found that 4 in 10 respondents reported that people have acted afraid of them because of their race. Consistent with the results reported by Lewis and colleagues, higher-income blacks were more likely to report this experience than lower-income blacks.

Following the killing of Trayvon Martin in Florida in 2013 and the subsequent acquittal of his killer, activists within the African American community formed the Black Lives Matter movement. The subsequent killing by police of Michael Brown in Ferguson, Missouri, and Eric Garner in New York City brought increased national attention to the problem of police interactions with black civilians ending in the death of the civilian.

In 2015 the *New York Times* reported on a speech given by F.B.I. Director James B. Comey about the growing national attention to race relations between police and African Americans (Schmidt 2015). As reported in the story, "Mr. Comey said that some officers scrutinize African-Americans more closely using a mental shortcut that 'becomes almost irresistible and maybe even rational by some lights' because black men are arrested at much higher rates than white men." In his speech Mr. Comey cited research showing that unconscious race bias was widespread, including among police officers.

Using data compiled by the *Washington Post*, Nix and colleagues (2017) were able to evaluate the circumstances involved in 990 fatal police shootings occurring in 2015. They looked for evidence of two principal characteristics of the shooting: whether the civilian had not been attacking the officer at the time of the shooting, and whether the civilian had been unarmed at the time of the shooting. As described by the authors, "Our findings showed that citizens in the other racial/ethnic group were significantly more likely than Whites to have not been attacking the officer(s) or other civilians and that Blacks were more than twice as likely as Whites to have been unarmed when they were shot and killed by police" (p. 328). These findings lead the authors to conclude: "These findings suggest evidence of implicit bias . . . officers subconsciously perceived minority civilians to have been a greater threat than they were" (p. 329).

Researchers at Stanford University have established a collaborative relationship with the police department in Oakland, California. Oakland has a racially diverse population, and was one of the principal cities included in the Alameda County Study cited in Chapter 3. The researchers were provided access to transcribed body camera footage from vehicle stops with 682 black motorists and 299 white motorists. Based on their analysis of the quality and intonation of the words and phrases used by the police in their interaction with the motorist they had stopped, they reported that "officers speak with consistently less respect toward black versus white community members, even after controlling for the race of the officer, the severity of the infraction, the location of the stop, and the outcome of the stop" (Voigt et al. 2017, p. 6521). This differential pattern of speaking to black motorists as compared to white motorists was evident even before the motorist had a chance to respond to the police officer. From the analysis of these interactions, the researchers were able to conclude that "experiences of respect or disrespect in personal interactions with police officers play a central role in community members' judgments of how procedurally fair the police are as an institution, as well as the community's willingness to support or cooperate with the police" (p. 6524).

Earlier in this chapter I described the outcomes of the study by van Ryn and Burke (2000) of cardiologists' impression of the patients they had recently treated. Compared to their white patients, the physicians in the study perceived their black patients as less intelligent, less well educated, and less likely to have the personal characteristics most conducive to a successful rehabilitation from a cardiac procedure, even when the patients' actual levels of education, income, and personal desire to participate in rehabilitation were identical to that of white patients.

I concluded that unconscious race bias, rather than explicit racism, was the most likely cause of this outcome. Again, the higher rate at which the parents of black children treated in the emergency room were reported for possible child abuse, as well as the high levels of race bias experienced by American Indian children treated in the emergency room, reflect an unconscious stereotyping of minority patients by physicians. Addressing the issue of unconscious race bias as a central and continuing issue of American society, Purdie-Vaughns and Williams (2015) write that "Unlike explicit bias, which reflects people's attitudes and beliefs that they consciously endorse, implicit bias results from cognitive processes that operate at a level below conscious awareness and without intentional control" (p. 341). Citing the growing research documenting the role of implicit bias in affecting interpersonal interactions, they offer an important conclusion about the role of this bias in impacting the lives of black Americans. "[P]sychologists have repeatedly demonstrated a strong and persistent finding: blackness in the U.S. is linked to perceptions of crime and danger. . . . Decades of research using more sophisticated methods reveals that blackness leads people to evaluate (without intent) ambiguously assertive behavior as aggressive, quickens the speed at which people decide to shoot someone holding a weapon, and increases the probability that someone would discharge a weapon at all" (p. 342).

Police officers as well as physicians treat black citizens and black patients differently based largely on the role of unconscious bias, often with tragic outcomes for black lives. Understanding how to end that bias remains a central question of social policy.

In 2015 Dr. Mary Bassett, Commissioner of the New York City Department of Health and Mental Hygiene, described a meeting she had with a group of medical students shortly after a New York grand jury had decided not to indict the police officer involved in the death of Eric Garner while in police custody. The medical students wanted to know how they could support the Black Lives Matter movement as part of their medical education and subsequent medical practice. Dr. Bassett subsequently published an article in the *New England Journal of Medicine* offering her response (Bassett 2015). "Should health professionals be accountable not only for caring for individual black patients but also for fighting the racism? . . . I believe that the dearth of critical thinking and writing on racism and health in mainstream medical journals represents a disservice to the medical students who approached me—and to all of us" (pp. 1085–86).

An accompanying article by Ansell and McDonald (2015) concurred with Dr. Bassett, especially in the context of medical education. "For the sake of not only black lives but all lives, we should heed our students' call to examine the implicit biases in our academic medical centers . . . most important, we should talk about bias, with our students, our faculties, our staff, our administrations, and our patients. Maybe then we'll have a chance to finally eliminate the racial health care disparities that persist in the United States" (p. 1089).

Differentiating among the Forms of Racial Bias

After exhaustive study, the authors of the IOM report on racial and ethnic disparities in health care concluded that "bias, stereotyping, prejudice, and clinical uncertainty on the part of healthcare providers may contribute to racial and ethnic disparities in healthcare" (Smedley et al. 2003, p. 12). We now are able to see that the racial bias the report is referring to may come in many forms. It is important to consider what the implications are of the various forms of bias, and to do so from the point of view of both the patient and the physician.

From the point of view of the patient, different forms of racial bias on the part of the physician will have similar outcomes, regardless of the type or source of the bias. Not surprisingly, when black patients perceive that they have experienced race-based discrimination in their care, they also perceive the quality of the care they have received to be lower (Sorkin and colleagues 2010). Patients who perceive physician race bias will often be less forthcoming with their physician and less likely to adhere to the treatment that physician recommends (Peek et al. 2010). They will trust that physician less, and as a consequence be less likely to adhere to recommended treatment for conditions such as hypertension and diabetes, and less likely to follow through with recommendations for cancer screening (Elder et al. 2012; Lee and Lin 2009; Yang et al. 2011).

If a black patient is denied treatment that a white patient in similar circumstances would have received, it makes relatively little difference if the bias that generated the disparity was intended or unintended, conscious or unconscious. My colleague who was treated poorly by the dermatologist knew enough about the roots of racial bias to realize that the aversion shown on the physician's face as he entered the room was probably unconscious. Despite this realization, my colleague was furious at the way he had been treated. In subsequent conversations I had with my patient with the sore knee, it was clear that he understood that his regular doctor had accused him of theft based on an unconscious negative stereotype of blacks. This understanding did little to buffer the pain and embarrassment he felt at being unjustly accused of being a thief.

If the outcomes of treatment are disparate for a black and a white patient based on race, it makes little difference if their physician was a conscious racist or a self-described "color-blind" individual who abhors explicit racism, yet nonetheless harbors unconscious aversion to blacks based on persisting cultural norms internalized as a child. It is understandable that, from the perspective of the patient, they have been the victim of racism. As summarized by Dovidio and Gaertner (1998), "Even though these negative feelings . . . may be unconscious and rooted in normal processes, this does not imply that this bias is either excusable or immutable. . . . Racial bias, whether subtle or blatant, is inconsistent with standards of fairness and justice" (p. 31).

From the point of view of physicians, however, it may be very important to differentiate among the various forms of bias, for without doing so, it may be difficult or impossible to eliminate bias of all types. If, as patients may understandably do, we dichotomize racism—that is, turn it into a category in which you either are a racist or you are not, with no middle ground—then it is unlikely that physicians who disavow conscious racism yet harbor unconscious biases will be willing to acknowledge their own tendency toward bias. Acknowledgment of that bias is of course a necessary precursor to eliminating it.

If I simply call a medical colleague a racist when I see them make clinical decisions I feel confident would not have been made if the patient had been white instead of black, they will simply close their ears and stop listening. My colleagues know who Bull Connor was. By calling them racist, I am in essence saying that they are no different from Bull Connor. If, on the other hand, I address the issue in ways that raise the possibility that a patient's race or ethnicity may have influenced a colleague's clinical judgment, without labeling my colleague as racist, I may be able to assist them to see how unconscious bias had entered into the decision process. I will illustrate this principle with a description of two patients I treated within a few months of each other.

The first patient was a well-known (white) professor in his sixties who had fallen onto his outstretched wrist while playing tennis. The fracture in his wrist extended into the joint, and had created an uneven area on what is supposed to be the perfectly smooth joint surface. When I called the orthopedist and described the fracture, he said, "That sounds like a nasty break. He'll probably need surgery to reduce his chances of developing arthritis in that wrist." The surgery worked reasonably well, and the professor went back to playing tennis.

The second patient was a professional landscaper (Mexican American) in his fifties who had fallen onto his outstretched wrist while playing soccer with his family. The fracture in his wrist extended into the joint and had created an uneven area on what is supposed to be the perfectly smooth joint surface. When I called the orthopedist on call and described the fracture, he said, "That sounds like a nasty break." As it was a Sunday, he instructed me to apply a splint to the wrist and have the patient see the on-call orthopedist the next day. After about a week, I checked the patient's chart to see how things had gone. The orthopedist he had seen had recommended a cast instead of surgery.

What was striking to me about these two cases was that the fractures were nearly identical. You could have laid one set of x-rays over the other and the bones would have lined up nearly exactly. I am not an orthopedist, so I did not have the training to second-guess an orthopedist's judgment as to when surgery is appropriate and when it is not. So, I sent a simple note to the chair of the orthopedic department, posing the following question: "If the patient had been a white professor rather than a Mexican American laborer, would he have been placed in a cast rather than undergoing surgery?" The only word I ever heard back was a week or so later, when

I received a copy of the operative report of the surgical repair of the laborer's wrist fracture. Rather than discussing whether the treating orthopedist had been biased, he and the department chief simply reviewed the case from a new perspective. The result of this review was a recommendation that the landscaper receive surgery.

If instead I had accused my orthopedic colleague of being a racist, harboring stereotypes or biases toward Mexican Americans, my letter would have been rejected out of hand. By asking the question of whether the patient would have received the same treatment if he were of a different racial/ethnic group and had a different occupation, I appear to have been able to avert a potential disparate outcome.

I will repeat here the quote from Dr. Sally Satel from the debate about the role of racial bias as a source of disparities in the treatment of heart disease. In response to the question, "Is racial bias one of the reasons for disparities?" Satel replied, "Possibly. It's certainly a hypothesis that people can entertain; but thus far, virtually every study that has been held up as an example of bias, I have found unconvincing" (American Heart Association 2001, p. 13). Satel appears to be rejecting out of hand the possibility that physicians exhibit racial bias. In a book she wrote addressing the cause of racial disparities in care, she concludes that "the race-related differences that do exist in both access to health care and in health status are better understood—and remedied—from the vantage points of clinical need and health care financing—not race politics" (Satel 2000, p. 157). Elsewhere she states, "We must remain clear-eyed about the fact that uneven access to medical services, disparate knowledge of good health practices, and patients' own attitudes about their health—not discrimination and bias—underlie the vast majority of differences in health outcomes" (Satel 2001, p. 64).

When physicians categorically dismiss racial bias as a source of disparities in care, they are often responding defensively to their perception that to admit bias is tantamount to admitting being a racist. It is crucially important for physicians to understand the nature of negative stereotypes and feelings of discomfort that are triggered unconsciously in many circumstances when a white physician who grew up in the United States encounters a patient who is black, Mexican American, or of another racial or ethnic minority.

I remember the way racial epithets were woven into the children's games and jargon I learned from my parents and grandparents. I can still get a vague sense of discomfort when I encounter a black person unexpectedly. I have learned to recognize it and to know where it comes from.

Physicians generally are well respected members of our society. Our high level of education and willingness to take responsibility for the health of our patients often place us in a position of deep trust. Respect and trust as professionals do not, however, make us immune to the lingering effects of beliefs and attitudes learned and internalized through growing up in a racially diverse and often racially divided society. This fundamental truth—that physicians are prone to the same unconscious racial beliefs and attitudes as others—was reflected in the conclusions of the IOM's *Unequal Treatment* report: "While it is reasonable to assume that the vast majority of healthcare providers find prejudice morally abhorrent and at odds with their professional values, healthcare providers, like other members of society, may not recognize manifestations of prejudice in their own behavior" (Smedley et al. 2003, p. 162).

Holding unconscious negative stereotypes of and associations with black and other minority racial/ethnic groups is an expected outcome of growing up in a society with a long history of racial exclusion and discrimination. Without conscious intent and awareness, these biases do not make the person who holds them a Bull Connor racist. Before they can be disempowered, however, and the disparate outcomes that stem from them eliminated, these biases must first be acknowledged and understood.

When, if Ever, Is It Appropriate to Use a Patient's Race/Ethnicity to Help Guide Medical Decisions?

In the previous chapters, I have come to a number of conclusions, grounded in the research literature on SES, race/ethnicity, and health.

- Most health disparities among groups are caused by differences in SES. These disparities are caused by a combination of the material effects of lower SES and the adverse physiologic effects of lower SES that accumulate over time.
- Blacks, Hispanics, and other minority racial/ethnic groups typically have worse health status across a wide range of health status measures. Most of these disparities can be explained by parallel disparities in SES. However, there are many instances of continuing disparities after taking into account SES.
- The racial categories originally proposed by scientists in the 1700s and still in use today have little biologic basis; instead, they reflect principally social convention as to how to categorize the human species. Evidence consistently demonstrates that there is more biologic variation within groups categorized as races than there is among these groups.
- For a range of medical conditions and treatments, there is continuing racial/ethnic disparity in the quality and availability of medical care, with blacks and other minority groups receiving lower quality and less care. These disparities are caused by a combination of differences in patient preferences and differences in the way physicians respond to individuals of different race/ethnicity.

From the knowledge we have gained studying these issues, it may seem problematic whether the race or ethnicity of a patient should *ever* be used in making a clinical decision. Certainly other demographic characteristics should be and are used in making treatment choices. Gender is often highly relevant to the evaluation of risk and the selection of treatment. Similarly, it is not only appropriate but often mandatory to consider age in the clinical context. In the face of overwhelming evidence that race and ethnicity are social constructions with little biologic basis, is it ever appropriate for a physician or other health care practitioner to use race to predict the expected risks of disease or the expected outcomes of treatment? I refer to this as "the practitioner's dilemma" (Barr 2005).

Especially among physicians and other practitioners who are acutely aware of the issues of racial bias discussed in the previous chapter, it is essential not to use a patient's race or ethnicity in ways that may result in a discriminatory outcome. In focus group discussions with primary care physicians in five metropolitan areas of the United States, Bonham and colleagues (2009) explored this issue. The physicians they spoke with were generally aware of the complexity of using a patient's race in a clinical context. They found, however, that for many of the physicians, "race in the clinical setting is a confusing and poorly defined construct. Although most physicians believed patients' race had important clinical implications, no consensus emerged regarding why race was useful in the clinical encounter. . . . Furthermore, some physicians expressed discomfort with explicitly talking with patients about their race and how the physician was incorporating the patient's race into their clinical recommendations" (p. 284).

This issue is crucially important, yet substantially complex. To explore it, I consider the following hypothetical patients with differing medical conditions:

- A white researcher such as myself who arrives in equatorial Africa for an extended period of field research
- Whites and blacks with glaucoma, a chronic disease of the eyes
- Three women—one a white Ashkenazi Jew, one a white who is not Jewish, and a black who is not Jewish—all concerned about breast cancer risk
- Whites and blacks with high blood pressure who need to be started on medication for their blood pressure
- Whites and blacks with congestive heart failure, caused by chronic weakening of the heart muscle
- Two women—one white and one black—both with a college education and both in the early stages of pregnancy

Race and the Prevention of Skin Cancer

Imagine a white professor from Stanford University who undertakes a 12-month research project in a country such as Kenya, situated on the equator. After arriving in Kenya, the researcher consults a Kenyan doctor about any special medical risks associated with field research in that country. Knowing the deleterious effects of ultraviolet rays and the increased risk of skin cancer associated with them, as well as the extreme intensity of ultraviolet sunlight in equatorial areas, the doctor recommends that the researcher apply a high-grade sun block to all exposed areas on a regular basis. Of course, the doctor does not make this recommendation to most of his patients, but is concerned about the researcher because of the relative scarcity of melanin in his skin cells (that is, his "white" skin).

Recall from Chapter 5 that, from the *Oxford English Dictionary*, a principal definition of *race* is "one of the great divisions of mankind, having certain physical peculiarities in common." One of the physical peculiarities of white people is that their skin, while not actually white, is nonetheless quite pale due to the relatively low melanin content in the skin cells. (Melanin absorbs many ultraviolet rays, thus protecting the skin from cancer risk.) From an evolutionary perspective, paler skin with less melanin has a distinct advantage in northern climates where there is relatively little sunlight. The lower melanin content facilitates the production of vitamin D and in turn the creation of bone. The farther from the equator one is, the less the annual sunlight, and the lower the associated risk of skin cancer; the closer to the equator, the larger the sun exposure, with accordingly higher risks of skin cancer. Thus, differences in skin melanin content, and corresponding differences in skin color, are one of the "physical peculiarities" used over the centuries to divide racial groups. Of course, as we have seen, those divisions based on skin pigmentation are often quite imprecise. Those with dark skin in sub-Saharan Africa are considered black by race; those with often equally dark skin in New Guinea or parts of Australia, also areas close to the equator, were historically considered Asian but now are classified as Native Hawaiian or Other Pacific Islander by race. Finally, those with deeply pigmented skin in areas of India have historically been considered to be Asian, even though their genetic ancestry is closer to that of white Europeans than to East Asians.

The complexities of racial classification aside, to the physician in Kenya the researcher from Stanford is white and needs to be treated with extra care in matters of skin cancer risk. I doubt I or any other white researcher would take issue with the Kenyan physician's use of my race in recommending treatment to prevent skin cancer. The physician was responding simply to a physical characteristic (or "peculiarity" as the dictionary refers to it) typical of my race that has both a well-defined biological basis (less melanin in the skin cells) and a directly relevant medical outcome (higher risk of skin cancer), without attaching any further meaning to the concept of race. Under these circumstances, I would not feel as though I had been stigmatized in any way by the physician's use of race in recommending treatment.

Race and the Treatment of Glaucoma

Glaucoma is a condition affecting the eyes, in which the pressure of the fluid inside the eye builds up to abnormal levels. Over time this increased pressure (referred to as increased intraocular pressure) can cause permanent damage to the eyes, including causing permanent blindness. One study from 1991 found that "glaucoma is four to six times more prevalent among blacks" and that "glaucoma-related blindness is between six and eight times more common among black Americans than among whites" (Javitt et al. 1991, p. 1418). The authors concluded that one of the reasons for the higher rate of blindness was because older blacks were not receiving treatment for their glaucoma at the same rate as older whites.

A series of medications can be used to reduce intraocular pressure, thereby reducing the chances of blindness caused by glaucoma. One of those medicines is travoprost, which is applied as eyedrops. It was originally sold under the brand name of Travatan, with detailed prescribing information provided by its manufacturer (Alcon Laboratories 2006b). As part of that information, the manufacturer advised physicians using it, "in clinical studies, patients with open-angle glaucoma or ocular hypertension and baseline pressure of 25–27 mm Hg [normal being less than 20 mm Hg] who were treated with Travatan˚ ophthalmic solution 0.004% dosed once daily in the evening demonstrated 7–8 mm Hg reductions in intraocular pressure [IOP]. In subgroup analyses of these studies, mean IOP reduction in black patients was up to 1.8 mm Hg greater than in non-black patients. It is not known at this time whether this difference is attributed to race or to heavily pigmented irides [irides is the plural of iris—the circular part of the eye that gives it its color]." Based on findings such as this, Travatan was marketed to physicians and to the public as "the first glaucoma drug to demonstrate greater effectiveness in black patients" (Alcon Laboratories 2006a).

The prescribing information also cautioned physicians that Travatan may cause permanent darkening of the color of the eyes and eyelids as a side effect. "Travatan˚ may gradually change eye color, increasing the amount of brown pigmentation in the iris by increasing the number of melanosomes (pigment granules) in melanocytes."

If a physician has a black patient with glaucoma and, cognizant of the historic undertreatment of glaucoma in blacks, wants to give this patient the best possible care, should the physician choose Travatan based on the patient's race? Similarly, should the physician avoid Travatan in a white patient with glaucoma? There are two aspects to these questions, one having to do with the effectiveness of the drug and one having to do with its chances of permanent eye and skin darkening as a side effect.

While the drug was somewhat more effective in blacks as a group than in whites as a group, it apparently is clinically effective in both groups. It lowered the average pressure in whites by between 5 and 7 mm Hg, bringing the average pressure close to the normal range of less than 20 mm Hg. The reduction in blacks was 1–1.8 mm Hg greater, lowering the average pressure to slightly below 20 mm Hg.

The mechanism by which the drug reduces pressure within the eye appears to have something to do with the amount of melanin pigment in the iris. The drug often causes the amount of melanin in the iris to increase in association with its clinical effect. The manufacturer appropriately points out that blacks, on average, are more likely to have dark brown eyes with more melanin in them than whites. Those individuals with blue eyes (a condition much more common among whites than among blacks) have essentially no melanin in their iris. Thus, it cannot be determined if the apparent clinical advantage for black patients is because they are black, or because they have brown eyes. There are substantial numbers of white patients with dark brown eyes. It seems more likely that the clinical advantage of Travatan is for those with dark brown eyes, regardless of their race. Similarly, the drug might be expected to be less effective in patients, white or black, with blue eyes. Thus, in deciding whether to use this drug in patients with glaucoma, a physician might be mistaken to use this drug based on race rather than on the color of the patient's eyes (a characteristic that is associated with race but is not the same as race).

There is a second factor the physician must consider in choosing whether to prescribe Travatan—its propensity to cause permanent darkening of the iris and eyelids through the production of increased amounts of melanin. If a patient is black, with the dark skin that is the "peculiar characteristic" of the black race and the dark brown eye pigment that usually goes along with dark skin, the implications of increased melanin production may be less of an issue than for a white patient, with the light skin that is the "peculiar characteristic" of the white race. In this case, as in the case of the white researcher in equatorial Africa, it seems quite appropriate to avoid the medication in whites because of its risk of skin darkening. This choice, based on skin color alone and without secondary meaning attached to the issue of race, seems quite appropriate. Before making the reverse choice, and automatically selecting the drug for blacks, the physician should first look at the patient's eyes as well as the patient's skin. Due to the extensive racial admixture that has occurred in the United States, persons who consider themselves to be black may actually have levels of melanin in the skin that are closer to the average white person's skin than the average black person's skin. The implications of the risk of permanent skin darkening around the eyes should be fully disclosed and discussed with a person categorized as black before selecting Travatan as the optimal treatment of glaucoma.

Race/Ethnicity and Breast Cancer

In 2015 242,476 women in the United States were newly diagnosed with breast cancer (CDC 2018). Among white women the rate per 100,000 population of newly identified cancer was 125.6, while it was 123.3 among black women and 93.6 among Hispanic women. Historically the incidence of breast cancer has been higher among white women than among black women. However, over the period 2008–12, the incidence rates converged (DeSantis et al. 2015).

Despite roughly comparable rates of occurrence, the death rate from breast cancer is significantly higher among blacks than among either whites or Hispanics. In 2015 the breast cancer death rate per 100,000 population was 27.6 among black women as compared to 19.8 among white women and 13.6 among Hispanic women. This disparity in death rates is due largely to the fact that, when breast cancer is diagnosed in a black woman, it is often at a later stage of development, having already spread to other parts of the body. When breast cancer is diagnosed, it can be localized to the breast without having spread to other parts of the body; it can have spread to regional lymph nodes located adjacent to the breast; or it can have spread to distant sites in the body such as the lung or the bone marrow. The survival rate for women newly diagnosed with breast cancer depends largely on the stage at which it was first identified. For the period 2007–13, 65 percent of white women were newly diagnosed with local disease, 27 percent were diagnosed with regional disease, and 5 percent were diagnosed with distant metastases. The comparable rates for black women were 55 percent local, 34 percent regional, and 9 percent distal (DeSantis et al. 2017).

While most cases of breast cancer develop in women who do not have a history of breast cancer in their family, as many as one woman in five who develops breast cancer will have either a mother, sister, or other close relative who also had breast cancer. A woman with a close relative who has had breast cancer has a risk of developing cancer in one of her breasts that is more than twice the risk of a woman without such a family history of breast cancer (National Cancer Institute 2006).

Given the increased risk among women with a family history of breast cancer, scientists have tried to identify specific genetic mutations that can be passed from mother to daughter, carrying with them an increased risk of breast cancer. While several of these mutations have been identified, the two most frequently identified are referred to as breast cancer genes 1 and 2, typically referred to by their acronyms BRCA1 and BRCA2.

In the US population as a whole, BRCA mutations occur in the range of once per 300 to 500 women. A woman who does have either BRCA1 or BRCA2 has a

60 to 85 percent chance of developing breast cancer at some time in her life (Nelson et al. 2005). Understandably, there has been considerable interest in identifying those women who have inherited a BRCA mutation before they develop breast cancer. While the precise benefits of early awareness of a BRCA mutation in terms of preventing death from breast cancer are not clear, nevertheless there is interest in developing and making widely available tests to identify BRCA gene mutations.

From the study of the BRCA genes, we have become aware that the frequency with which a mutation is present (especially the BRCA1 gene) is especially high among women of Ashkenazi Jewish ancestry. As I discussed in Chapter 5, Ashkenazi Jewish ancestry is not a race in itself, but rather identifies an ethnic group within the white race. Either a BRCA1 or BRCA2 gene is present in 2.5 percent of Ashkenazi Jewish women in the United States—a rate of 1 in 40—as compared to the 1 in 400 rate for the overall population. Knowing that a woman is of Ashkenazi Jewish ancestry identifies her as having a tenfold greater chance of carrying a BRCA mutation (Rubinstein 2004).

A physician who treats women for general health maintenance issues will include routine breast cancer screening in their practice. Routinely this will include mammography screening for women between the ages of 50 and 74, with screening for women aged 40–49 that is appropriate after women have been fully informed of the risks and benefits of screening for this age group (US Preventive Services Task Force 2016). However, if a woman in the physician's practice is found to have a BRCA gene, an entirely different series of issues arise: genetic counseling, possibly testing other family members, and consideration of the prophylactic removal of the breasts at a relatively young age in light of the extremely high incidence of cancer in women carrying a BRCA mutation.

Imagine that a physician has three women in their practice, all approximately the same age and all with the same level of health insurance: a white woman who identifies herself as an Ashkenazi Jew, a white woman who does not identify herself as an Ashkenazi Jew, and a black woman who does not identify herself as an Ashkenazi Jew. Should the physician recommend BRCA testing for all three women, or, given the tenfold higher risk, only for the Ashkenazi Jewish woman? Will the answer to this question change if it turns out that all three women have two relatives who had either breast cancer or ovarian cancer (a form of cancer also associated with the presence of a BRCA mutation)?

Nanda and colleagues (2005) addressed this question by testing 155 women, each from a family with a clear history of breast or ovarian cancer. Three of the women were Hispanic and two were Asian; none of these five women were found to have a BRCA mutation. Of the remaining women, 29 were Ashkenazi Jewish and white,

78 were white and not Jewish, and 43 were black and not Jewish. Among these subjects, they found:

- 20 of 29 (69 percent) Ashkenazi Jewish women had a BRCA mutation
- 36 of 78 (46 percent) white non-Jewish women had a BRCA mutation
- 12 of 43 (28 percent) black non-Jewish women had a BRCA mutation

These tests also showed that an additional 19 (44 percent) of the black women in the study had atypical sequencing in the gene involved in BRCA1 and BRCA2. These atypical gene sequences were neither characteristic of the BRCA mutation common to Ashkenazi Jewish women nor were they normal. The researchers were unable to determine precisely whether these atypical genes were the cause of the breast and ovarian cancers that had developed in the women's families. In their discussion of these findings, the researchers pointed out that, if they had only focused their genetic testing on racial or ethnic groups with high documented rates of BRCA1 and BRCA2 mutations, they would have missed the atypical gene mutations in the black women. Based on these considerations, the researchers concluded, "Irrespective of ancestry, early age at diagnosis and a family history of breast and ovarian cancer are the most powerful predictors of mutation status and should be used to guide clinical decision making" (p. 1925).

This conclusion was reinforced in research by Armstrong and colleagues (2005), who looked to see how often genetic counseling was recommended for women with a known family history of breast or ovarian cancer. They found that, even after taking into account SES and the availability of health insurance, "African American women with a family history of breast or ovarian cancer were significantly less likely to undergo genetic counseling for *BRCA1/2* testing than were white women with a family history of breast or ovarian cancer" (p. 1729).

In order to determine the factors that explain the pattern of later stage at diagnosis among black women, Iqbal and colleagues (2015) evaluated a large database of women newly diagnosed with breast cancer between 2004 and 2011. They looked specifically at women for whom the newly diagnosed breast cancer tumor had not grown to be larger than 2 cm. For most women, when the tumor is picked up at this size or smaller, it will not have spread to other parts of the body. However, for breast tumors with certain genetic mutations, these tumors can spread even before the tumor has grown to be 2 cm or greater. The authors found that black women with these small tumors were significantly more likely than white women to have had the tumor spread, and as a result had higher death rates than white women. Black women were also more likely to have a genetic mutation unrelated to the BRCA gene that increased their risk of early spread of the disease. These findings are consistent with earlier data showing that, for women between the ages of 20 and 50, black women have a breast cancer mortality rate that is higher than that of white women, with much of that difference due to certain types of aggressive cancer associated with genetic abnormalities (McCarthy et al. 2015).

The authors indicated that they were unable to determine the extent to which the higher rates of disease spread at the time of diagnosis was due to these genetic factors. As they described, "In our study, survival was associated with biological differences in tumor characteristics . . . but factors such as socioeconomic status, access to and use of health care, adherence to treatment, and comorbidity might also contribute to breast cancer disparities" (p. 172). In an editorial response to the article by Iqbal and colleagues, Daly and Olopade (2015) underscore the importance of considering both genetic and socioeconomic factors in seeking ways to reduce disparities in breast cancer mortality. "The biological differences in breast cancer by race/ethnicity, and failures in the US health care delivery system that lead to suboptimal care for black women and women of other races/ethnicities, can now begin to be addressed" (p. 141).

These results suggest that, in looking for possible genetic mutations that are tied to breast cancer and can be passed from mother to daughter, physicians should pay closest attention to the history of cancer in a woman's family. However, the fact remains that approximately 1 in 40 women of Ashkenazi Jewish ancestry may carry either the BRCA1 or the BRCA2 gene.

In addition to recommending genetic testing to all women, regardless of ancestry, who have a strong family history of breast or ovarian cancer, should they also recommend that all women of Ashkenazi Jewish ancestry undergo testing, regardless of family history? This question remains controversial, as it is still unclear whether early knowledge that the gene mutation is present will change the risk of dying from breast cancer. By the time a cancer caused by a BRCA mutation is detected, it may already have spread beyond the breast, substantially increasing the chances of death. In addition, there is an argument that singling out Ashkenazi Jewish women for testing may result in discrimination against them in things such as the cost of health or life insurance. Some have also expressed concern that, in light of the history of anti-Semitism related to the Holocaust, it would not be desirable to develop lists of women who are Jewish.

Knowledge that a certain genetic mutation that has been clearly connected to a specific illness is more common in a certain racial/ethnic group does not necessarily imply that physicians should focus their attention on testing for that mutation in that group alone. Other groups may have similar problems, identifiable from clinical history rather than ancestry, which could benefit from testing.

Focusing on a single racial/ethnic group may also trigger stigma or potential discrimination.

Others have argued that to ignore race/ethnicity completely in studying patterns of diseases in society is equally problematic. Burchard and colleagues (2003) argued that it is important for researchers to consider patterns of disease in different racial/ethnic groups in order to better understand those diseases. They argue that "excessive focus on racial or ethnic differences runs the risk of undervaluing the great diversity that exists among persons within groups. However, this risk needs to be weighed against the fact that in epidemiologic and clinical research, racial and ethnic categories are useful for generating and exploring hypotheses about environmental and genetic risk factors, as well as interactions between risk factors, for important medical outcomes" (p. 1171). In the clinical context, these authors suggest that "ignoring race and ethnic background would be detrimental to the very populations and persons that this approach allegedly seeks to protect . . . knowledge of a person's ancestry may facilitate testing, diagnosis, and treatment when genetic factors are involved" (p. 1174).

The physician is thus in the position of needing to know how race/ethnicity may affect patterns of disease and average outcomes from treatment, while at the same time taking care not to focus inappropriately on an individual's race/ethnicity to the exclusion of other pertinent factors. This need to balance group-level data with individual circumstances is further illustrated in the following section.

Race/Ethnicity and the Treatment of High Blood Pressure

In Chapter 5 we saw that blacks in the United States have higher rates of high blood pressure than whites. In Table 5.3 we saw that 41.8 percent of black men and 42.9 percent of black women have high blood pressure. The rate of high blood pressure in blacks is 35–50 percent higher than the rate for whites or Hispanics. From these data we might conclude that there is a racial predisposition to high blood pressure. However, cross-national data have shown that blacks from sub-Saharan Africa have one of the lowest rates of hypertension in the world, substantially lower than whites in either Europe or the United States (Cooper et al. 2005). Thus, the first lesson to be learned in assessing the risk of a black person for high blood pressure is how closely descended they are from sub-Saharan Africa. A black man or woman who has recently emigrated from Africa may be at no more risk—and possibly at substantially less risk—than a white man or woman living in this country.

Keeping this fact in mind, it is nonetheless extremely important to identify and treat high blood pressure when it exists in blacks in this country, to lessen the chances of complications such as heart disease, kidney failure, or stroke. As also described in Chapter 5, when researching which treatments are most effective in patients with high blood pressure, several studies have shown that two of the most important classes of drugs for high blood pressure—beta blockers and angiotensin-converting enzyme inhibitors (ACE-I)—often show less of an effect in blacks than in whites. Much of this racial variation in drug effect was found to be due to factors that are largely independent of race, such as underlying rates of diabetes, kidney disease, and obesity.

Knowing that research has shown that certain drugs are less effective in blacks as a group than they are in whites as a group, should physicians avoid those drugs or use them at a different dosage if a patient is black than if a patient is white? Satel suggests that they should: "In practicing medicine, I am not colorblind. I always take note of my patient's race. . . . When I prescribe Prozac to a patient who is African-American, I start at a lower dose, 5 or 10 milligrams instead of the usual 10- to 20-milligram dose. I do this in part because clinical experience and pharmacological research show that blacks metabolize antidepressants more slowly than Caucasians and Asians" (2002, p. 56).

To be able to answer this question, we must understand how comparisons of drug effectiveness are done. Rather than using a drug in one or two patients to see how well it works, researchers undertake trials of drug efficacy in large comparison groups, often with hundreds of patients in each group. They measure the drug's effect in each patient, and then compare the average effect across all groups, using standard statistical tests to identify differences in the average level of response. If the measured difference in drug effectiveness between two groups meets these statistical tests, then it is fair to conclude that the drug's average effect is different. Studies of this type led Materson (2003) and others to recommend against using beta blockers or ACE-I in blacks with high blood pressure.

Sehgal (2004) pointed out the potential flaw in this reasoning. He reviewed the results of 15 different research studies involving more than 10,000 patients. He was able to conclude that the differences in the effect of beta blockers and ACE-I in blacks and whites were real, but of questionable use in the setting of a single physician evaluating a single patient with high blood pressure. To illustrate his conclusion, he drew a schematic graph, shown in Figure 10.1.

When measuring the response of several hundred patients to a particular drug, we will typically find wide variation in that response. While a majority of them may have a similar response, some will have a substantially larger response and some will have a substantially smaller response. If one group has a few more patients with a substantially larger response, and the comparison group has a few more patients with a

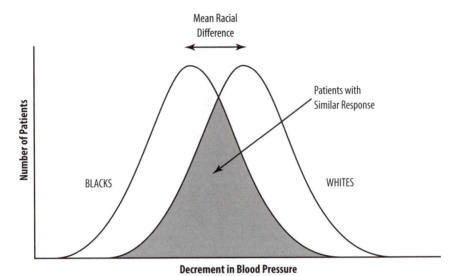

Figure 10.1. Reduction in blood pressure among whites and blacks after administration of a drug for high blood pressure. Shaded area represents whites and blacks who have similar responses. *Source*: A. R. Sehgal, "Overlap between whites and blacks in response to antihypertensive drugs," *Hypertension* 43 (2004):566–72, used by permission of Wolters Kluwer Health.

substantially smaller response, these "outliers" as they are referred to may skew the distribution of individual responses for both groups, such that the average response for one group is lower than the average response for the comparison group, even though the majority of patients in both groups have the same or similar responses. This is precisely what Sehgal found. Between 80 and 95 percent of patients treated with one of these two medications will show a similar response, even though the average response of the two groups differs by statistical tests of difference. Sehgal concluded that "race has little value in predicting antihypertensive drug response, because whites and blacks overlap greatly in their response to all categories of drugs" (p. 570).

Thus, well-meaning physicians who say, "The research shows that black patients don't respond to this medication as well as white patients, so whenever I have a black patient I don't use this medicine" misunderstand fundamental principles of statistical methodology. As described by Armstrong (2012), "even when evidence exists, uncertainty arises about the effect of that evidence on the individual patient. The gap between the average effect in a population and the effect in a specific patient can be substantial, in part because of differences between patients in practice and trial participants and in part because the average effect in a trial masks substantial variation among trial participants" (p. 1979).

It is technically accurate to say that, on average, the antihypertensive effect of beta blockers and ACE inhibitors is smaller for blacks than for whites. However, small differences across hundreds or thousands of patients, despite meeting tests of statistical significance, say little about how a particular patient will respond. To use such differences to decide that all blacks should not get these drugs would risk treating more than 9 out of 10 black patients with hypertension inappropriately by withholding drugs that are as likely to have a beneficial effect as in a white patient.

Race and the Treatment of Congestive Heart Failure: The First "Blacks Only" Medication

Research on the treatment of congestive heart failure has brought up the issues of selecting medicines based on the race of the patient. Some researchers have suggested that certain drugs are useful in whites but not in blacks. Others have suggested that there are drugs that are effective in blacks but not in whites. It is understandable that many physicians find these issues confusing.

Congestive heart failure is caused when the heart muscle becomes weakened to the point that it is incapable of adequately pumping the blood throughout the body. As a result of the weakness in the heart, blood returning to the heart in the venous system backs up. This increased venous pressure causes fluid to leak out of the blood vessels into the surrounding tissue, principally the lungs. This fluid leakage causes the lungs to become congested, impairing the exchange of oxygen—thus the term *congestive* heart failure, often referred to by its acronym CHF. There are two principal causes of CHF:

1. Damage to the heart muscle from chronic ischemia (lack of oxygen delivered to the muscle) as a result of clogged coronary arteries (ischemic CHF)
2. Damage to the kidneys and blood vessels as a result of chronic diseases, principally diabetes and high blood pressure, with increased strain on the heart as a secondary effect (nonischemic CHF)

Given the higher rates of ischemic heart disease among whites as compared to blacks and the higher rates of high blood pressure and diabetes among blacks as compared to whites, there is also a racial division in the most common cause of CHF. CHF in blacks is more likely to be nonischemic, while CHF in whites is more likely to be ischemic (Dries et al. 1999; Small et al. 2002).

Blacks with CHF are much more likely to die from their disease than whites (Dries et al. 1999). Thus, it is important that blacks receive optimal treatment once they develop CHF. Two studies of the treatment of CHF appeared simultaneously, one suggesting that ACE-I medications were effective in whites but not in blacks (Exner et al. 2001). The other suggested that beta-blockers were equally effective in treating both whites and blacks with CHF (Yancy et al. 2001). The authors of the first study concluded that "therapeutic recommendations may need to be tailored according to racial background" (p. 1357). An accompanying editorial supported this view, stating that "racial differences in response to drugs not only have practical importance for the choice and dose of drugs but should also alert physicians to important underlying genetic determinants of drug response" (Wood 2001, p. 1395). Others took an opposing view, suggesting that such arguments "are based on non-significant findings or genetic variation that does not have an established association with the disease being studied" (Cooper et al. 2003, p. 1168).

From the results of studies such as these, it might appear that practitioners are acting in the best interest of their patients if they use ACE-I medication for whites with CHF, but not for blacks. As reasonable as this conclusion appears on the surface, to follow it may leave many blacks inadequately treated. There are two reasons this may be true. The first is that the study suggesting a lack of effectiveness of ACE-I in blacks relied on a single measure of effect—the rate of hospitalization. One of the authors of this study published a subsequent paper, using the same data set, that came to a different conclusion, but which received much less publicity. When they assessed the effect of ACE-I in any of three different ways that measure the progression of CHF to either more severe symptoms or death, they found that ACE-I therapy "was equally efficacious" in blacks and whites (Dries et al. 2002, p. 311).

The second reason to be cautious is the different pattern of causation of CHF in blacks and whites. The combination of higher rates of high blood pressure, diabetes, and kidney disease in blacks with CHF explains much of the higher death rate from CHF in all blacks, both those receiving treatment and those in placebo control groups (Exner et al. 2001; Yancy et al. 2001). The presence of chronic kidney disease substantially increases the chances of death from CHF (Fonarow et al. 2005). ACE-I medication has been shown to be effective in reducing the adverse effects of CHF in patients with diabetes and kidney disease (Barnett et al. 2004). To systematically avoid ACE-I treatment in blacks with CHF in the belief that race accurately predicts drug response risks leaving a substantial segment of patients—especially those with chronic kidney disease—inadequately treated and without the proven benefit of these drugs.

The issue of using a patient's race to select treatment for CHF has become even more complicated with the approval by the federal government of a new treatment for CHF—but only if that drug is used in blacks. Isosorbide dinitrate and hydralazine are both drugs for heart disease and high blood pressure that have been available—separately—for decades. A combination of these two drugs was studied in the 1980s and found possibly to benefit patients with CHF (Cohn et al. 1986, 1991). A subsequent reanalysis of the data suggested that this benefit was more pronounced for blacks than for whites (Carson et al. 1999). A follow-up study involving only black patients confirmed a beneficial effect in the treatment of CHF of a combination of isosorbide dinitrate and hydralazine (ISD-H) (Taylor et al. 2004). Based on the results of this study, the federal Food and Drug Administration (FDA) approved a new drug, under the patented brand name of BiDil. In addition, the government approved a new patent for this combination of previously available drugs—but approved it only for use in black patients.

ISD-H exerts its beneficial effect in CHF patients by increasing the level of a substance called nitric oxide (NO) in the cells lining blood vessels, thereby causing them to dilate and as a result reducing the level of congestion in the circulation. It is important to note that reduced levels of NO in the cells lining blood vessels is also a principal contributor to the damage of the circulatory system caused by diabetes. Because rates of diabetes are substantially higher among blacks in the United States than among whites (17.7 percent versus 9.3 percent in 2014 [CDC 2017]), it stands to reason that NO levels will be, on average, lower among blacks than among whites. However, that reduced level of NO is because a person has diabetes, not because they are black. Whites with diabetes also have reduced NO levels. The coexistence of diabetes and high blood pressure may further reduce the effect of NO.

If one combines the results of the Exner study, suggesting that ACE-I is effective for whites with CHF but not blacks, with the Taylor study suggesting that ISD-H is effective for blacks with CHF but not whites, it may seem reasonable to conclude that we have established race-based treatment for a disease. This is the message of the company marketing BiDil to doctors and patients. In multipage, glossy ads in medical journals and on its website, that company stated, "BiDil is indicated for the treatment of heart failure in addition to standard therapy in self-identified black patients to improve survival, prolong time to first hospitalization for heart failure, and to improve patient-reported functional status" (Nitromed 2013).

The Taylor study compared the effectiveness of ISD-H in a randomized sample of 518 blacks with CHF, comparing the outcomes to 532 blacks given a placebo instead. Both groups continued to receive standard therapy in addition to ISD-H. The study was stopped early when it was found that the death rate for patients receiving ISD-H was significantly lower than that for patients receiving the placebo (10.2 percent versus 6.2 percent). Because ISD-H had not worked nearly as well in previous studies of mostly whites, this study led many to conclude that the reason ISD-H worked in these patients was because the patients were black.

At the time of the BiDil study, the rate of diabetes in the general population among black adults was 14.8 percent. Among blacks with CHF, the rate was 28.5 percent (Dries et al. 1999). Of the 512 blacks treated with ISD-H in the Taylor study, 44.8 percent had diabetes, compared to 37.0 percent of the patients receiving a placebo. Thus, the patients in the Taylor study, based on which the FDA approved the use of BiDil in black patients only, had a rate of coexisting diabetes that was significantly greater than the control group against which the effectiveness of the drug was measured, and substantially greater than the rate among all patients with CHF, black or white.

It is reasonable to expect ISD-H to be of benefit in a targeted population of CHF patients with high rates of coexistent diabetes, regardless of race. Similarly, as discussed above, ISD-H may be less useful in patients—black or white—with isolated ischemic CHF who do not have the added damage to blood vessels associated with diabetes. It is problematic to say with any certainty that the reason ISD-H was effective in the Taylor study was because the patients were black. An alternative explanation of the apparent benefit of ISD-H is because so many of the patients had nonischemic CHF and diabetes.

ISD-H may be a potentially useful medication for some patients with CHF who are not black, but who have the pattern of nonischemic CHF and diabetes that is so common among blacks. Similarly, a black person with ischemic CHF but without underlying diabetes may get little benefit from ISD-H treatment. The patient's race may alert physicians to look for underlying diabetes when selecting the optimal treatment for CHF, but it would be dangerous for the physician to assume that they may safely decide treatment based on the patient's race alone.

College-Educated Women in the Early Stages of Pregnancy

From the discussion in Chapter 6 and from the data in Tables 6.1 and 6.2, we learned that the infant mortality rate for infants born to black mothers in the United States is more than twice that of infants born to white mothers. Much of this difference is due to the substantially higher percentage of black babies born prematurely and weighing less than 1,500 grams. However, this risk of low birth weight was only seen in black mothers born in the United States, and not nearly so much in black mothers born in Africa but living in the United States (David and Collins 1997). The risk of premature birth and infant death seems to be associated principally with the SES of the mother giving birth, not her race.

There is one study that complicates this picture. Schoendorf and colleagues (1992) found that there continued to be a significantly higher rate of infant death among black mothers with a college education as compared to white mothers with a college education—two groups at comparably high levels of SES. The increased risk of infant death in the black mothers was due solely to a higher rate of low and very low birth weight infants. For some reason black mothers at high levels of SES had more premature, underweight babies than white mothers with comparable SES, and as a result a higher rate of infant mortality.

How should an obstetrician who provides prenatal care to women incorporate this finding into their practice? If a black woman comes in for early prenatal care, should the obstetrician treat her differently than a white woman? The first thing to do may be to determine the mother's level of education and other similar markers of SES, to assess for the known risk factors for premature birth associated with low SES. Once the physician determines that the woman is college educated, should they incorporate the patient's race into the plan for prenatal care? This can present a complex situation, one in which the patient should be directly involved in addressing. As suggested by Krumholz (2010), "the need to incorporate patient preferences even in such circumstances must be appreciated. . . . The estimate of the risks and anticipated benefits should consider each patient's unique characteristics. When the benefit is uncertain, the patient should be so informed" (p. 1190).

While the discussion of race in the treatment of breast cancer, high blood pressure, and CHF made it clear that it is often problematic to use a patient's race to decide treatment, the discussion of the white researcher in equatorial Africa suggested that it was perfectly appropriate to use race. Essentially all whites will be at increased risk for skin cancer from excess exposure to ultraviolet radiation. The use of the patient's race in that case seems perfectly appropriate, especially because the manner in which the physician used it had two fundamental aspects:

1. The physician used race to increase the protection of the patient's health, based on clear scientific evidence, and without attaching social meaning to racial categories.
2. The physician clearly explained to the patient how and why they were incorporating the patient's race into the recommended care.

In the case of the black, college-educated mother in the early stages of pregnancy, it may be equally appropriate to use her race in the same manner—at least until we have a better understanding of precisely why black women with a college education are at higher risk of having a premature baby. After explaining to the mother how and why her race is being incorporated into the treatment plan and that the change in treatment based on her race will be a heightened scrutiny for any risk factors that may contribute to prematurity, I would expect most mothers in this situation to be fully accepting of this use of race in medical care.

It seems then that the answer to the question posed at the beginning of this chapter—is it ever appropriate to use a patient's race/ethnicity to help guide medical decisions?—is yes, under certain limited and carefully considered circumstances. Those circumstances will be based on clear scientific evidence and with the full knowledge and consent of the person on whose behalf the medical decision is being made. Sweeping generalizations about using drug A for blacks and drug B for whites do not appear to meet these circumstances. It is crucially important for physicians and other health care professionals to understand these distinctions.

CHAPTER ELEVEN

What Should We Do to Reduce Health Disparities?

In 1979 the US Department of Health and Human Services created *Healthy People 2000*, a national program with the objective of improving the health of the American people by the beginning of the twenty-first century across a range of indicators and conditions. Building on that program, in 2010 the federal government launched an updated version titled *Healthy People 2020*, described as providing "science-based, 10-year national objectives for improving the health of all Americans" (HealthyPeople.gov 2010). The first stated goal of that program is to improve the length and quality of life of the American public. Its second goal is to "achieve health equity, eliminate disparities, and improve the health of all groups."

While this second goal has broad public and political support, it is important to understand the implications of such a sweeping objective. Consider, for example, the following facts:

- In 2016 the life expectancy for a white baby was 78.5 years, while that for a black baby was 74.8 years, a difference of 3.7 years.
- In 2016 the life expectancy for a female baby of any race was 81.1 years, while that for a male baby was 76.1 years, a difference of 5 years (National Center for Health Statistics 2018).

Both gaps in life expectancy represent a disparity. In nearly all developed societies, girl babies live longer on average than boy babies. The principal source of this disparity is the genetic and biological differences between females and males, although gender-based behaviors also play a role. Few would argue that the goal of the federal government should be to equalize the life expectancy of males and females.

Disparities in life expectancy between white and black babies are different from those between female and male babies. As we saw in Chapter 5, there are few meaningful genetic or biological differences between white babies and black babies, and certainly none that can explain a disparity of 3.7 years in life expectancy. The black/white disparity in life expectancy is instead the result of a combination of social and economic factors that affect living conditions, preferences, behaviors, and access to health care. There is broad consensus that it is the responsibility of the federal government to address these issues and, as a matter of public policy, to reduce the health disparities that they generate.

As defined by the *Oxford English Dictionary*, a *disparity* is an "inequality or dissimilarity in respect of age, amount, number, or quality; want of parity or equality." The health of an 80-year-old is, in most cases, unequal or dissimilar to the health of an eight-year-old. This difference represents a disparity, but not one that necessarily must be reduced as a matter of public policy. It is essential to identify those disparities in health status or access to health care that should, as a matter of public policy, be reduced or eliminated. To do so, I will delineate a framework by which I can separate out those disparities.

This book has, by design, not addressed the many health disparities that exist based on gender. There is substantial evidence that women receive a lower level of treatment for heart disease and other conditions in a way that is analogous to the racial differences in care we have seen. This book also has not considered disparities based on age, and issues of age in the allocation of health care resources. Nor has it considered disparities associated with sexual orientation. This is not to imply that these disparities are unimportant; rather, those issues exist in a different context, and are caused by a different combination of biologic and social factors. This book has instead focused on health disparities that can be explained by underlying disparities in SES, on one hand, and race or ethnicity, on the other. In doing so, I am adopting an approach that is consistent with the Secretary of Health and Human Services' Advisory Committee for Healthy People 2020, which defined health disparities as "systematic, plausibly avoidable health differences adversely affecting socially disadvantaged groups" (Braveman et al. 2011, p. S149).

A central message of this book is that there is a complex relationship between SES and race/ethnicity in creating the disparities that are the focus of our concerns. Throughout history, those in a disadvantaged social or economic position have, on average, had shorter lives and lives with greater levels of illness and disability than those in a position of social advantage. Part of this difference is due to the material benefits of social and economic advantage—better nutrition, better housing, better sanitation, and better health care. An additional part is due to the deleterious effect a position of social disadvantage has on individual attitudes and behaviors, with much of that effect translating over time into illness and premature death.

Beyond the effects of a position of disadvantaged SES, there is a second effect of being a member of a racial or ethnic group that faces discrimination that extends beyond SES. The experience of discrimination, especially when accompanied by a sense of powerlessness to confront that discrimination, is associated with measurable differences in cellular and physiologic functioning that, over time, lead to increased illness in a way that is analogous to the effects of SES disadvantage. When the effects of SES disadvantage and racial/ethnic discrimination are combined, as they so often are, the inevitable result is a marked disparity in health. A black baby can expect to live 3.7 years less than a white baby not because of any inherent qualities associated with being black, but because of the different ways our social and economic system impacts babies who are black.

The first aspect, then, of my framework to assess health disparities is to separate out those that have, principally, a biologic cause from those that have a social or economic cause, and to focus my attention on the latter.

When the plague was ravaging Europe in the fourteenth century, those in a position of SES disadvantage were more likely to die. When tuberculosis was endemic in Europe at the turn of the twentieth century, a seamstress with low SES was more likely to die from it than was the son of a wealthy family—as we saw from Chapter 1 in the discussion of Mimi and Hans. Throughout history, political and economic systems have struggled with the issue of economic inequality. As we observed in Chapter 4, the level of inequality within a society, measured in any number of ways, is strongly associated with the overall health within that society. We will not be solving any time soon the inequalities of social or economic position that have existed within societies for millennia. Nor will we be able to eliminate the disparities in health status that stem from those inequalities. We can, however, focus our attention on reducing those disparities in health that are due to a fundamental inadequacy of the social or economic resources that are necessary for human existence, resources that are well within the capability of modern, industrialized societies to provide. These resources were defined in 1948 at the time of the creation of the United Nations, as part of its Universal Declaration of Human Rights: "Everyone has the right to a standard of living adequate for the health and well-being of himself and of his family, including food, clothing, housing and medical care and necessary social services, and the right to security in the event of unemployment, sickness, disability, widowhood, old age or other lack of livelihood in circumstances beyond his control" (United Nations 1948, Article 25).

Nobel Prize–winning economist Amartya Sen describes what he refers to as the "instrumental freedoms" necessary to unfettered human existence. These include basic political freedoms, as well as social and economic freedoms, "which influence the individual's substantive freedom to live better. These freedoms are important not only for the conduct of private lives (such as living a healthy life and avoiding preventable morbidity and premature mortality), but also for more effective participation in economic and political activities" (1999, p. 39).

The second aspect of my framework to assess health disparities is to identify those disparities that are based on SES inequality and reflect the absence of the basic resources and opportunities that are fundamental to human existence—the "instrumental freedoms" described by Sen. It is well within the capability of industrialized societies to provide the minimum level of resources required to live adequately and to pursue the opportunity for full participation in society. Health disparities that stem from a lack of these fundamental human rights and freedoms should be included within our focus.

As part of this focus, I include an examination of disparities in access to health care. A basic level of health care is essential for the prevention of avoidable illness and the treatment of illness and injury when they occur. It remains the subject of intense social and political debate within the United States as to what is that basic level of health care. Few, though, argue that there is no obligation for our society to provide at least a basic level of care. Federal and state programs such as Medicare, Medicaid, and the Children's Health Insurance Program have provided for a basic level of care for our most vulnerable groups—children, the poor, and the elderly. Yet as we have seen throughout this book, there remain instances when illness is not prevented, and serious medical conditions are not adequately treated due to the lack of economic resources on the part of the patient. All too often those without the resources to pay for that treatment are black, Hispanic, or of another racial/ethnic minority group.

In 1999 Congress instructed the federal Agency for Health Care Research and Quality (US Department of Health and Human Services, Agency for Health Care Research and Quality 2005) to identify and monitor "prevailing disparities in health care delivery as it relates to racial factors and socioeconomic factors in priority populations" (p. 13). In establishing this political mandate, the federal government has helped us to define a third aspect of my framework to assess those disparities that are based on race or ethnicity alone, without an underlying basis in SES.

As I have discussed in this book, a principal source of health care disparities based on race/ethnicity stems from differences in the way physicians and other providers treat people from differing racial or ethnic backgrounds. The elimination of discrimination based on race or ethnicity continues to be one of the top social and political priorities of our society. There is a disturbing level of scientific evidence that our national legacy of racial and ethnic discrimination still lingers in the ways physicians incorporate race and ethnicity into their decisions, with resulting disparities in either access to care or quality of care. These disparities are not due to continued racial intolerance and explicit racism, as discussed in Chapter 9. They are much more likely to be caused by unconscious responses to individuals of certain racial or ethnic groups or by the unconscious but inappropriate uses of racial stereotypes. In this context, the Institute of Medicine report on *Unequal Treatment* defined the racial or ethnic disparities we should focus on eliminating as "racial or ethnic differences in the quality of healthcare that are not due to access-related factors or clinical needs, preferences, and appropriateness of intervention" (Smedley et al. 2003, p. 3).

Based on the framework I have described, I can summarize those disparities on which we should focus our attention for reduction or elimination:

1. Those disparities that have, principally, a social or economic cause rather than a biologic cause
2. As described by the *Unequal Treatment* report, those disparities that are due to racial or ethnic differences in health care that are unrelated to access, clinical appropriateness, or patient preferences
3. Those disparities based in SES inequality that reflect the absence of the basic resources and opportunities fundamental to human existence

It is possible to identify five basic steps we as a society can take to address and reduce these disparities:

1. Take explicit measures to eliminate unconscious race bias and ethnic bias as a cause of health disparities.
2. Monitor patterns of care to identify any of these disparities that continue to exist.
3. Strengthen the physician-patient relationship, especially when physician and patient are from differing backgrounds.
4. Increase the racial and ethnic diversity of the medical profession and other health professions.
5. Assure access to care through universal health insurance.

Eliminate Unconscious Racial Bias and Ethnic Bias as a Cause of Health Disparities

While we may never be able to eliminate all health disparities that stem from differences in SES, we certainly should be able to eliminate health disparities that are due to the way in which our system of health care responds differently to people of differing race or ethnicity. Those in minority racial or ethnic groups often face disparities caused by economic barriers to care. Those barriers are primarily due to differences in SES. Beyond disparities caused by differences in SES, a disturbing pattern of disparities persists, apparently as a result of racial/ethnic biases that persist among physicians and other health care providers. As discussed in Chapter 9, these residual biases are unconscious and unintended, and do not represent the type of explicit racism that characterized much of the history of the United States.

How are we to consciously change psychological processes that are invoked on an unconscious level? This is a dilemma that has faced those who study the psychology of bias for years, if not decades. Piper (1990) described how unconscious race bias exists in "thoughtful, well-intentioned, and conscientious individuals who nevertheless have failed adequately to confront and work through their own prejudices. . . . Such individuals are being neither disingenuous nor hypocritical when they deny that a person's race . . . affects their judgment of her competence or worth" (p. 299). Piper goes on to suggest that the only way to prevent unconscious biases from influencing our actions is to "scrutinize our social behavior even in situations in which we sincerely believe ourselves to be above . . . discrimination" (p. 289).

Stangor and colleagues (2001) summarized the research of others and demonstrated in their own research that openly confronting and discussing unconscious racial stereotypes can go a long way toward reducing those stereotypes. Their research showed that it is more effective for whites to discuss with other whites the effects of unconscious stereotypes of blacks, rather than for whites to discuss those stereotypes with blacks. Through a process of joint learning, those who hold negative stereotypes can safely reduce the impact of those stereotypes. As summarized by the authors, "withdrawing the social backing from an idea, in this case a social stereotype, goes a long way toward undermining the power of that idea over an individual thinker" (p. 494).

Geiger (2001) summarized the role of stereotyping and unconscious bias in contributing to health disparities. He emphasizes the incorrect attribution of data gathered from large epidemiologic studies to the case of an individual, an issue discussed in Chapter 9. "It is important to note that in the vast majority of cases these documented disparities in diagnosis and treatment do not reflect conscious racial bias or calculated cultural insensitivity. Time pressure and cognitive complexity (the need to think about many tasks at once) stimulate stereotyping and what has been called 'application error,' that is, the inappropriate application of epidemiological data to every individual in a group" (p. 1700).

Geiger goes on to suggest that cultural gaps that exist between the physician and the patient, based on either differences of SES or differences of race/ethnicity, are a major contributor to perpetuating the inappropriate use of stereotypes. To bridge this cultural gap, he recommends that physicians and other health care providers receive formal training to develop "cultural competence"—a catchphrase that has been widely adopted to describe skills in cultural awareness, sensitivity, and cross-cultural communication that are necessary to bridging the cultural gap between physician and patient. Betancourt and colleagues (2005) described the rapid adoption of training programs in cultural competence and emphasized that "the goal of cultural competence is to create a health care system and workforce that are capable of delivering the highest-quality care to every patient regardless of race, ethnicity, culture, or language proficiency" (p. 499).

The Association of American Medical Colleges (AAMC) (2005), an organization that sets national standards for medical education in the United States, designed a curriculum to provide medical students and physicians with the skills of cultural competence. It defines cultural and linguistic competence as "a set of congruent behaviors, knowledge, attitudes, and policies that come together in a system, organization, or among professionals that enables effective work in cross-cultural situations. . . . 'Competence' implies having the capacity to function effectively as an individual or an organization within the context of the cultural beliefs, practices, and needs presented by patients and their communities" (p. 1). In collaboration, the Liaison Committee on Medical Education (2013), the organization tasked with inspecting and certifying medical schools, established the following as one of its standards: "ED-21. The faculty and medical students of a medical education program must demonstrate an understanding of the manner in which people of diverse cultures and belief systems perceive health and illness and respond to various symptoms, diseases, and treatments. Instruction in the medical education program should stress the need for medical students to be concerned with the total medical needs of their patients and the effects that social and cultural circumstances have on patients' health" (p. 11). The AAMC (2013) developed a "Tool for Assessing Cultural Competence Training" to assist medical schools in meeting this standard.

Sociologist and ethicist Reneé Fox (2005) reemphasized that cultural competence involves more than developing an awareness of the cultural characteristics of others. Supporting the position of the AAMC, Fox emphasizes the point that physicians and other health care providers need to appreciate and accept "that their own culture also merits enlightened examination, for it is far from a neutral background against which other cultures are measured" (p. 1316). To become fully competent to work in cross-cultural situations, including the situation in which the patient grew up in the same country, speaks the same language, but comes from a different racial or ethnic background, a physician must recognize the risk that they may invoke unconscious stereotypes or feelings of aversion and that those unconscious biases may affect clinical decisions in ways that perpetuate unjustified health disparities.

Monitor Patterns of Care to Identify and Eliminate Unconscious Racial/Ethnic Bias

Once we acknowledge that unconscious racial and ethnic bias continues to exert an influence on clinical decision making and adopt the goal of eliminating the effects of that bias through education, it becomes essential to have a means of monitoring the process of care to be able to identify the disparities that may have bias as a contributing factor. Historically, many issues pertaining to alleged racial discrimination have been addressed through the courts as possible violations of civil rights laws.

Because of discriminatory outcomes from the perspective of blacks or other minorities confronting racial/ethnic bias, it is understandable that they would feel that the manner in which they had been treated had been a violation of their civil rights. Consider the patient with bone marrow cancer described in the Preface and the patient with the sore knee described in Chapter 9. I spoke personally with each of them following their medical treatment. Each was understandably angry. Both had the clear sense that, had they been white instead of black, their treatment would have been different—they would have been provided rapid access to the care their clinical condition warranted. To them, they had been victims of unwarranted and illegal racial discrimination. It makes little difference to the victim of racial discrimination if that discrimination was enacted consciously or unconsciously (see Chapter 9).

There are two principal ways to address disparities in health care that may violate federal civil rights laws. The first is through the Office of Civil Rights of the Department of Justice. The second is through the Office of Civil Rights of the US Department of Health and Human Services.

Addressing possible racial discrimination in health care as a matter to be resolved through the courts is extremely difficult, due to an interpretation of civil rights laws by the US Supreme Court in the case of *Washington v. Davis* (426 U.S. 229 1974). In a case involving employment rather than health care, the Court held that, to find that an action had violated the civil rights of an individual or a group, the person or group alleging the violation must prove that the person who had acted in a discriminatory manner had intended to discriminate. Without proving the intent to discriminate, documenting a discriminatory outcome usually is not enough to prove that an action had violated federal civil rights laws.

This doctrine, often referred to as the "intent doctrine," makes it extremely difficult to approach possible civil rights violations through the courts. As described by the Equal Justice Society (2004), a national civil rights advocacy organization, "The doctrine requires plaintiffs to prove the near-impossible: a decisionmaker's specific intent to discriminate. If a plaintiff cannot overcome this hurdle, the law will not recognize the discrimination he or she has experienced, even though some form of discrimination has come into play."

The Office of Civil Rights (OCR) of the US Department of Health and Human Services addresses the issue of racial discrimination in health care from a different context, uses different remedies, and applies somewhat different standards. Rather than addressing instances of possible discrimination through the courts, OCR has the authority to recommend that a provider—either an individual, hospital, or other health care organization—be denied federal funds through programs such as Medicare and Medicaid. OCR was able to use this remedy extremely effectively in the 1960s to desegregate hospitals and health care facilities, both in the South and elsewhere in the United States. While the issue of school desegregation was often fought out in the courts, that of health care desegregation was redressed fairly smoothly, without substantial court intervention.

OCR publishes guidelines it uses in evaluating cases of possible discrimination in health care. In defining what constitutes illegal discrimination, OCR stated that health care providers who receive any federal health care funding "may not, based on race, color, or national origin: Deny services or other benefits provided as a part of health or human service programs. Provide a different service or other benefit, or provide services or benefits in a different manner from those provided to others under the program" (US Department of Health and Human Services, Office of Civil Rights 2018). These restrictions were reinforced with passage of the Affordable Care Act (ACA), which states that "an individual shall not be excluded from participation in, be denied the benefits of, or be subjected to discrimination on the grounds prohibited under, among other laws, Title VI of the Civil Rights Act of 1964, under any health program or activity, any part of which is receiving federal financial assistance, or under any program or activity that is administered by an Executive Agency or any entity established under Title I of the Affordable Care Act or its amendments" (Affordable Care Act Section 1557 2010). OCR acknowledges that discrimination in health care may be intentional or unintentional, and that not all disparities in care are due to discrimination by the provider.

For the purposes of OCR enforcement, determination of a civil rights violation involves a balancing of intent and outcomes. Nonetheless, it would still be extremely difficult for individual patients such as those we have discussed here to successfully claim that their civil rights had been violated because of the care they had received.

However, there is another approach to unconscious discrimination in health care that a growing number of people support. Rather than approaching racial or ethnic discrimination in care as an issue of legal rights, it may be substantially more effective to approach it as an issue of quality. The federal government's 2005 National Health Care Disparities Report (US Department of Health and Human Services, Agency for Healthcare Research and Quality 2005) indicated that these disparities constitute disparities in quality as much as they may raise issues of civil rights. By defining care that continues to result in racial/ethnic disparities as poor-quality care, it becomes possible to address those disparities without raising issues of individual blame, but rather by looking at the outcomes of care at the level of the organization or the system.

Fiscella, with a group of colleagues that included Carolyn Clancy of the US Agency for Healthcare Research and Quality, proposed that we address issues of socioeconomic, racial, and ethnic disparities in health care as fundamental issues of health care quality. They proposed five principles to be used in modifying quality review procedures to address disparities in care (Fiscella et al. 2000, p. 2579):

1. Disparities represent a significant quality problem.
2. Current data collection efforts are inadequate to identify and address disparities.
3. Clinical performance measures should be stratified by race/ethnicity and socioeconomic position for public reporting.
4. Population-wide monitoring should incorporate adjustment for race/ethnicity and socioeconomic position.
5. Strategies to adjust payment for race/ethnicity and socioeconomic position should be considered to reflect the known effects of both on morbidity.

Rather than racial disparities in care, consider the analogous issue of a high rate of postoperative infections occurring in a hospital. It would be possible to look at the care of each individual surgeon to determine why their patients were getting infections as a complication of surgery. It has proven more effective, however, to look at the entire system within the hospital, and to define key measures to monitor. By reemphasizing the need for quality care in the process of surgery, from the patient being admitted to the hospital to the patient's eventual discharge, one can often reduce infection rates. The way instruments are sterilized or bandages changed may prove to be equally as important as the surgeon's technical skill in affecting the rate of infection. If, through careful scrutiny of the process, it becomes clear that an individual surgeon is contributing disproportionately to the infection rate, the peer review system within the hospital can address issues of professional competence and quality. The success or failure of the intervention will be measured by the overall infection rate for all the patients undergoing surgery at the hospital.

If a hospital or system of care were to monitor the patterns of care for racial or ethnic groups proven historically to be at risk for discrimination in care in the same way it monitored infection rates in patients undergoing surgery, it could identify disparate outcomes when they occur. By applying the same level of attention to improving the processes of care, the hospital or care system could identify what the OCR refers to as the "red flag for discrimination"—the finding that patients may not have received the same quality of care because of their race or ethnicity.

The Kaiser Permanente health care system in California provides an example of how a coordinated system of care can successfully address the issue of racial disparities in care. A study by Ayanian and colleagues (2014) evaluated the care provided for seniors by Medicare Advantage plans nationally. They looked at the extent to which patients in the plans were successful in controlling their blood pressure, cholesterol levels, and glycated hemoglobin levels (a measure of diabetes control). Each of these factors increases a patient's risk of cardiovascular disease if not well controlled. The authors found substantial black/white disparities nationally in the control of these risk factors among Medicare Advantage plans, except for the Kaiser Permanente plan in northern California. The authors reported that "disparities in risk-factor control for blacks have been eliminated in the West among Kaiser health plans . . . The elimination of racial disparities in control of blood pressure, LDL cholesterol, and glycated hemoglobin between black enrollees and white enrollees in Kaiser health plans in the West may reflect systematic efforts by the health plans to improve control of these risk factors over the past decade" (p. 2294). The experience at Kaiser has demonstrated that, given sufficient organizational commitment, the elimination of racial disparities in the quality of care is possible.

Miranda and colleagues (2003) demonstrated that addressing racial/ethnic disparities in mental health care as an issue of quality of care can also be very effective. Working with providers in 46 primary care practice groups and six managed care organizations, they used standard quality improvement methods to improve the treatment of depression among a group of 398 Hispanic, 93 black, and 778 white patients. Interestingly, they showed that focusing on improving the quality of care for racial/ethnic minority patients "can improve the quality of care for whites and underserved minorities alike, while minorities may be especially likely to benefit clinically" (p. 613).

Lavizzo-Mourey and Mackenzie (1996) argued that the issue of improving cultural competence among physicians and other providers should also be addressed as one of quality improvement. In addition to encompassing issues of access to treatment, they suggested that quality review and assessment mechanisms should include an evaluation of the cultural sensitivity and cultural appropriateness of care, in particular as those qualities affect the quality of the physician-patient interaction.

Rather than relying on courts to address the issue of health care disparities that have unintended racial or ethnic bias as a contributor, it may be preferable, as well as more effective, to work with organizations such as the Joint Commission, the organization that monitors the quality of care provided by hospitals and health plans nationally, to incorporate the issue of racial disparities into their assessment of the quality of care. By defining as issues of quality rather than violations of law, the presence of racial or ethnic disparities in care that are unrelated to economic access, clinical appropriateness, or patient preferences, it becomes unnecessary to prove blame in order to redress those disparities. Congress or other governmental agencies may need to take the lead in some circumstances in establishing this definition, but once there is wide acceptance of approaching racial disparities as issues of quality, the issue of eliminating them becomes much more straightforward.

In adopting a quality-improvement approach to the elimination of racial/ethnic disparities in care, it is crucially important to point out a basic issue that must first be overcome. In 2005 Lurie noted that "until very recently, the bulk of the delivery system had no data on race and ethnic background, so it has been virtually impossible to examine, let alone publicly report, data on the quality of care for various racial and ethnic groups . . . we cannot make progress without being able to measure and monitor that progress, which means that they need information about the race and ethnic background of enrollees" (2005, pp. 727–28). Before being able to implement a quality-improvement approach to eliminating racial/ethnic health care disparities, it will first be necessary to make universal the gathering of data about the race or ethnicity of patients treated. A study published in 2011 (Robert Wood Johnson Foundation) found that 80 percent of hospitals nationally collected data on the race and ethnicity of the patients they served, while 60 percent collected data on language. Among health plans, however, the gathering of race/ethnicity data is less consistent, as compliance is voluntary (except in California and Massachusetts, both of which require health plans to collect and report race and ethnicity data).

Section 4302 of the Affordable Care Act initiated a process of establishing national standards for the collection of patient data on race, ethnicity, sex, language, and disability status (US Department of Health and Human Services 2011). The widespread use of these standards will hopefully contribute to continuing decline and eventual elimination in racial and ethnic disparities in the quality of care nationally.

Strengthen the Physician-Patient Relationship, Especially When Physician and Patient Are from Differing Backgrounds

As discussed in Chapter 7, there are numerous instances in which two principal factors contribute to patients who otherwise are clinically appropriate for care nonetheless not receiving that care:

1. The physician recommends the care, but the patient chooses not to undergo the care.
2. The physician does not recommend the care.

The discussion so far in this chapter has focused on reducing or eliminating disparities stemming from the second reason. To fully eliminate these disparities, we must also address the causes of the first reason—racial/ethnic differences in patients' understanding of and preference for alternative treatment approaches.

Trust is central to the quality of the physician-patient interaction and is a major determinant of the treatment decisions that come out of it. As described by Hall and colleagues (2001), "trust is the core, defining characteristic that gives the doctor-patient relationship meaning, importance, and substance" (p. 613). Unfortunately, since the 1972 disclosure of the Tuskegee Study of Untreated Syphilis in the Negro Male, mistrust of the medical care system increased substantially among African Americans (Alsan and Wanamaker 2017).

When seeing a physician, racial/ethnic minorities and those from lower SES approach the encounter with lower levels of trust than whites (Long and Bart 2017). When patients approach an encounter with a physician with a sense of distrust, they often come away from the encounter with lower levels of satisfaction with the care they have received. Doescher and colleagues (2000) documented this in a study of nearly 30,000 patients in a nationally representative sample. Much of the decrement in satisfaction had to do with the minorities' perceptions of the physician's thoroughness, how well the physician listened, and how well the physician explained things.

Mistrust of one's physician due to past experience of racial discrimination has been shown to weaken the physician-patient interaction for patients being treated for cancer by a nonblack oncologist. Penner and colleagues (2017) reviewed surveys completed by 113 black cancer patients before their upcoming visit with their oncologist, assessing patients' perceptions of past discrimination in a health care context and their general level of trust or mistrust in physicians. Based on videotapes of the subsequent physician-patient interaction and surveys of the physician following the visit, those patients who had expressed greater levels of mistrust tended to talk more during the visit and to use more of a negative tone in the words they used. The greater this response, the more negative was the physician's subsequent description of their interaction with the patient.

This type of negative physician-patient interaction also presents a potential impediment to black women receiving optimal screening for breast cancer (see Chapter 10). When women undergo a mammogram, some women are found to have breasts with increased tissue density. This increased breast density does not in itself indicate the presence of cancer, but it does indicate that the woman is at increased risk of developing breast cancer as a consequence of the tissue density. Manning and colleagues (2017) surveyed 211 white and 241 black women who had undergone screening mammograms and were found to have increased breast density. Each woman was informed of her increased breast density as part of the mammogram results, and each was given information about the increased cancer risk associated with breast density. The black women reported greater levels of anxiety and greater levels of suspicion regarding this information. These negative reactions were partially explained by previous experiences of racial discrimination and associated mistrust. Fortunately, the black women who expressed increased anxiety about the mammogram results also expressed a stronger intent to discuss this new information with a physician in order to gain a better understanding.

LaVeist and colleagues (2000) looked into the impact of mistrust in the physician-patient relationship in a study of 781 blacks and 1,003 whites with a chronic heart condition that required frequent visits to a physician. They surveyed these patients about their satisfaction with the care they received from the physicians, their perceptions of trust in the health care system, and their perceptions of racial bias inherent in the health care system. They then used multivariate analysis to determine which of the factors they measured, including the patient's age, race, gender, educational level, and type of insurance, were associated with the reported satisfaction with care. The results of their analysis are shown in Figure 11.1.

When looking only at the association between race and satisfaction, they found that blacks were significantly less satisfied with the care they received than whites. However, when they included in the analysis all measured variables, they found that only the patient's age, perceptions of racial bias, and trust in the physician were associated with the level of reported satisfaction. Understandably, the higher the level of the patient's trust in the physician, the higher the reported satisfaction. Conversely, the greater the perceived racial bias, the lower the satisfaction.

After including measures of perceived bias and trust in the analysis, race no longer had a significant association with satisfaction. In separate analyses, the authors

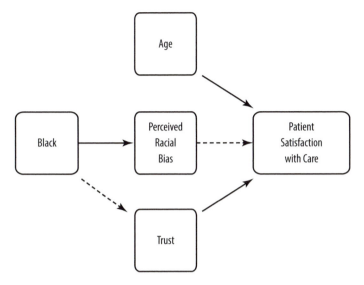

Figure 11.1. Determinants of patient satisfaction with care. Solid arrow indicates a direct relationship; dashed arrow indicates an inverse relationship. *Source:* Based on LaVeist et al. (2000).

were able to determine that blacks approached the physician encounter with lower levels of trust and higher levels of perceived bias. An individual's perceptions of trust and bias were associated most strongly with satisfaction, independent of race.

The authors did one final analysis: they followed the patients to see which ones actually received a referral to undergo cardiac catheterization. The results of this analysis are shown in Figure 11.2.

Patients with greater perceptions of racial bias in the health care system were less likely to end up with a referral for catheterization. Those who reported higher levels of trust in the system were more likely to end up with a referral. The strongest relationship of all involved patients' satisfaction with the care they were receiving for their heart conditions: the more satisfied the patient, the more likely the receipt of a referral. Knowing from the previous analysis that blacks report lower levels of trust and greater perceptions of bias, and as a result lower levels of satisfaction, it is understandable why blacks typically undergo cardiac catheterization less frequently than whites, other things being equal. Some of the difference can be explained by patients' preexisting perceptions of trust and racial bias in the health care system.

Communication between physician and patient seems to be a key factor in determining whether a patient refuses or avoids a treatment recommended by a physician. In a study of 1,106 adult patients from the Detroit area, Moore and colleagues

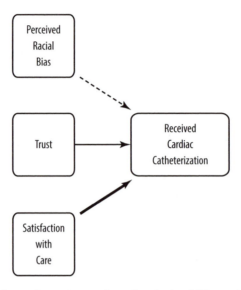

Figure 11.2. Factors that predict receiving cardiac catheterization. Solid arrow indicates a direct relationship; dashed arrow indicates an inverse relationship. The width of the line indicates the strength of the relationship. *Source*: Based on LaVeist et al. (2000).

(2004) found that "[patients] who felt their physicians listened more to their concerns were less likely to avoid treatment" (p. 421). In support of this finding, Tucker and colleagues (2003), from the results of focus group interviews with 135 white, black, and Hispanic, low-income patients, found that all three racial/ethnic groups agreed on which factors characterized a high-quality and culturally sensitive interaction between physician and patient: good people skills, effective communication, and a sense of individualized care, in addition to evidence of technical competence.

For many black patients, access to a culturally sensitive physician is often not available. This issue is of particular concern for black men, who face one of the highest risk profiles for cardiovascular disease of any group in the United States (Mainous et al. 2018). To address this issue, a group of mostly black medical students at the University of Pennsylvania tried a new approach (Ha et al. 2018). They were aware of a common cultural pattern among black men of going to the barbershop every 2 to 3 weeks for a haircut. Most men consistently go to the same barbershop each visit and get to know both the barbers and the other patrons at the shop. The students began going to a barbershop in Philadelphia every Saturday afternoon and, with the barbers' permission, began talking to the men waiting to get their hair cut about the issue of high blood pressure. The students took the men's blood pressure, advised them of the risk of untreated hypertension, and provided advice on how to obtain treatment. Previous studies have indicated that black men often believe that changes in diet and exercise are sufficient to treat high blood pressure and that medication is not necessary (Campbell et al. 2015). Hearing from these students in a culturally sensitive way about the importance of treatment led many of these clients to seek treatment they might otherwise have foregone.

Victor and colleagues (2018) built on this model in a study of black male barbershop patrons in Los Angeles County. The researchers identified 52 black-owned barbershops and, with the barbers' permission, began a controlled study of a new model of treatment of hypertension. In approximately half of the barbershops, the barbers encouraged their clients to meet with a pharmacist with special training in the treatment of hypertension. The pharmacist would talk to the clients about the importance of blood pressure control and then take the client's blood pressure.

For those clients with elevated blood pressure, the pharmacist would initiate treatment with prescription medication, following a protocol approved either by the client's own physician or, for those clients with no regular physician, by a collaborating physician. The pharmacist followed up with the client monthly and provided financial assistance in purchasing medications when necessary. In the control group of barbershops, clients received written information about controlling high blood pressure and encouragement to follow up with a physician for evaluation and treatment. Both sets of clients received vouchers to pay for their haircuts as compensation for their participation.

After six months of follow-up, the clients with elevated blood pressure who had received direct treatment from the pharmacist had reduced their blood pressure significantly more than the clients in the control group. An editorial published in response to this study concluded that "Victor et al. provide persuasive evidence that we can succeed in reaching treatment-resistant hypertensive populations with powerful yet simple treatment algorithms . . ." (Margolis 2018, p. 1346). The more we can create new treatment algorithms that emphasize cultural sensitivity, communication, and trust between provider and patient, the more we will be able to reduce disparities such as these.

Ashton and colleagues (2003) reviewed an extensive literature on factors that contribute to racial and ethnic disparities in health care. From this review, they developed a model of the relationship between the patient and the physician, acknowledging that both bring to the clinical encounter factors that may predispose to racial/ethnic differences in care. They suggest that communication is the linchpin in this relationship, with two key aspects to its effect (p. 146):

1. Communication during the medical interaction plays a central role in decision making about subsequent interventions and health behaviors.
2. Doctors have poorer communication with minorities than with others, but problems in doctor-patient communication have received little attention as a potential cause, a remediable one, of health disparities.

Johnson and colleagues (2004) provide support for the latter effect—that doctors tend to have worse communication with minorities. They evaluated videotapes from 458 physician-patient encounters, which included 256 blacks and 202 whites. Using standardized measurement tools to evaluate the content of these videotapes, they found that physicians tended to be more verbally dominant with their black patients, and to have more "patient-centered" communication with their white patients.

Malat (2001) suggests that minority race and lower SES combine to define a "social distance" between physician and patient, each acting independently. Patients with lower SES, independent of race, tend to feel more distant from their physician than those with higher SES. Similarly, blacks and other nonwhites tend to feel more distant from white physicians than from physicians of their own race or ethnicity. Racial/ethnic concordance—the situation in which the patient and the physician are of the same race or ethnicity—contributes substantially to reducing the sense of social distance between patient and physician, and in turn leads to higher levels of satisfaction and trust.

The opposite of a racially concordant relationship is referred to as a racially (or ethnically) discordant relationship. This term does not imply discord between physician and patient, but rather signifies simply a difference in the race or ethnicity of the dyad. Cooper and Powe (2004) reviewed the research on the implications of racial/ethnic discordance in the physician-patient relationship. They confirm that this discordance contributes to lower levels of patient satisfaction and ultimate racial/ethnic disparities in care. Cooper-Patrick and colleagues (1999) also found strong evidence for a positive effect of racial concordance between physician and patient. In a survey of 1,816 adult patients (43 percent white and 45 percent black) treated by one of 64 physicians (56 percent white and 25 percent black), they found that

- the average perceived quality of the physician-patient interaction was no different for white physicians and black physicians

- patients (white or black) in a racially concordant physician-patient relationship rated the quality of their interaction with the physician as higher than those patients in a racially discordant relationship

Increase Diversity of the Health Professions to Reduce Disparities

It seems clear that having a medical profession with a level of racial/ethnic diversity that is similar to the racial/ethnic diversity in the general population will optimize the chances of racial/ethnic concordance between physician and patient, which in turn will increase patient satisfaction and trust. This is not to suggest that we should assign patients arbitrarily to a physician of the same race/ethnicity, but rather that we should strive to maintain a profession that reflects the racial/ethnic diversity of the general population.

The Institute of Medicine released two reports in support of this conclusion. The first report, titled *The Right Thing to Do, the Smart Thing to Do: Enhancing Diversity in Health Professions* (Smedley et al. 2001), underscored the importance of enhanced racial/ethnic diversity among physicians. The second report, issued three years later, offered an explicit acknowledgment of the importance of increasing racial/ethnic diversity among physicians as a means of reducing health disparities. "A preponderance of scientific evidence supports the importance of increasing racial and ethnic diversity among health professionals. This evidence . . . demonstrates that greater diversity among health professionals is associated with improved access to care for racial and ethnic minority patients, greater patient choice and satisfaction, better patient-provider communication, and better educational experiences for *all* students while in training" (Smedley et al. 2004, p. 5).

The Association of American Medical Colleges (2013) publishes data on the racial/ethnic composition of practicing physicians in the United States as well as students graduating each year from US medical schools. Information about race/ethnicity is available for 471,408 physicians who graduated from a US medical school between 1978 and 2008. Figure 11.3 compares the racial/ethnic diversity of those physicians, the racial/ethnic diversity of students graduating in 2012 from a US medical school, and the US population as a whole in 2012.

We can see that whites and Asians make up a larger share of practicing physicians than their respective share in the population. Whites make up approximately the same percentage of medical school graduates as of the population, while Asians make up a percentage of medical school graduates that is more than four times their percentage of the population. Blacks, Hispanics, and Native Americans each make

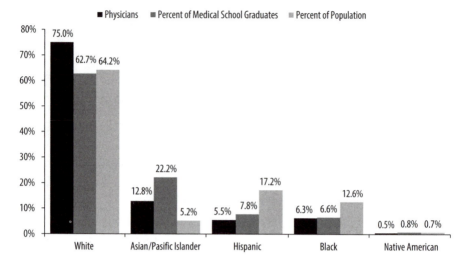

Figure 11.3. Racial/ethnic diversity of practicing physicians, medical school graduates, and the general population, 2012. *Source*: Based on population data from US Census Bureau and Association of American Medical Colleges 2013.

up substantially smaller shares of practicing physicians and medical school graduates than their respective share in the general population. Data on the racial composition of recent medical school graduates show relatively little change in the diversity of young physicians. In 2015, 6 percent of US medical school graduates were black and 5 percent were Hispanic—about the same percentages as among practicing physicians (Association of American Medical Colleges 2016). In order to attain the levels of racial/ethnic diversity in the US medical profession called for in the Institute of Medicine reports and other policy documents, there will have to be a substantial increase in the number of medical students coming from the three racial/ethnic groups that are underrepresented in medicine (URM): blacks, Hispanics, and Native Americans.

In the 1960s a number of medical schools nationwide began programs of affirmative action to increase the racial/ethnic diversity of entering medical students. Within the University of California system, several medical schools adopted specific targets to increase the number of URM students in their entering class, and used the race/ethnicity of applicants, along with standard measures of academic achievement, to meet that target. Allan Bakke was a white premedical student who had applied twice for admission to the medical school at the University of California, Davis, and was rejected for admission both times. In each year that he had applied, there were URM students who were admitted to Davis with lower college grades and standardized test scores than Bakke's. Bakke filed suit, asserting that his civil rights had been violated because of the racial/ethnic preference given to the URM students who were accepted. His suit was eventually heard by the US Supreme Court, which ruled in 1978 (*Regents of the University of California v. Bakke*, 438 U.S. 265) that UC Davis could not use race/ethnicity as the sole or principal criterion on which to admit students. However, the Court indicated that race/ethnicity could be used as one of a number of criteria for admissions. The constitutionality of this use of race as one factor among many was reaffirmed in 2003 in another Supreme Court case involving the University of Michigan Law School (*Grutter v. Bollinger*, 539 U.S. 306). The Court ruled that the goal of achieving diversity among students admitted to law school, and as a consequence the diversity of the legal profession, presented a "compelling interest" that permitted the use of race/ethnicity, so long as it is one of a number of factors used in the admissions process.

It seems equally compelling that the medical profession attain a substantially increased level of racial/ethnic diversity, in order to improve the quality of care and contribute to the reduction or elimination of the disparities faced by patients of minority race or ethnicity. Medical schools nationwide are taking another look at the policies they use in selecting students for admission. The predominant model of premedical education was established in 1910, as part of the Flexner Report (Flexner 1910). Writing in 2006, Emanuel suggested that much within the premedical curriculum established by Flexner in 1910 was "irrelevant to future medical education and practice" (p. 1128) and therefore no longer appropriate to select future physicians for the twenty-first century. As a principal means of reducing racial and ethnic disparities in health status and health care, medical schools and the medical profession will need to undertake a thorough reexamination of the criteria by which students are chosen for medical school. The need for increased racial and ethnic diversity within the medical profession is compelling.

The Association of American Medical Colleges (2013) has studied the issue of diversity among the students selected for admission to medical schools, and encourages medical schools to look beyond a narrow focus on grades in science classes and standardized test scores in selecting students. They have called for a "Holistic Review" process in which students are evaluated on their academic ability as well as on factors such as commitment to service, cultural sensitivity, empathy, capacity for growth, emotional resilience, strength of character, interpersonal skills, and the life choices they have made. In describing the need for a shift to Holistic Review, Witzburg and Sondheimer (2013) emphasize the role of diversity. "The imperative for a diverse physician workforce in an increasingly diverse society is one important driver of the move to take a more expansive view of excellence in medical student selection. This more comprehensive approach to considering a multitude of factors in evaluating all applicants provides a context for the inclusion of race, ethnic background, language, culture, and heritage, among other factors, in a way that is educationally sound and legally viable" (p. 1565).

The need for racial and ethnic diversity goes beyond the medical profession. The same need is seen for a wide range of health professionals, including dentists, pharmacists, physician assistants, registered nurses, nurse practitioners, and licensed practical nurses (Grumbach et al. 1993). In our own research on factors affecting patients' perceptions of what constitutes culturally competent care in the primary care setting, patients from racial and ethnic minority groups cited the diversity of the nonphysician staff as equally important as (and in some cases more important than) the diversity of the physician staff (Barr and Wanat 2005).

Access to Care as a First Step to Reducing Health Disparities

Throughout most of the twentieth century, the United States approached the provision of medical care as largely an issue to be left to private markets. The federal government, in taking a largely hands-off approach, supported the views of Sade, published in the *New England Journal of Medicine*: "Medical care is neither a right nor a privilege: it is a service that is provided by doctors and others to people who wish to purchase it" (1971, p. 1289). Only in the 1960s did the federal government adopt the Medicare and Medicaid programs, assuring a basic level of health care for elderly and/or poor people. While Medicare has consistently provided for a high level of care, the Medicaid program has faced continuing financial obstacles to providing a high level of care to poor families and children. As described by economist Uwe Reinhardt, "Americans have . . . decided to treat health care as essentially a private consumer good of which the poor might be guaranteed a basic package, but which is otherwise to be distributed more and more on the basis of ability to pay" (Reinhardt and Relman 1986, p. 23).

As a supplement to Medicare and Medicaid, in 1997 Congress passed the Children's Health Insurance Program to provide coverage to limited numbers of children in working families earning too much to qualify for Medicaid. Together these three programs provide tax-financed health insurance for the most vulnerable segments of our society. However, a growing number of Americans who are ineligible for these programs face severely restricted access to health care as a consequence of being uninsured. They lack any form of health insurance to assist in paying for needed care. The federal government's National Health Disparities Report summarized the extensive research literature about the health effects of going without health insurance: "The uninsured are more likely to die early and have poor health status. . . . The uninsured report more problems getting care, are diagnosed at later disease stages, and get less therapeutic care. They are sicker when hospitalized and more likely to die during their stay" (US Department of Health and Human Services, Agency for Healthcare Research and Quality 2005, p. 89).

As the costs of health care were rising in the United States, the number of uninsured Americans rose in concert. Between 1987 and 2010, the proportion of the population who were uninsured grew from just under 12 percent to about 16 percent (US Census Bureau 2018). This increase came largely among working families. Seventy-nine percent of uninsured families had at least one adult who worked on a regular basis throughout the year. Of those who were working, 80 percent worked full-time. Sixty-two percent of uninsured adults and children lived in families with incomes greater than the federal poverty level (Kaiser Family Foundation 2013). The principal cause of going without health insurance is not poverty or unemployment but the lack of affordable health insurance for working adults and families.

In Chapter 6 we saw that nonwhite racial and ethnic groups are disproportionately represented among lower SES groups. The same is true for health insurance. Using data for 2017, Figure 11.4 compares the racial/ethnic makeup of the US population with the racial/ethnic makeup of the uninsured.

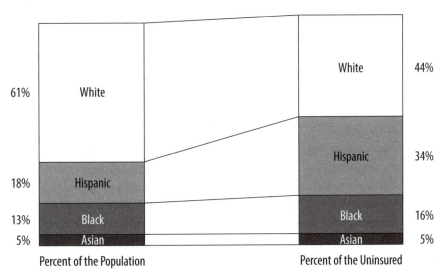

Figure 11.4. Comparing the racial/ethnic composition of the US population with the racial/ethnic composition of the uninsured for the four largest racial/ethnic groups, 2017. *Source*: US Census Bureau: Population Quick Facts; Health Insurance Coverage in the United States, 2017.

Blacks and Hispanics are overrepresented among the population of those without health insurance, compared to their percentage in the general population. While health disparities due to economic barriers to obtaining needed health care fall disproportionately on those in lower SES groups, they also fall disproportionately on Hispanics and blacks.

Without health insurance, a low-income individual or family has available only basic health care, typically focused on emergencies. When someone places a call to 911, the paramedics will respond and treat any person with an emergency medical condition, regardless of income or ability to pay. Similarly, all hospital emergency rooms are required, as a matter of federal law, to provide care to any person with a life-threatening condition, a condition causing severe pain, or a woman who is in active labor.

Access to emergency services, while crucially important, is not the principal driver of the health disparities we have discussed. Many if not most of those health disparities—whether for those in lower SES groups or those from minority racial/ethnic groups—are due to the effects of chronic illnesses such as heart disease, high blood pressure, or diabetes. These conditions are best treated before they have done their damage, and certainly before they have led to an emergency situation. If we are to fulfill the mandate of the Universal Declaration of Human Rights and if we are to provide all members of our society with the instrumental freedoms described by Sen, then we will need to take steps to see that all people have access to a basic level of health care that provides for the identification and treatment of chronic conditions as well as emergency conditions. Until we do so, we will have little chance of attaining a meaningful reduction in those health disparities that fall within the framework I have established.

Identifying the need to provide a basic level of health care to all people that includes prevention, health promotion, and the treatment of chronic diseases as well as emergency coverage is a task that is complicated by the intense politics surrounding health care policy. The United States has considered adopting universal health insurance at a number of times throughout its history. In the 1930s the original architects of the Social Security program had hoped to include universal health insurance as part of it, but they were thwarted by the political implications of doing so. The United States again considered universal health insurance following World War II, when the United Kingdom was establishing its National Health Service and other European countries were incorporating universal coverage into their reconstruction plans. The political fear of any program that seemed to imply a movement toward socialism was sufficient to thwart that effort. Universal health insurance was again considered in the 1960s, at the time of the creation of the Medicare

and Medicaid programs; in the 1970s as part of the movement to health maintenance organizations; and in the 1990s as part of President Bill Clinton's national
agenda.

Each time universal health insurance was considered, the politics of special in-
terests were able to prevent the adoption of a national program to provide the basic
level of care called for by the Universal Declaration of Human Rights. In 2010 Congress passed the ACA, and in so doing took a major step in the direction of providing universal health insurance to its residents. As described by President Obama on
the signing of the ACA, "We have enshrined the core principle that everybody
should have some basic security when it comes to their health care" (Obama 2010).
As the sometimes harsh political debate that has followed enactment of the ACA
suggests, by enshrining a "core principle" we may have taken a significant step toward
universal coverage, but we have not gotten there yet. If we are ever to adopt the
policy—previously adopted by *all* other developed countries—of providing for the
basic level of care necessary to support the opportunity for all people to fully participate in society, we will have to set aside partisan politics and focus on what is
best for the health and well-being of the American people.

Addressing the Social Determinants of Health as Part of the Health Care System

Gail Wilensky was the Director of Medicare and Medicaid from 1990 to 1992 under
President George H. W. Bush, and subsequently chaired the Medicare Payment
Advisory Commission from 1997 to 2001. In 2016 she published an article in the
Journal of the American Medical Association titled "Addressing Social Issues Affecting Health to Improve US Health Outcomes" (Wilensky 2016). In that article
Dr. Wilensky offered advice on how to improve the health outcomes of those facing socioeconomic or racial/ethnic disadvantage. "I want to use a different rationale
in advocating more attention to the social determinants of health: they reflect our
best opportunity to improve health outcomes reported for the United States that are
relatively poor, despite how much we spend on medical care . . . There is substantial evidence that addressing social or nonmedical determinants of health such as
early childhood development, economic opportunities, and education is more
important than medical care per se for better health outcomes and avoiding premature death" (pp. 1552–53).

The National Academy of Medicine (formerly the Institute of Medicine) is one
of the principal advisors to the federal government on issues of health policy. The
National Academy created a collaborative, nationwide effort titled "Vital Directions

for Health and Health Care," with the goal of identifying policy priorities for improving the health of Americans. The Steering Committee for this effort published a summary of the recommendations developed by the more than 150 policy experts participating in the effort (Dzau et al. 2017). One of their central priorities for action to improve both health and health care was to "remove barriers to integration of social services with medical services. Treatments are frequently prescribed without consideration of the social, behavioral, and environmental factors that are important determinants of health" (p. 1464).

The Health and Public Policy Committee of the American College of Physicians has published recommendations on how to incorporate consideration of the social determinants of health into the existing medical care system (Daniel et al. 2018). One of their central policy recommendations is that "Health care professionals should be knowledgeable about screening and identifying social determinants of health and approaches to treating patients whose health is affected by social determinants throughout their training and medical career . . ." (p. 578). Based on this knowledge and awareness, they recommend that physicians and other providers establish "increased interprofessional communication and collaborative models that encourage a team-based approach to treating patients at risk to be negatively affected by social determinants of health" (p. 578).

Onie and colleagues (2018) describe an exploratory project titled "Health Leads" undertaken by a group of medical care providers in Boston with the goal of integrating the social needs of patients into the delivery of medical care. With support from a range of philanthropic sources, they established a screening process to identify patients with unmet social needs. Those patients identified as having such needs were referred to a "help desk," where a trained staff member could help the patient to prioritize the additional resources they need to access, and then to act as an advocate to assist the patient in accessing these resources. The advocates would follow up with the patient over time and then report back to the provider on the progress they had made.

Between 2009 and 2011 these advocates provided assistance and support to more than 18,000 patients. As the news of the success of this program spread, increasing numbers of providers and payers referred patients to the program for social needs assessment and advocacy. Between 2012 and 2014 the program served more than 33,000 patients. Based on the success of the model and the growing number of patients in the Boston area with unmet social needs, the model was fundamentally changed. Rather than having an independent referral agency address unmet social needs, the decision was made to integrate these processes into the routine provision of care by existing medical care providers.

Building on this model, in 2017 the federal Centers for Medicare and Medicaid Services (CMS) established the Accountable Health Communities Model of primary care delivery. As described on the program's website (United States Centers for Medicare and Medicaid Services 2017), the goal of the new model of care is "testing whether systematically identifying and addressing the health-related social needs of Medicare and Medicaid beneficiaries through screening, referral, and community navigation services will impact health care costs and reduce health care utilization." In 2018 CMS published a "Health-Related Social Needs Screening Tool" to be used as a central part of the program (United States Centers for Medicare and Medicaid Services 2018). It makes available a screening survey health care providers can administer to their patients. It includes five core issues: housing instability, food insecurity, transportation problems, utility help needs, and interpersonal safety, with additional questions asking about issues such as employment, education, substance use, and mental health.

As part of the Medicaid program, CMS allows state Medicaid programs to be granted what is referred to as an 1115 waiver (pronounced "eleven-fifteen") to try new ways of enhancing the quality of the care provided to Medicaid beneficiaries (Artiga and Hinton 2018). Examples of the waiver programs states have been able to enact to address social determinants of health include a program in Oregon, similar to the Health Leads program, that created community advisory councils to work with Medicaid providers to develop and administer a community health needs assessment to patients and to offer supplemental support services for those patients facing unmet social needs. Under an 1115 waiver, California allows certain county Medicaid programs to use Medicaid funds to pay the costs of permanent supportive housing with supportive services for chronically homeless individuals. Research has shown that providing housing and supportive services can substantially reduce local government expenditures related to responding to chronic homelessness on the streets (Larimer et al. 2009).

Given the administrative complexity often associated with addressing the social determinants of health, the federal government has enabled federally qualified health centers that treat poor and uninsured patients to include the costs of civil legal services in their approved budget. This support has led to the expansion of medical-legal partnerships nationally that assist medical care providers to address "the complexities of patients' lives" (Regenstein et al. 2018, p. 378).

Once a provider has completed a health needs assessment that includes the social determinants of health, an important question arises as to how this information should be incorporated into the patient's medical record. Both federal and private payer standards require physicians and other providers to maintain electronic health records (EHR) that record data about each patient treated. These records include direct patient interactions, laboratory results, x-ray test results, and other relevant information. Much of this information is stored with a code indicating the condition for which a patient is being treated. These codes are determined according to the International Statistical Classification of Diseases and Related Health Problems (ICD). The most recent version of these codes, referred to as ICD-10, now includes a series of new codes, referred to as Z codes, that identify social determinants of health that are relevant to a specific patient (Torres et al. 2017). Examples of Z codes include social determinants such as problems related to education and literacy, problems related to housing, and problems related to family circumstances. A growing number of providers and policy scholars are calling for establishing national standards to assure that information relevant to social determinants is included in a patient's health record in a way that can be applied both to the care the patients receive and to gathering data about the social determinants affecting a population of patients (Cantor and Thorpe 2018). These data can then be used to monitor the quality of care offered by specific providers in addressing relevant social determinants (Gottlieb et al. 2016). Aggregate data from specific patient populations could also be made available to local public health professionals and to public health scholars to facilitate the development of policies and procedures to reduce the impact of social determinants of health (Narain and Zimmerman 2018).

In addition to storing data on social determinants as reported by individual patients, it is also possible to do the reverse—to gather relevant environmental data from specific communities and, when a localized environmental risk is identified, enter that information into the record of individual patients living within those communities (Beck et al. 2017). An example would be integrating data on air pollution levels and housing quality within certain neighborhoods into the EHR of children with asthma.

Researchers at the Kaiser Family Foundation have published a review of the new policies and programs intended to improve health by addressing the social determinants of health (Artiga and Hinton 2018). They provide the following summary of their review: "With growing recognition of the importance of social factors to health outcomes, an increasing number of initiatives have emerged to address social determinants of health by bringing a greater focus on health within non-health sectors and increasingly recognizing and addressing health-related social needs through the health care system" (p. 8). Addressing social determinants of health will be a central component of ongoing efforts to reduce health disparities nationally.

How Far Have We Come in Reducing Health Disparities?

The research documenting health disparities among different groups in the United States spans more than a quarter of a century. As described in this book, there have been numerous government and private reports on the progress we have made and the problems that remain. In 2012 Professor David R. Williams of Harvard School of Public Health, one of the leading national voices in the effort to reduce health disparities, published a paper, the title of which carries a poignant message: *Miles to Go Before We Sleep: Racial Inequities in Health*. As described by Williams, "Despite thousands of published studies, our current knowledge is limited with regard to the most effective strategies to reduce health inequities, and there is an urgent need to develop a science base to guide societal interventions" (p. 279). While it seems clear that we still don't know the optimal means to eliminate health disparities that are based on inequality of socioeconomic position and race/ethnicity, I hope that the material we have covered in this book will support you in your own effort to work toward attaining this important goal.

Abbasi, J. 2017. Emergency department opioid misuse diagnoses increasing in adolescents and young adults. *JAMA* 318(24): 2416–17.

Abel, T. D., White, J. 2011. Skewed riskscapes and gentrified inequities: Environmental exposure disparities in Seattle, Washington. *American Journal of Public Health* 101 (Suppl. 1): S246–54.

Acevedo-Garcia, D., Soobader, M. J., and Berkman, L. F. 2005. The differential effect of foreign-born status on low birth weight by race/ethnicity and education. *Pediatrics* 115(1): 20–30 (Web version only).

Adam, E. K., Heissel, J. A., Zeiders, K. H., et al. 2015. Developmental histories of perceived racial discrimination and diurnal cortisol profiles in adulthood: A 20-year prospective study. *Psychoneuroendocrinology* 62: 279–91.

Adler, N. A., Boyce, T., Chesney, M. A., et al. 1994. Socioeconomic status and health: The challenge of the gradient. *American Psychologist* 49: 15–24.

Adler, N. E., Epel, E., Castallazzo, G., Ickovics, J. 2000. Relationship of subjective and objective social status with psychological and physiological functioning in preliminary data in healthy white women. *Health Psychology* 19(6): 586–92.

Adler, N., and Ostrove, J. 1999. Socioeconomic status and health: What we know and what we don't. *Annals of the New York Academy of Sciences* 896: 3–15.

Affordable Care Act, Section 1557. 2010. Available at http://www.hhs.gov/healthcare/rights/law/index.html.

Ahnquist, J., Wamala, S. P., Lindstrom, M. 2012. Social determinants of health—a question of social or economic capital? Interaction effects of socioeconomic factors on health outcomes. *Social Science and Medicine* 74: 930–39.

Akincigil, A., Olfson, M., Siegel, M., et al. 2012. Racial and ethnic disparities in depression care in community-dwelling elderly in the United States. *American Journal of Public Health* 102: 319–28.

Alcon Laboratories, Inc. 2006a. Alcon's New Anti-Glaucoma Drug Shows Greater Effectiveness in Black Patients. Available at www.alconlabs.com/corporate/newsreleases/travatan.jhtml.

Alcon Laboratories, Inc. 2006b. Travatan® (travoprost ophthalmic solution) prescribing information. Available at http://myglaucomasupport.com/travatan-z-solution.shtml.

Alexander, G. C., and Sehgal, A. R. 1998. Barriers to cadaveric renal transplantation among blacks, women, and the poor. *JAMA* 280: 1148–52.

Alsan, M., Wanamaker, M. 2017. Tuskegee and the Health of Black Men. National Bureau of Economic Research Working Paper 22323. Available at http://www.nber.org/papers/w22323.pdf, accessed August 30, 2018.

American Academy of Pediatrics. 2012. Policy Statement—Early Childhood Adversity, Toxic Stress, and the Role of the Pediatrician: Translating Developmental Science into Lifelong Health. *Pediatrics* 129(1): e224–e231.

American Community Survey. 2016. Tables for Health Insurance Coverage, 2013–2016. Available at https://www.census.gov/data/tables/time-series/demo/health-insurance/acs-hi.2016.html, accessed July 3, 2018.

American Heart Association and American College of Cardiology. 2001. Controversial Issues in Quality: Race/Gender/Ethnicity/SES—Are There Disparities in the Quality of Care? Panel discussion held October 1, 2001, Washington, D.C. Transcript available at www.kaisernetwork.org/health_cast/uploaded_files/ACFD7A.pdf.

American Medical Association, Council on Ethical and Judicial Affairs. 1990. Black-white disparities in health care. *JAMA* 263: 2344–46.

American Public Health Association. 2018. Chronic Stress and the Risk of High School Dropout. Available at https://www.apha.org/-/media/files/pdf/sbhc/chronic_stress.ashx, accessed August 14, 2018.

American Society of Hematology. 2018. Sickle Cell Trait. Available at http://www.hematology.org/Patients/Anemia/Sickle-Cell-Trait.aspx, accessed September 23, 2018.

Andrews, R. M., and Elixhauser, A. 2000. Use of major therapeutic procedures: Are Hispanics treated differently than non-Hispanic whites? *Ethnicity and Disease* 10: 384–94.

Ansell, D. A., McDonald, E. K. 2015. Bias, black lives, and academic medicine. *New England Journal of Medicine* 372(12): 1087–89.

Appiah, K. A. 1990. Racisms. In Goldberg, D. T., ed. *Anatomy of Racism*, pp. 3–17. Minneapolis: University of Minnesota Press.

Arias, E., Xu, J., Jim, M. A. 2014. Period Life Tables for the Non-Hispanic American Indian and Alaska Native Population, 2007–2009. *American Journal of Public Health* 104(S3): S312–S319.

Armstrong, K. 2012. Genomics and health care disparities: The role of statistical discrimination. *JAMA* 308: 1979–80.

Armstrong, K., Micco, E., Carney, A., Stopfer, J., and Putt, M. 2005. Racial differences in the use of BRCA1/2 testing among women with a family history of breast or ovarian cancer. *JAMA* 293: 1729–36.

Artiga, S., Hinton, E. 2018. Beyond Health Care: The Role of Social Determinants in Promoting Health and Health Equity. Kaiser Family Foundation. Available at https://www.kff.org/disparities-policy/issue-brief/beyond-health-care-the-role-of-social-determinants-in-promoting-health-and-health-equity/, accessed September 5, 2018.

Ashton, C. M., Haidet, P., Paterniti, D. A., et al. 2003. Racial and ethnic disparities in the use of health services: Bias, preferences, or poor communication? *Journal of General Internal Medicine* 18: 146–52.

Association of American Medical Colleges. 2005. Cultural Competence Education for Medical Students. Available at https://www.aamc.org/download/54338/data/culturalcomped.pdf.

Association of American Medical Colleges. 2013. Diversity in Medical Education: Facts and Figures 2012. Available at https://members.aamc.org/eweb/upload/Diversity%20in%20Medical%20Education_Facts%20and%20Figures%202012.pdf.

Association of American Medical Colleges. 2013. Diversity in the Physician Workforce: Facts and Figures 2010. Available at https://members.aamc.org/eweb/upload/Diversity%20in%20the%20Physician%20Workforce%20Facts%20and%20Figures%202010.pdf.

Association of American Medical Colleges. 2013. Tool for Assessing Cultural Competence Training. Available at https://www.aamc.org/initiatives/tacct/.

Association of American Medical Colleges. 2016. Diversity in Medical Education—Facts and Figures 2016. Available at http://www.aamcdiversityfactsandfigures2016.org/, accessed September 27, 2018.

Ayanian, J. Z., Landon, B. E., Newhouse, J. P., Zaslavsky, A. M. 2014. Racial and ethnic disparities among enrollees in Medicare Advantage Plans. *New England Journal of Medicine* 371: 2288–97.

Ayanian, J. Z., Cleary, P. D., Weissman, J. S., and Epstein, A. M. 1999. The effect of patients' preferences on racial differences in access to renal transplantation. *New England Journal of Medicine* 341: 1661–69.

Babey, S. H., Wolstein, J., Diamant, A. L. 2011. Food Environments Near Home and School Related to Consumption of Soda and Fast Food. Available at http://healthpolicy.ucla.edu/publications/search/pages/detail.aspx?PubID=8.

Bach, P. B., Cramer, L. D., Warren, J. L., and Begg, C. B. 1999. Racial differences in the treatment of early-stage lung cancer. *New England Journal of Medicine* 341: 1198–205.

Bach, P. B., Pham, H. H., Schrag, D., Tate, R. C., and Hargraves, J. L. 2004. Primary care physicians who treat blacks and whites. *New England Journal of Medicine* 351: 575–84.

Bancks, M. P., Kershaw, K., Carson, A. P., et al. 2017. Association of modifiable risk factors in young adulthood with racial disparity in incident type 2 diabetes during middle adulthood. *JAMA* 318(24): 2457–65.

Bandura, A. 1997. *Self-Efficacy—The Exercise of Control.* New York: W. H. Freeman and Company.

Barnett, A. H., Bain, S. C., Bouter, P., et al. 2004. Angiotensin-receptor blockade versus converting enzyme inhibition in type 2 diabetes and nephropathy. *New England Journal of Medicine* 351: 1952–61.

Barr, D. A. 2005. The practitioner's dilemma: Can we use a patient's race to predict genetics, ancestry, and the expected outcomes of treatment? *Annals of Internal Medicine* 143: 809–15.

Barr, D. A. and Wanat, S. F. 2005. Listening to patients: Cultural and linguistic barriers to health care access. *Family Medicine* 37: 199–204.

Barr, D. A. 2017. The childhood roots of cardiovascular disease disparities. *Mayo Clinic Proceedings* 92(9): 1415–21.

Barr, D. A. 2018. When trauma hinders learning. *Phi Delta Kappan* 99(6): 39–44.

Bassett, M. T. 2015. #BlackLivesMatter—A challenge to the medical and public health communities. *New England Journal of Medicine* 372(12): 1085–87.

Beck, A. F., Sandel, M. T., Ryan, P. H., Kahn, R. S. 2017. Mapping neighborhood health geomarkers to clinical care decisions to promote equity in child health. *Health Affairs* 36(6): 999–1005.

Bellinger, D. C. 2016. Lead contamination in Flint—An abject failure to protect public health. *New England Journal of Medicine* 374: 1101–3.

Berchick, E. R., Hood, E., Barnett, J. C. 2018. Health Insurance Coverage in the United States: 2017. Available at https://www.census.gov/library/publications/2018/demo/p60-264.html, accessed September 30, 2018.

Berg, M. T., Simons, R. L., Ashley Barr, A., et al. 2017. Childhood/adolescent stressors and allostatic load in adulthood: Support for a calibration model. *Social Science and Medicine* 193: 130–39.

Bergstrom, N., Horn, S. D. 2011. Racial disparities in rates of pressure ulcers in nursing homes and site of care. *JAMA* 306: 211–12.

Berhane, K., Chang, C-C., McConnell, R., et al. 2016. Association of changes in air quality with bronchitic symptoms in children in California, 1993–2012. *JAMA* 315(14): 1491–1501.

Besser, L. M., Rodriguez, D. A., McDonald, N., et al. 2018. Neighborhood built environment and cognition in non-demented older adults: The multi-ethnic study of atherosclerosis. *Social Science and Medicine* (200): 27–35.

Betancourt, J. R., Green, A. R., Carrillo, J. E., and Park, E. R. 2005. Cultural competence and health care disparities: Key perspectives and trends. *Health Affairs* 24(2): 499–505.

Births: Final Data for 2010. National Vital Statistics Reports 61, no. 1, August 28, 2012.

Blackstock, A. W., Herndon, J. E. II, Paskett, E. D., et al. 2006. Similar outcomes between African American and non-African American patients with extensive-stage small-cell lung carcinoma: Report from the Cancer and Leukemia Group B. *Journal of Clinical Oncology* 24: 407–12.

Blair, I. V., Havranek, E. P., Price, D. W., et al. 2013. Assessment of biases against Latinos and African Americans among primary care providers and community members. *American Journal of Public Health* 103: 92–98.

Blalock, H. M. 1979. *Social Statistics.* 2nd ed. New York: McGraw Hill.

Blendon, R. J., Benson, J. M. 2018. The public and the opioid-abuse epidemic. *New England Journal of Medicine* 378: 407–11.

Bloche, M. G. 2004. Health care disparities: Science, politics, and race. *New England Journal of Medicine* 350: 1568–70.

Blumenthal, D., Seervai, S. 2017. To Combat the Opioid Epidemic, We Must Be Honest About All Its Causes. *Harvard Business Review*, October 26, 2017. Available at https://hbr.org/2017/10/to-combat-the-opioid-epidemic-we-must-be-honest-about-all-its-causes?autocomplete=true, accessed July 26, 2018.

Bogart, L. M., Elliott, M. N., Kanouse, D. E., et al. 2013. Association between perceived discrimination and racial/ethnic disparities in problem behaviors among preadolescent youths. *American Journal of Public Health* 103: 74–81.

Bonham, V. L., Sellers, S. L., Gallagher, T. H., et al. 2009. Physicians' attitudes toward race, genetics, and clinical medicine. *Genetics in Medicine* 11: 279–86.

Bor, J., Cohen, G. H., Galea, S. 2017. Population health in an era of rising income inequality: USA, 1980–2015. *Lancet* 389(10077): 1475–90.

Boyce, W. T., Obradovi, J., Bush, N. R., et al. 2012. Social stratification, classroom climate, and the behavioral adaptation of kindergarten children. *Proceedings of the National Academy of Sciences U S A.* 109 (Suppl. 2): 17168–73.

Bradby, H. 2010. What do we mean by 'racism'? Conceptualising the range of what we call racism in health care settings: A commentary on Peek et al. *Social Science and Medicine* 71(1): 10–12.

Braveman, P. 2017. A New Definition of Health Equity to Guide Future Efforts and Measure Progress. Available at https://www.healthaffairs.org/do/10.1377/hblog20170622 .060710/full/, accessed July 12, 2018.

Braveman, P. 2012. Health inequalities by class and race in the US: What can we learn from the patterns? *Social Science and Medicine* 74: 665–67.

Braveman, P. A., Kumanyika, S., Fielding, J., et al. 2011. Health disparities and health equity: The issue is justice. *American Journal of Public Health* 101 (Suppl. 1): S149–55.

Braveman, P., Barclay, C. 2009. Health disparities beginning in childhood: A life-course perspective. *Pediatrics* 124 (Suppl. 3): S163–S175.

Brawley, O. W. 2006. Lung cancer and race: Equal treatment yields equal outcome among equal patients, but there is no equal treatment. *Journal of Clinical Oncology* 24: 332–33.

Brent, D. A., Silverstein, M. 2013. Shedding light on the long shadow of childhood adversity. *JAMA* 309: 1777–78.

Bridget, M., Kuehn, B. M. 2016. Pediatrician sees long road ahead for Flint after lead poisoning crisis. *JAMA* 315(10): 967–69.

Brooks, D. 2006. Marshmallows and public policy. *New York Times,* May 7.

Brown, C. M., Copeland, K. A., Sucharew, H., Kahn, R. S. 2012. Social-emotional problems in preschool-aged children: Opportunities for prevention and early intervention. *Archives of Pediatric and Adolescent Medicine* 166: 926–32.

Brown, E. R., Ojeda, V. D., Wyn, R., and Levan, R. 2000. Racial and ethnic disparities in access to health insurance and health care. UCLA Center for Health Policy Research, Henry J. Kaiser Family Foundation. Available at www.healthpolicy.ucla.edu/pubs /publication.asp?pubID=31.

Browne, A. J. 2017. Moving beyond description: Closing the health equity gap by redressing racism impacting Indigenous populations. *Social Science and Medicine* 184: 23–26.

Brunkard, J., Namulanda, G., Ratard, R. 2008. Hurricane Katrina Deaths, Louisiana, 2005. *Disaster Medicine and Public Health Preparedness* 2(4): 215–23.

Brunner, E., Davey Smith, G., Marmot, M., et al. 1996. Childhood social circumstances and psychosocial and behavioural factors as determinants of plasma fibrinogen. *Lancet* 347(9007): 1008–13.

Brunner, E., Marmot, M. G., Nanchahal, K., et al. 1997. Social inequality in coronary risk: Central obesity and the metabolic syndrome; Evidence from the Whitehall II study. *Diabetologia* 40: 1341–49.

Burchard, E. G., Ziv, E., Coyle, N., et al. 2003. The importance of race and ethnic background in biomedical research and clinical practice. *New England Journal of Medicine* 348: 1170–75.

Byrd, W. C., Hughey, M. W. 2015. Biological determinism and racial essentialism—The ideological double helix of racial inequality. *Annals of the American Academy of Political and Social Science* 661(1): 8–22.

Cadar, D., Lassale, C., Davies, H., et al. 2018. Individual and area-based socioeconomic factors associated with dementia incidence in England: Evidence from a 12-year follow-up in the English longitudinal study of ageing. *JAMA Psychiatry* 75(7): 723–32.

Cai, S., Feng, Z., Fennell, M. L., Mor, V. 2011. Despite small improvement, black nursing home residents remain less likely than whites to receive flu vaccine. *Health Affairs (Millwood)* 30(10): 1939–46.

Campbell, K. M., Rodríguez, J. E., Nowakowski, A. C. H., Gotrace, P. 2015. Attitudes and perceptions about hypertension among churchgoing blacks. *Journal of Health Care for the Poor and Underserved* 26(1): 260–65.

Canto, J. G., Every, N. R., Magid, D. J., et al. 2000. Relation of race and sex to the use of reperfusion therapy in Medicare beneficiaries with acute myocardial infarction. *New England Journal of Medicine* 342: 1094–1100.

Cantor, M. N., Thorpe, L. 2018. Integrating data on social determinants of health into electronic health records. *Health Affairs* 37(4): 585–90.

Carroll-Scott, A., Gilstad-Hayden, K., Rosenthal, L., et al. 2013. Disentangling neighborhood contextual associations with child body mass index, diet, and physical activity: The role of built, socioeconomic, and social environments. *Social Science and Medicine* 95: 106–14.

Carson, P., Ziesche, S., Johnson, G., and Cohn, J. N. 1999. Racial differences in response to therapy for heart failure: Analysis of the vasodilator–heart failure trials. *Journal of Cardiac Failure* 5: 178–87.

Case, A., Deaton, A. 2015. Rising morbidity and mortality in midlife among white non-Hispanic Americans in the 21st century. *Proceedings of the National Academy of Sciences of the United States* 112(49): 15078–83.

Case, A., Deaton, A. 2017. Mortality and morbidity in the 21st century. Available at https://www.brookings.edu/wp-content/uploads/2017/03/6_casedeaton.pdf, accessed July 3, 2018.

CDC (Centers for Disease Control and Prevention)—See US Department of Health and Human Services, Centers for Disease Control and Prevention.

Center on the Developing Child at Harvard University. 2011. Building the Brain's "Air Traffic Control" System: How Early Experiences Shape the Development of Executive Function: Working Paper No. 11. Available at www.developingchild.harvard.edu, accessed August 14, 2018.

Chatterjee, N. A., He, Y., Keating, N. L. 2013. Racial differences in breast cancer stage at diagnosis in the mammography era. *American Journal of Public Health* 103: 170–76.

Cisternas, M. G., Murphy, L., Croft, J. B., Helmick, G. C. 2009. Racial disparities in total knee replacement among Medicare enrollees—United States, 2000–2006. *MMWR* 58(06): 133–38.

Clancy, C. 2003. Letter concerning Health Disparities Report. Available at www.qualitytools.ahrq.gov/disparitiesreport/2003/documents/DisparitiesLtr.htm.

Clark, C. R., Coull, B., Berkman, L. F., Buring, J. E., Ridker, P. M. 2011. Geographic variation in cardiovascular inflammation among healthy women in the Women's Health Study. *PLoS One* 6(11): e27468.

Cohen, S., Doyle, W. J., Skoner, D. P., Rabin, B. S., and Gwaltney, J. M. 1997. Social ties and susceptibility to the common cold. *JAMA* 277: 1940–44.

Cohen, S., Janicki-Deverts, D., Doyle, W. J., et al. 2012. Chronic stress, glucocorticoid receptor resistance, inflammation, and disease risk. *Proceedings of the National Academy of Sciences U S A.* 109(16): 5995–99.

Cohn, J. N., Archibald, D. G., Ziesche, S., et al. 1986. Effect of vasodilator therapy on mortality in chronic congestive heart failure: Results of a Veterans Administration Cooperative Study. *New England Journal of Medicine* 314: 1547–52.

Cohn, J. N., Johnson, G., Ziesche, S., et al. 1991. A comparison of Enalapril with Hydralazine-isosorbide Dinitrate in the treatment of chronic congestive heart failure. *New England Journal of Medicine* 325: 303–10.

Colen, C. G., Ramey, D. M., Cooksey, E. C., Williams, D. R. 2018. Racial disparities in health among nonpoor African Americans and Hispanics: The role of acute and chronic discrimination. *Social Science and Medicine* 199: 167–80.

Collins, F. S., Koroshetz, W. J., Volkow, N. D. 2018. Helping to end addiction over the long-term: The research plan for the NIH HEAL Initiative. *JAMA* 320(2): 129–30.

Congressional Budget Office. 2008. Growing Disparities in Life Expectancy. April 17, 2008. Available at http://cbo.gov/publication/41681, accessed June 26, 2013.

Cooper-Patrick, L., Gallo, J. J., Gonzales, J. J., et al. 1999. Race, gender, and partnership in the patient-physician relationship. *JAMA* 282: 583–89.

Cooper, L. A., and Powe, N. R. 2004. Disparities in Patient Experiences, Health Care Processes, and Outcomes: The Role of Patient-Provider Racial, Ethnic, and Language Concordance. Commonwealth Fund. Available at www.cmwf.org/publications/publications _show.htm?doc_id=231670.

Cooper, R. C., Wolf-Maier, K., Luke, A., et al. 2005. An international comparative study of blood pressure in populations of European vs. African descent. *BMC Medicine* 3(2). Available at www.biomedcentral.com/1741-7015/3/2.

Cooper, R. S., Kaufman, J. S., and Ward, R. 2003. Race and genomics. *New England Journal of Medicine* 348: 1166–70.

Creighton, M. J., Goldman, N., Pebley, A. R., Chung, C. Y. 2012. Durational and generational differences in Mexican immigrant obesity: Is acculturation the explanation? *Social Science and Medicine* 75: 300–310.

Crimmins, E. M., Kim, J. K., Alley, D. E., Karlamangla, A., Seeman, T. 2007. Hispanic paradox in biological risk profiles. *American Journal of Public Health* 97: 1305–10.

Cullen, M. R., Cummins, C., Fuchs, V. R. 2012. Geographic and racial variation in premature mortality in the U.S.: Analyzing the disparities. *PLoS One* 7(4): e32930.

Cunningham, P. J., Green, T. L., Braun, R. T. 2018. Income disparities in the prevalence, severity, and costs of co-occurring chronic and behavioral health conditions. *Medical Care* 56(2): 139–45.

Cunningham, T. J., Croft, J. B., Liu, Y., et al. 2017. Vital signs: Racial disparities in age-specific mortality among blacks or African Americans—United States, 1999–2015. *Morbidity and Mortality Weekly Report* 66(17): 444–56.

Cykert, S., Dilworth-Anderson, P., Monroe, M. H., et al. 2010. Factors associated with decisions to undergo surgery among patients with newly diagnosed early-stage lung cancer. *JAMA* 303: 2368–76.

Cykert, S., Phifer, N. 2003. Surgical decision for early stage non–small cell lung cancer: Which racially sensitive perceptions of cancer are likely to explain racial variations in surgery? *Medical Decision Making* 23: 167–76.

D'Angelo, H., Ammerman, A., Gordon-Larsen, P., et al. 2016. Sociodemographic disparities in proximity of schools to tobacco outlets and fast-food restaurants. *American Journal of Public Health* 106(9): 1556–62.

Daly, B., Olopade, O. I. 2015. Race, ethnicity, and the diagnosis of breast cancer. *JAMA* 313(2): 141–42.

Daniel, H., Bornstein, S. S., Kane, K. C. 2018. Addressing social determinants to improve patient care and promote health equity: An American College of Physicians Position Paper. *Annals of Internal Medicine* 168(8): 577–78.

Das, A. 2013. How does race get "under the skin"?: Inflammation, weathering, and metabolic problems in late life. *Social Science and Medicine* 77: 75–83.

Dasgupta, N., Beletsky, L., Ciccarone, D. 2018. Opioid crisis: No easy fix to its social and economic determinants. *American Journal of Public Health* 108(2): 182–86.

David, R. J., and Collins, J. W. 1997. Differing birth weight among infants of U.S.-born blacks, African-born blacks, and U.S.-born whites. *New England Journal of Medicine* 337: 1209–14.

Davis, M. A., Guo, C., Sol, K., et al. 2017. Trends and disparities in the number of self-reported healthy older adults in the United States, 2000 to 2014. *JAMA Internal Medicine* 177(11): 1683–84.

Davis, S. K., Liu, Y., Quarells, R. C., Din-Dzietharn, R. 2005. Metro Atlanta Heart Disease Study Group. Stress-related racial discrimination and hypertension likelihood in a population-based sample of African Americans: The Metro Atlanta Heart Disease Study. *Ethnicity and Disease* 15: 585–93.

Deaton, A., Lubotsky, D. 2003. Mortality, inequality and race in American cities and states. *Social Science and Medicine* 56: 1139–53.

Debbink, M. P., Bader, M. D. 2011. Racial residential segregation and low birth weight in Michigan's metropolitan areas. *American Journal of Public Health* 101(9): 1714–20.

DeSantis, C. E., Fedewa, S. A., Goding Sauer, A., et al. 2015. Breast cancer statistics, 2015: Convergence of incidence rates between black and white women. *CA: A Cancer Journal for Clinicians* 66(1): 31–42.

DeSantis, C. E., Ma, J., Goding Sauer, A., et al. 2017. Breast cancer statistics, 2017, racial disparity in mortality by state. *CA: A Cancer Journal for Clinicians* 67(6): 439–48.

Detrano, R., Guerci, A. D., Carr, J. J., et al. 2008. Coronary calcium as a predictor of coronary events in four racial or ethnic groups. *New England Journal of Medicine* 358: 1336–45.

Devine, P. G. 1989. Stereotypes and prejudice: Their automatic and controlled components. *Journal of Personality and Social Psychology* 56: 5–18.

Diez Roux, A. V., Merkin, S. S., Arnett, D., et al. 2001. Neighborhood of residence and incidence of coronary heart disease. *New England Journal of Medicine* 345: 99–106.

Dimick, J., Ruhter, J., Sarrazin, M. V., Birkmeyer, J. D. 2013. Black patients more likely than whites to undergo surgery at low-quality hospitals in segregated regions. *Health Affairs (Millwood)* 32(6): 1046–53.

Din-Dzietham, R., Nembhard, W. N., Collins, R., and Davis, S. K. 2004. Perceived stress following race-based discrimination at work is associated with hypertension in African-Americans: The Metro Atlanta Heart Disease Study, 1999–2001. *Social Science and Medicine* 58: 449–61.

Do, D. P., Frank, R., Iceland, J. 2017. Black-white metropolitan segregation and self-rated health: Investigating the role of neighborhood poverty. *Social Science and Medicine* 187: 85–92.

Do, D. P. 2009. The dynamics of income and neighborhood context for population health: Do long-term measures of socioeconomic status explain more of the black/white health disparity than single-point-in-time measures? *Social Science and Medicine* 68(8): 1368–75.

Doescher, M. P., Saver, B. G., Franks, P., and Fiscella, K. 2000. Racial and ethnic disparities in perceptions of physician style and trust. *Archives of Family Medicine* 9: 1156–63.

Douglas, J. C., Bakris, G. L., Epstein, M., et al. 2003. Management of high blood pressure in African Americans. *Archives of Internal Medicine* 163: 525–41.

Dovidio, J. F. 2001. On the nature of contemporary prejudice: The third wave. *Journal of Social Issues* 57: 829–49.

Dovidio, J. F., and Gaertner, S. L. 1998. On the nature of contemporary prejudice. In Eberhardt, J. L., and Fiske, S. T., eds., *Confronting Racism: The Problem and the Response,* 3–32. Thousand Oaks: Sage.

Dowell, D., Noonan, R. K., Houry, D. 2017. Underlying factors in drug overdose deaths. *JAMA* 318(23): 2295–96.

Dries, D. L., Exner, D. V., Gersh, B. J., Cooper, H. A., Carson, P. E., and Domanski, M. J. 1999. Racial differences in the outcome of left ventricular dysfunction. *New England Journal of Medicine* 340: 609–16.

Dries, D. L., Strong, M. H., Cooper, R. S., and Drazner, M. H. 2002. Efficacy of angiotensin-converting enzyme inhibitor in reducing progression from asymptomatic left ventricular dysfunction to symptomatic heart failure in black and white patients. *Journal of the American College of Cardiology* 40: 311–17.

Dunlay, S. M., Lippmann, S. J., Greiner, M. A., et al. 2017. Perceived discrimination and cardiovascular outcomes in older African Americans: Insights from the Jackson Heart Study. *Mayo Clinic Proceedings* 92(5): 699–709.

Durham, A. L., Wiegman, C., Adcock, I. M. 2011. Epigenetics of asthma. *Biochimica et Biophysica Acta* 1810: 1103–9.

Durkheim, E. 1997. *Suicide: A Study in Sociology.* New York: Free Press; repr. of 1951 ed., originally published in French, 1897.

Dwyer-Lindgren, L., Bertozzi-Villa, A., Stubbs, R. W., et al. 2017. Inequalities in life expectancy among US counties, 1980 to 2014—Temporal trends and key drivers. *JAMA Internal Medicine* 177(7): 1003–11.

Dwyer-Lindgren, L., Bertozzi-Villa, A., Stubbs, R. W., et al. 2018. Trends and patterns of geographic variation in mortality from substance use disorders and intentional injuries among US counties, 1980–2014. *JAMA* 319(10): 1013–23.

Dzau, V. J., McClellan, M., McGinnis, J. M., et al. 2017. Vital directions for health and health care—Priorities from a National Academy of Medicine Initiative. *JAMA* 317(14): 1461–70.

Ebbeling, C. B., Ludwig, D. S. 2008. Tracking pediatric obesity: An index of uncertainty? *JAMA.* 299: 2442–43.

Egen, O., Beatty, K., Blackley, D. J., et al. 2017. Health and social conditions of the poorest versus wealthiest counties in the United States. *American Journal of Public Health* 107(1): 130–35.

Elder, K., Ramamonjiarivelo, Z., Wiltshire, J., et al. 2012. Trust, medication adherence, and hypertension control in Southern African American men. *American Journal of Public Health* 102: 2242–45.

Ellsworth, M. A., Stevens, T. P., D'Angio, C. T. 2010. Infant race affects application of clinical guidelines when screening for drugs of abuse in newborns. *Pediatrics* 125: e1379–85.

Elo, I. T., Culhane, J. F. 2010. Variations in health and health behaviors by nativity among pregnant black women in Philadelphia. *American Journal of Public Health* 100: 2185–92.

Emanuel, E. 2006. Changing premed requirements and the medical curriculum. *JAMA* 296: 1128–31.

Emerging Risk Factors Collaboration. 2012. C-reactive protein, fibrinogen, and cardiovascular disease prediction. *New England Journal of Medicine* 367: 1310–20.

Epstein, A. M., Ayanian, J. Z., Keogh, J. H., et al. 2000. Racial disparities in access to renal transplantation: Clinically appropriate or due to underuse or overuse? *New England Journal of Medicine* 343: 1537–44.

Equal Justice Society. 2004. Protecting Equally: Dismantling the Intent Doctrine and Healing Racial Wounds. Available at www.equaljusticesociety.org/protectingequally/.

Evans, R. G., Stoddart, G. L. 1994. Producing health, consuming health care. In Evans, R. G., Barer, M. L., and Marmor, T. R., eds., *Why Are Some People Healthy and Others Not?* 27–54. New York: Aldine De Gruyter.

Evans, R. G., Barer, M. L., and Marmor, T. R., eds. 1994. *Why Are Some People Healthy and Others Not?* New York: Aldine De Gruyter.

Exner, D. V., Dries, D. L., Domanski, M. J., and Cohn, J. N. 2001. Lesser response to angiotensin-converting-enzyme inhibitor therapy in black as compared with white patients with left ventricular dysfunction. *New England Journal of Medicine* 344: 1351–57.

Fang, J., Madhavan, S., and Alderman, M. 1996. The association between birthplace and mortality from cardiovascular causes among black and white residents of New York City. *New England Journal of Medicine* 335: 1545–51.

Farmer, M. M., Ferraro, K. F. 2005. Are racial disparities in health conditional on socioeconomic status? *Social Science and Medicine* 60: 191–204.

Federal Interagency Forum on Child and Family Statistics. 2017. America's Children: Key National Indicators of Well-Being, 2017. Available at https://www.childstats.gov/americaschildren/index.asp, accessed August 13, 2018.

Fedewa, S. A., Edge, S. B., Stewart, A. K., et al. 2011. Race and ethnicity are associated with delays in breast cancer treatment (2003–2006). *Journal of Health Care for the Poor and Underserved* 22: 128–41.

Feinberg, A. P. 2018. The key role of epigenetics in human disease prevention and mitigation. *New England Journal of Medicine* 378(14): 1323–34.

Fiscella, K., Franks, P., Gold, M. R., and Clancy, C. M. 2000. Inequality in quality: Addressing socioeconomic, racial, and ethnic disparities in health care. *JAMA* 283: 2579–84.

Fiske, S. T. 1998. Stereotyping, prejudice, and discrimination. In Gilbert, D. T., Fiske, S. T., and Lindzey, G. eds. *The Handbook of Social Psychology,* 357–411. 4th ed., vol. 1. Boston: McGraw Hill.

Fitzgerald, F. 1994. The tyranny of health. *New England Journal of Medicine* 331: 196–98.

Flexner, A. 1910. *Medical Education in the United States and Canada.* Carnegie Foundation for the Advancement of Teaching.

Fonarow, G. C., Adams, K. F., Abraham, W. T., Yancy, C. W., and Boscardin, W. J. 2005. Risk stratification for in-hospital mortality in acutely decompensated heart failure. *JAMA* 293: 572–80.

Fontanarosa, P. B., Bauchner, H. 2018. Race, ancestry, and medical research. *JAMA.* 320(15): 1539–40.

Fox, R. 2005. Cultural competence and the culture of medicine. *New England Journal of Medicine* 353: 1316–17.

Frank, J. W., Cohen, R., Irene Yen, I., Balfour, J., and Smith, M. 2003. Socioeconomic gradients in health status over 29 years of follow-up after midlife: The Alameda County study. *Social Science and Medicine* 57: 2305–23.

Franzini, L., Elliott, M. N., Cuccaro. P., et al. 2009. Influences of physical and social neighborhood environments on children's physical activity and obesity. *American Journal of Public Health* 99: 271–78.

Franzini, L., Taylor, W., Elliott, M. N., et al. 2010. Neighborhood characteristics favorable to outdoor physical activity: Disparities by socioeconomic and racial/ethnic composition. *Health Place* 16: 267–74.

Freedman, R. A., He, Y., Winer, E. P., Keating, N. L. 2013. Racial/ethnic differences in receipt of timely adjuvant therapy for older women with breast cancer: Are delays influenced by the hospitals where patients obtain surgical care? *Health Services Research,* May 13, 2013 (Epub ahead of print).

Fuchs, V. R. 1983. *Who Shall Live?* New York: Basic Books.

Fuchs, V. R. 1986. *The Health Economy.* Cambridge, MA: Harvard University Press.

Gaffin, J. M., Phipatanakul, W. 2009. The role of indoor allergens in the development of asthma. *Current Opinion in Allergy and Clinical Immunology* 9: 128–35.

Galea, S., Tracy, M., Hoggatt, K. J., Dimaggio, C., Karpati, A. 2011. Estimated deaths attributable to social factors in the United States. *American Journal of Public Health* 101: 1456–65.

Garcia, R. S. 2004. No come nada. *Health Affairs (Millwood)* 23(2): 215–19.

Gaskin, D. J., Dinwiddie, G. Y., Chan, K. S., McCleary, R. R. 2012. Residential segregation and the availability of primary care physicians. *Health Services Research* 47: 2353–76.

GBD 2015 Obesity Collaborators. 2017. Health effects of overweight and obesity in 195 countries over 25 years. *New England Journal of Medicine* 377(1): 13–27.

Gee, G. C., Ryan, A., Laflamme, D. J., and Holt, J. 2006. Self-reported discrimination and mental health status among African descendants, Mexican Americans, and other Latinos in the New Hampshire REACH 2010 Initiative: The added dimension of immigration. *American Journal of Public Health* 96: 1821–28.

Geiger, H. J. 1996. Race and health care: An American dilemma? *New England Journal of Medicine* 335: 815–16.

Geiger, H. J. 2001. Racial stereotyping and medicine: The need for cultural competence. *Canadian Medical Association Journal* 164: 1699–1700.

Geiger, H. J. 2004. Why is HHS obscuring a health care gap? *New York Times,* January 27.

Geronimus, A. T., Hicken, M., Keene, D., Bound, J. 2006. "Weathering" and age patterns of allostatic load scores among blacks and whites in the United States. *American Journal of Public Health* 96: 826–33.

Geserick, M., Vogel, M., Gausche, R., et al. 2018. Acceleration of BMI in early childhood and risk of sustained obesity. *New England Journal of Medicine* 379: 1303–12.

Giordano, G. N., Björk, J., Lindström, M. 2012. Social capital and self-rated health—a study of temporal (causal) relationships. *Social Science and Medicine* 75: 340–48.

Global Burden of Disease. 2018. About GBD. Available at http://www.healthdata.org/gbd/about, accessed July 20, 2018.

Goldfrank, L. R., Knopp, R. K. 2000. Racially and ethnically selective oligoanalgesia: Is this racism? *Annals of Emergency Medicine* 35: 79–82.

Gomes, T., Tadrous, M., Mamdani, M. M., et al. 2018. The burden of opioid-related mortality in the United States. *JAMA Network Open* 1(2): e180217.

Goode, E. 2002a. With video games, researchers link guns to stereotypes. *New York Times,* December 10.

Goode, E. 2002b. The heavy cost of chronic stress. *New York Times,* December 17.

Goodnough, A. 2018. When an Iowa family doctor takes on the opioid epidemic. *New York Times,* June 23, 2018.

Goodwin, J. S., Kuo, Y-F., Brown, D., et al. 2018. Association of chronic opioid use with presidential voting patterns in US counties in 2016. *JAMA Network Open* 1(2): e180431.

Gordon, H. S., Paterniti, D. A., and Wray, N. P. 2004. Race and patient refusal of invasive cardiac procedures. *Journal of General Internal Medicine* 19: 962–66.

Gornick, M. E., Eggers, P. W., Reilly, T. W., et al. 1996. Effects of race and income on mortality and use of services among Medicare beneficiaries. *New England Journal of Medicine* 335: 791–99.

Gottlieb, L., Tobey, R., Cantor, J., et al. 2016. Integrating social and medical data to improve population health: Opportunities and barriers. *Health Affairs* 35(11): 2116–23.

Graham, H. 2004. Social determinants and their unequal distribution: Clarifying policy understanding. *Milbank Quarterly* 82(1): 101–24.

Grayburn, P. A. 2012. Interpreting the coronary-artery calcium score. *New England Journal of Medicine* 366: 294–96.

Greenough, P. G., Lappi, M. D., Hsu, E. B., et al. 2008. Burden of disease and health status among Hurricane Katrina–displaced persons in shelters: A population-based cluster sample. *Annals of Emergency Medicine* 51(4): 426–32.

Greenwald, A. G., McGhee, D. E., Schwartz, J. L. K. 1998. Measuring individual differences in implicit cognition: The implicit association test. *Journal of Personality and Social Psychology* 74(6): 464–80.

Gregg, E. W., Shaw, J. E. 2017. Global health effects of overweight and obesity. *New England Journal of Medicine* 377(1): 80–81.

Griffith, D. M., Johnson, J. L., Zhang, R., Neighbors, H. W., Jackson, J. S. 2011. Ethnicity, nativity, and the health of American blacks. *Journal of Health Care for the Poor and Underserved* 22: 142–56.

Groeneveld, P. W., Laufer, S. B., and Garber, A. M. 2005. Technology diffusion, hospital variation, and racial disparities among elderly Medicare beneficiaries, 1989–2000. *Medical Care* 43: 320–29.

Grol-Prokopczyk, H. 2017. Sociodemographic disparities in chronic pain, based on 12-year longitudinal data. *Pain* 158(2): 313–22.

Gruenewald, T. L., Cohen, S., Matthews, K. A., Tracy, R., Seeman, T. E. 2009. Association of socioeconomic status with inflammation markers in black and white men and women in the Coronary Artery Risk Development in Young Adults (CARDIA) study. *Social Science and Medicine* 69: 451–59.

Grumbach, K., Coffman, J., Gándara, P., et al. 1993. Strategies for Improving the Diversity of the Health Professions. Center for California Health Workforce Studies, University of California, San Francisco. Available at www.futurehealth.ucsf.edu/pdf_files/StrategiesforImprovingFINAL.pdf.

Guralnik, J. M., Land, K. C., Blazer, D., Fillenbaum, G. G., and Branch, L. G. 1993. Educational status and active life expectancy among older blacks and whites. *New England Journal of Medicine* 329: 191–204.

Guthrie, L. C., Butler, S. C., Ward, M. M. 2009. Time perspective and socioeconomic status: A link to socioeconomic disparities in health? *Social Science and Medicine* 68: 2145–51.

Ha, Y. P., Seifu, L. D., Lewis, L. M., et al. 2018. Partnering medical students with barbers to cut hypertension in black men. *American Journal of Public Health* 108(6): 785–87.

Hackbarth, A. D., Romley, J. A., Goldman, D. P. 2011. Racial and ethnic disparities in hospital care resulting from air pollution in excess of federal standards. *Social Science and Medicine* 73(8): 1163–68.

Haffajee, R. L., Mello, M. M., Zhang, F., et al. 2018. Four states with robust prescription drug monitoring programs reduced opioid dosages. *Health Affairs* 37(6): 964–74.

Hager, E. R., Candelaria, M., Latta, L. W., et al. 2012. Maternal perceptions of toddler body size. *Archives of Pediatric and Adolescent Medicine* 166: 417–22.

Haider, A. H., Sexton, J., Sriram, N., et al. 2011. Association of unconscious race and social class bias with vignette-based clinical assessments by medical students. *JAMA* 306: 942–51.

Hales, C. M., Carroll, M. D., Fryar, C. D., Ogden, C. L. 2017. Prevalence of Obesity Among Adults and Youth: United States, 2015–2016. *NCHS Data Brief* No. 288. Available at https://www.cdc.gov/nchs/data/databriefs/db288.pdf, accessed August 15, 2018.

Haley, J. M., Kenney, G. M., Wang, R., et al. 2018. Uninsurance and Medicaid/CHIP Participation Among Children and Parents: Variation in 2016 and Recent Trends. Available at https://www.urban.org/research/publication/uninsurance-and-medicaidchip-participation-among-children-and-parents-variation-2016-and-recent-trends, accessed October 4, 2018.

Halfon, N. 2012. Addressing health inequalities in the US: A life course health development approach. *Social Science and Medicine* 74: 671–73.

Hall, M. A., Dugan, E., Zheng, B., Mishra, A. K. 2001. Trust in physicians and medical institutions: What is it, can it be measured, and does it matter? *Milbank Quarterly* 79(4): 613–39.

Hankerson, S. H., Suite, D., Bailey, R. K. 2015. Treatment disparities among African American men with depression: Implications for clinical practice. *Journal of Health Care for the Poor and Underserved* 26(1): 21–34.

Hanna-Attisha, M., LaChance, J., Sadler, R. C., Champney Schnepp, A. 2016. Elevated blood lead levels in children associated with the Flint drinking water crisis: A spatial analysis of risk and public health response. *American Journal of Public Health* 106(2): 283–90.

Hannan, E. L., van Ryn, M., Burke, J., et al. 1999. Access to coronary artery bypass surgery by race/ethnicity and gender among patients who are appropriate for surgery. *Medical Care* 37: 68–77.

Harrison, J. M., Lagisetty, P., Sites, B. D., et al. 2018. Trends in prescription pain medication use by race/ethnicity among US adults with noncancer pain, 2000–2015. *American Journal of Public Health* 108(6): 788–90.

Hasnain-Wynia, R., Baker, D. W., Nerenz, D., et al. 2007. Disparities in health care are driven by where minority patients seek care: Examination of the hospital quality alliance measures. *Archives of Internal Medicine* 167: 1233–39.

Hastert, T. A., Babey, S. H., Diamant, A. L. 2008. Low-Income Adolescents Face More Barriers to Healthy Weight. UCLA Center for Health Policy Research, Policy Brief. Available at http://healthpolicy.ucla.edu/publications/Documents/PDF/Low-Income%20Ad olescents%20Face%20More%20Barriers%20to%20Healthy%20Weight.pdf.

Hayanga, A. J., Zeliadt, S. B., Backhus, L. M. 2013. Residential segregation and lung cancer mortality in the United States. *JAMA Surgery* 148(1): 37–42.

Hayes, S. L., Radley, D. C., McCarthy, D. 2018. States of Despair: A Closer Look at Rising State Death Rates from Drugs, Alcohol, and Suicide. The Commonwealth Fund, To the Point August 9, 2018. Available at https://www.commonwealthfund.org/blog/2018/states -despair-closer-look-rising-state-death-rates-drugs-alcohol-and-suicide, accessed August 22, 2018.

HealthyPeople.gov. 2010. Available at http://www.healthypeople.gov/2020/about/default .aspx.

Heffernan, K. S., Jae, S. Y., Wilund, K. R., Woods, J. A., Fernhall, B. 2008. Racial differences in central blood pressure and vascular function in young men. *American Journal of Physiology—Heart and Circulatory Physiology* 295: H2380–87.

Helft, G., Worthley, S. G., and Chokron, S. 1999. Race, sex, and physicians' referrals for cardiac catheterization. *New England Journal of Medicine* 341: 285.

Hempstead, K., Phillips, J. 2019. Divergence in recent trends in deaths from intentional and unintentional poisoning. *Health Affairs* 38(1): 29–35.

Herzog, A. R., Ofstedal, M. B., and Wheeler, L. M. 2002. Social engagement and its relationship to health. *Clinics in Geriatric Medicine* 18: 593–609.

Himmelstein, D. U., Woolhandler, S. 2018. Determined action needed on social determinants. *Annals of Internal Medicine* 168(8): 596–97.

History of Hoyle. Available at http://www.hoylegaming.com/c-9-history-of-hoyle.aspx, accessed July 17, 2013.

Ho, S. M. 2010. Environmental epigenetics of asthma: An update. *Journal of Allergy and Clinical Immunology* 126: 453–65.

Holtby, S., Zahnd, E., Grant, D., Park, R. 2011. Children's Exposure to Secondhand Smoke: Nearly One Million Affected in California. UCLA Center for Health Policy Research. Available at http://healthpolicy.ucla.edu/publications/Documents/PDF /SmokePBREVISED11-2-11.pdf.

Huang, X., Keyes, K. M., Li, G. 2018. Increasing prescription opioid and heroin overdose mortality in the United States, 1999–2014: An age–period–cohort analysis. *American Journal of Public Health* 108(1): 131–36.

Indian Health Services. 2018. Disparities. Available at https://www.ihs.gov/newsroom /factsheets/disparities/, accessed August 10, 2018.

Institute for Health Metrics and Evaluation. 2018. Global Burden of Disease. Described at http://www.healthdata.org/gbd, accessed August 10, 2018.

Institute of Medicine. 2002. Unequal Treatment: What Healthcare Providers Need to Know about Racial and Ethnic Disparities in Healthcare. Available at www.iom.edu/CMS /3740/4475.aspx.

Iqbal, J., Ginsburg, O., Rochon, P.A., et al. 2015. Differences in breast cancer stage at di-agnosis and cancer-specific survival by race and ethnicity in the United States. *JAMA* 313(2): 165–73.

Isaacs, S. L., Schroeder, S. A. 2004. Class: The ignored determinant of the nation's health. *New England Journal of Medicine* 351: 1137–42.

Ivey-Stephenson, A. Z., Crosby, A. E., Jack, S. P. D., et al. 2017. Suicide trends among and within urbanization levels by sex, race/ethnicity, age group, and mechanism of death— United States, 2001–2015. *Morbidity and Mortality Weekly Report Surveillance Summaries* 66(18): 1–16.

James, C. V., Moonesinghe, R., Wilson-Frederick, S. M., et al. 2018. Racial/Ethnic Health Disparities Among Rural Adults—United States, 2012–2015. *MMWR Surveillance Summaries* 66(SS-23): 1–9. Available at https://www.cdc.gov/mmwr/volumes/66/ss/ss6623a1 .htm?s_cid=ss6623a1_w, accessed August 10, 2018.

James, P. A., Oparil, S., Carter, B. L., et al. 2014. 2014 Evidence-based guideline for the man-agement of high blood pressure in adults—Report from the Panel Members Appointed to the Eighth Joint National Committee (JNC 8). *JAMA* 311(5): 507–20.

James, S. A. 1994. John Henryism and the health of African-Americans. *Culture, Medicine and Psychiatry* 18(2): 163–82.

James, A., Daley, C. M., Greiner, K. A. 2011. "Cutting" on cancer: Attitudes about cancer spread and surgery among primary care patients in the U.S.A. *Social Science and Medicine* 73: 1669–73.

Japan, Statistics Bureau, Ministry of Internal Affairs and Communication. Concerning the 2005 Population Census. Available at www.stat.go.jp/English/data/kokusei/e_cen_en.htm.

Javitt, J. C., McBean, A. M., Nicholson, G. A., Babish, J. D., Warren, J. L., and Krakauer, H. 1991. Undertreatment of glaucoma among black Americans. *New England Journal of Medicine* 325: 1418–22.

Jay, C. L., Cigarroa, F. G. 2018. Disparities in live donor kidney transplantation related to poverty, race, or ethnicity? *JAMA* 319(1): 24–26.

Jemal, A., Ward, E., Hao, Y., and Thun, M. 2005. Trends in the leading causes of death in the United States, 1970–2002. *JAMA* 294: 1255–59.

Jha, A. K., Orav, E. J., Epstein, A. M. 2011. Low-quality, high-cost hospitals, mainly in South, care for sharply higher shares of elderly black, Hispanic, and Medicaid patients. *Health Affairs (Millwood)* 30(10): 1904–11.

Johnson, S. C., Cavallaro, F. L., Leon, D. A. 2017. A systematic review of allostatic load in relation to socioeconomic position: Poor fidelity and major inconsistencies in biomarkers employed. *Social Science and Medicine* 192: 66–73.

Johnson, R. L., Roter, D., Powe, N. R., and Cooper, L. A. 2004. Patient race/ethnicity and quality of patient-physician communication during medical visits. *American Journal of Public Health* 94: 2084–90.

Jorde, L. B., Wooding, S. P. 2004. Genetic variation, classification, and "race." *Nature Genetics* 36 (Suppl. 11): S28–33.

Journal of the American Medical Association. 2013. Theme issue on Child Health. 309(17): 1749–1843.

Joynt, K. E., Orav, E. J., Jha, A. K. 2011. Thirty-day readmission rates for Medicare beneficiaries by race and site of care. *JAMA* 305: 675–81.

Kaiser Family Foundation. 1999. Race, Ethnicity and Medical Care: A Survey of Public Perceptions and Experiences. Available at www.kff.org/minorityhealth/1529-index.cfm.

Kaiser Family Foundation. 2002. National Survey of Physicians, Part I: Doctors on Disparities in Medical Care. Available at www.kff.org/minorityhealth/20020321a-index.cfm.

Kaiser Family Foundation. 2013. Health Insurance Coverage in America, 2011. Available at http://kff.org/slideshow/health-insurance-coverage-in-america-2011/.

Kaiser Family Foundation. 2018. Overdose Deaths by Race/Ethnicity, 2016. Available at https://www.kff.org/state-category/health-status/opioids/, accessed July 26, 2018.

Kaplan, R. M., Howard, V. J., Safford, M. M., Howard, G. 2015. Educational attainment and longevity: Results from the REGARDS U.S. national cohort study of blacks and whites. *Annals of Epidemiology* 25(5): 323–28.

Kasiske, B. L., Neylan, J. F. III, Riggio, R. R., et al. 1991. The effect of race on access and outcome in transplantation. *New England Journal of Medicine* 324: 302–7.

Katz, J. 2017. Drug deaths in America are rising faster than ever. *New York Times,* June 5, 2017.

Kaufman, J. S., Dolman, L., Rushani, D., Cooper, R. S. 2015. The contribution of genomic research to explaining racial disparities in cardiovascular disease: A systematic review. *American Journal of Epidemiology* 181(7): 464–72.

Kawachi, I. 1999. Social capital and community effects on population and individual death. *Annals of the New York Academy of Sciences* 896: 120–30.

Kawachi, I., Berkman, L. 2000. Social cohesion, social capital, and health. In Berkman, L., Kawachi, I., eds. *Social Epidemiology*, 174–90. New York: Oxford University Press.

Kawachi, I., Kennedy, B. P. 1997. The relationship of income inequality to mortality: Does the choice of indicator matter? *Social Science and Medicine* 45: 1121–27.

Kawachi, I., Kennedy, B. P., Lochner, K., Prothrow-Stith, D. 1997. Social capital, income inequality, and mortality. *American Journal of Public Health* 87: 491–98.

Keita, S. O. Y., Kittles, R. A., Royal, C. D. M., et al. 2004. Conceptualizing human variation. *Nature Genetics* 36 (Suppl.11): S17–20.

Kershaw, K. N., Robinson, W. R., Gordon-Larsen, P., et al. 2017. Association of changes in neighborhood-level racial residential segregation with changes in blood pressure among black adults—The CARDIA Study. *JAMA Internal Medicine* 177(7): 996–1002.

Khullar, D. 2017. How prejudice can harm your health. *New York Times,* June 8, 2017.

Kids Count Data Center, available at https://datacenter.kidscount.org/, accessed October 22, 2018.

Kim, D., Baum, C. F., Ganz, M. L., Subramanian, S. V., Kawachi, I. 2011. The contextual effects of social capital on health: A cross-national instrumental variable analysis. *Social Science and Medicine* 73: 1689–97.

Kimbro, R. T., Bzostek, S., Goldman, N., Rodríguez, G. 2008. Race, ethnicity, and the education gradient in health. *Health Affairs (Millwood)* 27(2): 361–72.

Kimbro, R. T., Denney, J. T. 2013. Neighborhood context and racial/ethnic differences in young children's obesity: Structural barriers to interventions. *Social Science and Medicine* 95: 97–105.

Kimm, S. Y. S., Glynn, N. W., Kriska, A. M., et al. 2002. Decline in physical activity in black girls and white girls during adolescence. *New England Journal of Medicine* 347: 709–15.

Kind, A. J. H., Buckingham, W. R. 2018. Making neighborhood-disadvantage metrics accessible—The neighborhood atlas. *New England Journal of Medicine* 378(26): 2456–58.

Kirby, J. B., Taliaferro, G., and Zuvekas, S. H. 2006. Explaining racial and ethnic disparities in health care. *Medical Care* 44: I-64–I-72.

Kochanek, K. D., Murphy S. L., Xu J., Arias, E. 2017. Mortality in the United States, 2016. *NCHS Data Brief* No. 293 2017. Available at https://www.cdc.gov/nchs/products /databriefs/db293.htm, accessed July 13, 2018.

Koh, H. K., Parekh, A. K. 2018. Toward a United States of health: Implications of understanding the US burden of disease. *JAMA* 319(14): 1438–40.

Kontis, V., Bennett, J. E., Mathers, C. D., et al. 2017. Future life expectancy in 35 industrialised countries: Projections with a Bayesian model ensemble. *Lancet* 389(10076): 1323–35.

Kozhimannil, K. B., Henning-Smith, C. 2018. Racism and health in rural America. *Journal of Health Care for the Poor and Underserved* 29(1): 35–43.

Krieger, N., Sidney, S. 1996. Racial discrimination and blood pressure: The CARDIA Study of young black and white adults. *American Journal of Public Health* 86: 1370–78.

Krieger, N., Williams, D. R., Moss, N. E. 1997. Measuring social class in US public health research: Concepts, methodologies, and guidelines. *Annual Review of Public Health* 18: 341–78.

Krumholz, H. M. 2010. Informed consent to promote patient-centered care. *JAMA* 303: 1190–91.

Kum-Nji, P., Meloy, L. D., Keyser-Marcus, L. 2012. The prevalence and effects of environmental tobacco smoke exposure among inner-city children: Lessons for pediatric residents. *Academic Medicine* 87: 1772–78.

Kuriakose, J. S., Miller, R. L. 2010. Environmental epigenetics and allergic diseases: Recent advances. *Clinical and Experimental Allergy* 40: 1602–10.

Kutney-Lee, A., Smith, D., Thorpe, J., et al. 2017. Race/ethnicity and end-of-life care among veterans. *Medical Care* 55(4): 342–51.

Landler, M., Shear, M. D. 2013. President offers a personal take on race in U.S. *New York Times,* July 19.

Lane, W. G., Rubin, D. M., Monteith, R., Christian, C. W. 2002. Racial differences in the evaluation of pediatric fractures for physical abuse. *JAMA* 288: 1603–9.

Larimer, M. E., Malone, D. K., Garner, M. D., et al. 2009. Health care and public service use and costs before and after provision of housing for chronically homeless persons with severe alcohol problems. *JAMA* 301(13): 1349–57.

Lathan, C. S., Neville, B. A., Earle, C. C. 2006. The effect of race on invasive staging and surgery in non-small-cell lung cancer. *Journal of Clinical Oncology* 24: 413–18.

LaVeist, T. 2000. Minority health status in adulthood: The middle years of life. *Health Care Financing Review* 21(4): 9–21.

LaVeist, T. A., Nickerson, K. J., and Bowie, J. V. 2000. Attitudes about racism, medical mistrust, and satisfaction with care among African American and white cardiac patients. *Medical Care Research and Review* 57 (Suppl. 1): 146–61.

LaVeist, T., Pollack, K., Thorpe, R. Jr., Fesahazion, R., Gaskin, D. 2011. Place, not race: Disparities dissipate in southwest Baltimore when blacks and whites live under similar conditions. *Health Affairs (Millwood)* 30(10): 1880–87.

Lavizzo-Mourey, R., Mackenzie, E. R. 1996. Cultural competence: Essential measurements of quality for managed care organizations. *Annals of Internal Medicine* 124: 919–21.

Lawrence, C. R. 1987. The id, the ego, and equal protection: Reckoning with unconscious racism. *Stanford Law Review:* 317–88.

LeClere, F. B., Rogers, R. G., and Peters, K. D. 1997. Ethnicity and mortality in the United States: Individual and community correlates. *Social Forces* 76: 169–98.

Lee, S. M. 2001. Using the New Racial Categories in the 2000 Census. Annie E. Casey Foundation and Population Reference Bureau. Available at www.aecf.org/kidscount /racial2000.pdf.

Lee, S. S., Mountain, J., Koenig, B. A. 2001. The meanings of "race" in the new genomics: Implications for health disparities research. *Yale Journal of Health Policy, Law, and Ethics* 1: 33–75.

Lee, Y. Y, Lin, J. L. 2009. The effects of trust in physician on self-efficacy, adherence and diabetes outcomes. *Social Science and Medicine* 68: 1060–68.

Leitner, J. B., Hehman, E., Ayduk, O., Mendoza-Denton, R. 2016. Blacks' death rate due to circulatory diseases is positively related to whites' explicit racial bias—A nationwide investigation using Project Implicit. *Psychological Science* 27(10): 1299–1311.

Let's Move—America's Move to Raise a Healthier Generation of Kids. Available at http:// www.letsmove.gov/.

Lewis, T. T., Cogburn, C. D., Williams, D. R. 2015. Self-reported experiences of discrimination and health: Scientific advances, ongoing controversies, and emerging issues. *Annual Review of Clinical Psychology* 11: 407–40.

Li, J. Z., Absher, D. M., Tang, H., et al. 2008. Worldwide human relationships inferred from genome-wide patterns of variation. *Science* 319(5866): 1100–1104.

Li, Y., Yin, J., Cai, X., Temkin-Greener, J., Mukamel, D. B. 2011. Association of race and sites of care with pressure ulcers in high-risk nursing home residents. *JAMA* 306: 179–86.

Liaison Committee on Medical Education. June 2013. Standards for Accreditation of Medical Education Programs Leading to the M.D. Degree. Available at http://www .lcme.org/publications/functions.pdf.

Lillie-Blanton, M., Rushing, O. E., Sonia Ruiz, S., Mayberry, R., Boone, L. 2002. Racial/ ethnic differences in cardiac care: The weight of the evidence. Henry J. Kaiser Family Foundation and American College of Cardiology Foundation. Available at www.kff.org /whythedifference/6040summary.pdf.

Linnaeus, C. 1956. *Systema naturae.* Photographic facsimile of the first volume of the 10th ed. (1758), originally published under the name Carl von Linné. London: British Museum of Natural History.

Liu, C., Moon, M., Sulvetta, M., Chawla, J. 1992. International infant mortality rankings: A look behind the numbers. *Health Care Financing Review* 13(4): 105–18.

Liu, J. H., Zingmond, D. S., McGory, M. L., et al. 2006. Disparities in the utilization of high-volume hospitals for complex surgery. *JAMA* 296: 1973–80.

Lodge, H. C. 1897. Senate speech, February 2. Congressional Record, 54th Congress, 2nd Session, vol. 29, part 2, p. 1432.

Logan, T. D., Parman, J. M. 2017. Segregation and mortality over time and space. *Social Science and Medicine* 199: 77–86.

London Department of Health and Social Security. 1980. Inequalities in health: Report of a research working group.

Long, S. K., Bart, L. 2017. Do Patients Trust Their Providers? Urban Institute Health Policy Center Health Reform Monitoring Survey. Available at http://hrms.urban.org /briefs/do-patients-trust-their-providers.html, accessed August 30, 2018.

Lopez, R. 2004. Income inequality and self-rated health in US metropolitan areas: A multilevel analysis. *Social Science and Medicine* 59: 2409–19.

Loucks, E. B., Lynch, J. W., Pilote, L., et al. 2009. Life-course socioeconomic position and incidence of coronary heart disease: The Framingham Offspring Study. *American Journal of Epidemiology* 169: 829–36.

Loucks, E. B., Pilote, L., Lynch, J. W., et al. 2010. Life course socioeconomic position is associated with inflammatory markers: The Framingham Offspring Study. *Social Science and Medicine* 71(1): 187–95.

Louie, G. H., Ward, M. M. 2011. Socioeconomic and ethnic differences in disease burden and disparities in physical function in older adults. *American Journal of Public Health* 101: 1322–29.

Lozano, P., Connell, F. A., Koepsell, T. D. 1995. Use of health services by African-American children with asthma on Medicaid. *JAMA* 274: 469–73.

Lucas, F. L., Stukel, T. A., Morris, A. M., Siewers, A. E., Birkmeyer, J. D. 2006. Race and surgical mortality in the United States. *Annals of Surgery* 243: 281–86.

Lurie, N. 2005. Health disparities: Less talk, more action. *New England Journal of Medicine* 353: 727–29.

Lurie, N., Fremont, A., Jain, A. K., et al. 2005. Racial and ethnic disparities in care: The perspectives of cardiologists. *Circulation* 111: 1264–69.

Lynch, J. L., von Hippel, P. T. 2016. An education gradient in health, a health gradient in education, or a confounded gradient in both? *Social Science and Medicine* 154: 18–27.

Lynch, J. W., Kaplan, G. A., and Shema, S. J. 1997. Cumulative impact of sustained economic hardship on physical, cognitive, psychological, and social functioning. *New England Journal of Medicine* 337: 1889–95.

MacArthur Research Network on Socioeconomic Status and Health. Described at http://www.macses.ucsf.edu/about/, accessed July 3, 2013.

MacArthur Research Network on Socioeconomic Status and Health. Reaching for a Healthier Life—Facts on Socioeconomic Status and Health in the U.S. 2007. Available at http://www.macses.ucsf.edu/downloads/reaching_for_a_healthier_life.pdf, accessed July 3, 2013.

MacArthur Scale of Subjective Social Status. MacArthur Research Network on Socioeconomic Status and Health, Sociodemographic Questionnaire. Described at http://www.macses.ucsf.edu/research/psychosocial/subjective.php, accessed July 3, 2013.

Mainous, A. G., Tanner, R. J., Jo, A., et al. 2018. Trends in cardiovascular disease risk in the U.S., 1999–2014. *American Journal of Preventive Medicine* 55(3): 384–88.

Makaroun, L. K., Brown, R. T., Diaz-Ramirez, L. G., et al. 2017. Wealth-associated disparities in death and disability in the United States and England. *JAMA Internal Medicine* 177(12): 1745–53.

Malat, J. 2001. Social distance and patients' rating of healthcare providers. *Journal of Health and Social Behavior* 42: 360–72.

Manning, M., Albrecht, T. L., Yilmaz-Saab, Z., et al. 2017. Explaining between race differences in African-American and European-American women's responses to breast density notification. *Social Science and Medicine* 195: 149–58.

Margolis, K. L. 2018. Inventing a new model of hypertension care for black men. *New England Journal of Medicine* 378(14): 1345–47.

Margolis, M. L., Christie, J. D., Silvestri, G. A., Kaiser, L., Santiago, S., and Hansen-Flaschen, J. 2003. Racial differences pertaining to a belief about lung cancer surgery: Results of a multicenter survey. *Annals of Internal Medicine* 139: 558–63.

Marks, J. 1995. *Human Biodiversity: Genes, Race, and History.* New York: Aldine De Gruyter.

Marmot, M. 1999. Epidemiology of socioeconomic status and health: Are determinants within countries the same as between countries? *Annals of the New York Academy of Sciences* 896: 16–29.

Marmot, M. 2001. Inequalities in health. *New England Journal of Medicine* 345: 134–36.

Marmot, M. 2004. *The Status Syndrome: How Social Standing Affects Our Health and Longevity.* New York: Henry Holt.

Marmot, M. 2006. Status syndrome: A challenge to medicine. *JAMA* 295: 1304–7.

Marmot, M., Bobak, M., Smith, G. D. 1995. Explanation for social inequalities in health. In Amick, B., Levine, S., Tarlov, A. R., Walsh, D. C., eds. *Society and Health,* 172–210. New York: Oxford University Press.

Marmot, M. G., Shipley, M. J., Rose, G. 1984. Inequalities in death—specific explanations of a general pattern? *Lancet* 323 (Issue 8384): 1003–6.

Marmot, M., Theorell, T. 1988. Social class and cardiovascular disease: The contribution of work. *International Journal of Health Services* 18: 659–74.

Martin, J. A., Hamilton, B. E., Osterman, M. J. K., et al. 2018. Births: Final Data for 2016. *National Vital Statistics Reports* 67(1). Available at https://www.cdc.gov/nchs/data/nvsr /nvsr67/nvsr67_01.pdf, accessed August 13, 2018.

Martin, M. L. 2000. Ethnicity and analgesic practice: An editorial. *Annals of Emergency Medicine* 35: 77–79.

Martinson, M. L. 2012. Income inequality in health at all ages: A comparison of the United States and England. *American Journal of Public Health* 102: 2049–56.

Massey, D. S. 2004. Segregation and stratification: A biosocial perspective. *Du Bois Review* 1: 7–25.

Materson, B. J. 2003. High blood pressure in African Americans. *Archives of Internal Medicine* 163: 521–22.

Mathews, T. J., Menacker, F., and MacDorman, M. F. 2004. Infant mortality statistics from the 2002 period linked birth / infant death data set. *National Vital Statistics Reports* 53(10).

Matthews, K. A., Schwartz, J. E., Cohen, S. 2011. Indices of socioeconomic position across the life course as predictors of coronary calcification in black and white men and women: Coronary artery risk development in young adults study. *Social Science and Medicine* 73: 768–74.

Mays, V. M., Jones, A. L., Delany-Brumsey, A., et al. 2017. Perceived discrimination in health care and mental health / substance abuse treatment among blacks, Latinos, and whites. *Medical Care* 55(2): 173–81.

McCarthy, A. M., Yang, J., Armstrong, K. 2015. Increasing disparities in breast cancer mortality from 1979 to 2010 for US black women aged 20 to 49 years. *American Journal of Public Health* 105(S3): S446–S448.

McDonough, P., Duncan, G. J., Williams, D., House, J. 1997. Income dynamics and adult mortality in the United States, 1972 through 1989. *American Journal of Public Health* 87: 1476–83.

McEwen, B. S. 2012. Brain on stress: How the social environment gets under the skin. *Proceedings of the National Academy of Sciences U S A* 109, Suppl. 2: 17180–85.

McEwen, B. S., Seeman, T. 1999. Protective and damaging effects of mediators of stress. *Annals of the New York Academy of Sciences* 896: 30–47.

McGlade, M. S., Saha, S., and Dahlstrom, M. E. 2004. The Latina paradox: An opportunity for restructuring prenatal care delivery. *American Journal of Public Health* 94: 2062–65.

McKeown, T. 1979. *The Role of Medicine.* Princeton: Princeton University Press.

McKinlay, J., McKinlay, S. 1997. Medical measures and the decline of mortality. In Conrad, P., ed. *The Sociology of Health and Illness,* 10–23. New York: St. Martin's Press.

McLemore, M. R., Altman, M. R., Cooper, N., et al. 2018. Health care experiences of pregnant, birthing and postnatal women of color at risk for preterm birth. *Social Science and Medicine* 201: 127–35.

Mehra, R., Boyd, L. M., Ickovics, J. R. 2017. Racial residential segregation and adverse birth outcomes: A systematic review and meta-analysis. *Social Science and Medicine* 191: 237–50.

Mehta, N. K., Lee, H., Ylitalo, K. R. 2013. Child health in the United States: Recent trends in racial/ethnic disparities. *Social Science and Medicine* 95: 6–15.

Melanson, T. A., Hockenberry, J. M., Plantinga, L., et al. 2017. New kidney allocation system associated with increased rates of transplants among black and Hispanic patients. *Health Affairs* 36(6): 1078–85.

Meng, Y-Y., Rull, R. P., Wilhelm, M., et al. 2006. Living Near Heavy Traffic Increases Asthma Severity. UCLA Center for Health Policy Research. Available at www .healthpolicy.ucla.edu/pubs/files/Traffic_Asthma_PB.081606.pdf.

Mensah, G. A., Goff, D. C., Gibbons, G. H. 2017. Cardiovascular mortality differences— Place matters. *JAMA* 317(19): 1955–57.

Merrick, M.T., Guinn, A.S. 2018. Child abuse and neglect: Breaking the intergenerational link. *American Journal of Public Health* 108(9): 1117–18.

Michael, Y. L., Berkman, L. F., Colditz, G. A., Kawachi, I. 2001. Living arrangements, social integration, and change in functional health status. *American Journal of Epidemiology* 153: 123–31.

Miller, G. E., Chen, E., Fok, A. K., et al. 2009. Low early-life social class leaves a biological residue manifested by decreased glucocorticoid and increased proinflammatory signaling. *Proceedings of the National Academy of Sciences U S A* 106(34): 14716–21.

Miller, W., Robinson, L. A., Lawrence, R. S., eds. 2006. *Valuing Health for Regulatory Cost-Effective Analysis*. Washington, D.C.: National Academies Press.

Miranda, J., Duan, N., Sherbourne, C., et al. 2003. Improving care for minorities: Can quality improvement interventions improve care and outcomes for depressed minorities? Results of a randomized, controlled trial. *Health Services Research* 38: 613–30.

Mischel, W., Shoda, Y., Peake, P. K. 1988. The nature of adolescent competencies predicted by preschool delay of gratification. *Journal of Personality and Social Psychology* 54: 687–96.

Mohnen, S. M., Groenewegen, P. P., Völker, B., Flap, H. 2011. Neighborhood social capital and individual health. *Social Science and Medicine* 72: 660–67.

Mokwe, E., Ohmit, S. E., Nasser, S. A., et al. 2004. Determinants of blood pressure response to Quinapril in black and white hypertensive patients. *Hypertension* 43: 1202–7.

Molina, Y., Silva, A., Rauscher, G. H. 2015. Racial/ethnic disparities in time to a breast cancer diagnosis: The mediating effects of health care facility factors. *Medical Care* 53(10): 872–78.

Montez, J. K., Zajacova, A., Hayward, M. D. 2017. Disparities in disability by educational attainment across US states. *American Journal of Public Health* 107: 1101–8.

Montez, J. K., Zajacova, A. 2013. Trends in mortality risk by education level and cause of death among US white women from 1986 to 2006. *American Journal of Public Health* 103: 473–79.

Moore, P. J., Sickel, A. E., Malat, J., Williams, D., Jackson, J., Adler, N. E. 2004. Psychosocial factors in medical and psychological treatment avoidance: The role of the doctor-patient relationship. *Journal of Health Psychology* 9: 421–33.

Morales, L. S., Staiger, D., Horbar, J. D., et al. 2005. Mortality among very low–birthweight infants in hospitals serving minority populations. *American Journal of Public Health* 95: 2206–12.

Mueller, B. 2015. $25,000 fine proposed in taxi driver's snub of black family. *New York Times,* August 6, 2015.

Murphy, S. L., Xu, J., Kochanek, K. D., et al. 2017. Deaths: Final Data for 2015. *National Vital Statistics Reports* 66(6). Available at https://www.cdc.gov/nchs/data/nvsr/nvsr66 /nvsr66_06.pdf, accessed October 17, 2018.

Murphy, S. L., Xu, J., Kochanek, K. D., Arias, E. 2018. Mortality in the United States, 2017. NCHS Data Brief No. 328. Available at https://www.cdc.gov/nchs/products/databriefs /db328.htm, accessed January 24, 2019.

Nanda, R., Schumm, L. P., Cummings, S., et al. 2005. Genetic testing in an ethnically diverse cohort of high-risk women: A comparative analysis of BRCA1 and BRCA2 mutations in American families of European and African ancestry. *JAMA* 294: 1925–33.

Narain, K., Zimmerman, F. 2018. Advancing health equity: Facilitating action on the social determinants of health among public health departments. *American Journal of Public Health* 108(6): 737–38.

National Cancer Institute, Surveillance Epidemiology and End Results, Fact Sheet: Myeloma. Available at http://seer.cancer.gov/statfacts/html/mulmy.html, accessed October 17, 2018.

National Cancer Institute. 2006. Genetics of Breast and Ovarian Cancer. Available at www .cancer.gov/cancertopics/pdq/genetics/breast-and-ovarian/health professional.

National Center for Health Statistics—See US Department of Health and Human Services, Centers for Disease Control and Prevention.

National Institutes of Health. 2019. Definition of obesity. Available at https://www.niddk .nih.gov/health-information/weight-management/glossary-healthy-eating-obesity -physical-activity-weight-control#o, accessed February 20, 2019.

National Population Council of Mexico and the University of California. 2009. Migration and Health: The Children of Mexican Immigrants in the U.S. Available at http:// healthpolicy.ucla.edu/publications/search/pages/detail.aspx?PubID=98.

National Public Radio, the Robert Wood Johnson Foundation, and Harvard T.H. Chan School of Public Health. 2017. Discrimination in America—Experiences and Views of African Americans, October 2017. Available at https://www.rwjf.org/content/dam/farm /reports/reports/2017/rwjf441128, accessed August 24, 2018.

Nelson, H. D., Huffman, L. H., Fu, R., Harris, E. L. 2005. Genetic risk assessment and *BRCA* mutation testing for breast and ovarian cancer susceptibility: Systematic evidence review for the U.S. Preventive Services Task Force. *Annals of Internal Medicine* 143: 362–79.

Nitromed. 2013. BiDil. Available at www.bidil.com.

Nix, J., Campbell, B. A., Byers, E. H., Alpert, G. P. 2017. A bird's eye view of civilians killed by police in 2015. *Criminology & Public Policy* 16(1): 309–40.

Nobel, L., Jesdale, W. M., Tjia, J., et al. 2017. Neighborhood socioeconomic status predicts health after hospitalization for acute coronary syndromes: Findings from TRACE-CORE. *Medical Care* 55(12): 1008–16.

North, M. L., Ellis, A. K. 2011. The role of epigenetics in the developmental origins of allergic disease. *Annals of Allergy, Asthma and Immunology* 106: 355–61.

Nosek, B. A., Smytha, F. L., Hansena, J. J., et al. 2007. Pervasiveness and correlates of implicit attitudes and stereotypes. *European Review of Social Psychology* 18: 36–88.

Nunnelley, W. A. T. Eugene "Bull" Connor. 2006. Alabama Department of Archives and History, Alabama Moments in American History. Available at www.alabamamoments .state.al.us/sec62.html.

Obama, B. 2010. Remarks by the president at signing of the health insurance reform bill, March 23, 2010. Available at http://www.whitehouse.gov/the-press-office/remarks -president-and-vice-president-signing-health-insurance-reform-bill.

O'Donnell, J. K., Halpin, J., Mattson, C. L., et al. 2017. Deaths involving fentanyl, fentanyl analogs, and U-47700—10 states, July–December 2016. *MMWR Morbidity and Mortality Weekly Report* 66: 1197–1202.

Office of National Drug Control Policy. 2017. President's Commission. Described at https:// www.whitehouse.gov/ondcp/presidents-commission/, accessed July 25, 2018.

Ogden, C. L., Fryar, C. D., Hales, C. M., et al. 2018. Differences in obesity prevalence by demographics and urbanization in US children and adolescents, 2013–2016. *JAMA* 319(23): 2410–18.

Ogden, C., Carroll, M. 2010. Prevalence of obesity among children and adolescents: United States, trends 1963–1965 through 2007–2008. Available at http://www.cdc.gov/nchs/data /hestat/obesity_child_07_08/obesity_child_07_08.htm.

Olfson, M., Cherry, D. K., Lewis-Fernández, R. 2009. Racial differences in visit duration of outpatient psychiatric visits. *Archives of General Psychiatry* 66: 214–21.

Onie, R. D., Lavizzo-Mourey, R., Lee, T. H., et al. 2018. Integrating social needs into health care: A twenty-year case study of adaptation and diffusion. *Health Affairs* 37(2): 240–47.

Oquendo, M. A., Volkow, N. D. 2018. Suicide: A silent contributor to opioid-overdose deaths. *New England Journal of Medicine* 378: 1567–69.

Orchard, J., Price, J. 2017. County-level racial prejudice and the black-white gap in infant health outcomes. *Social Science and Medicine* 181: 191–98.

Organisation for Economic Co-operation and Development. Health Data 2017. Available at http://www.oecd.org/statistics/, accessed October 22, 2018.

Oxford English Dictionary. Available at www.oed.com.

Parsons, T. 1979. Definitions of health and illness in the light of American values and social structure. In Jaco, E. G., ed. *Patients, Physicians, and Illness*, 120–44. New York: Free Press.

Patrinos, A. 2004. "Race" and the human genome. *Nature Genetics* 36 (Suppl. 11): S1–2.

Peek, M. E., Odoms-Young, A., Quinn, M. T., Gorawara-Bhat, R., Wilson, S. C., Chin, M. H. 2010. Race and shared decision-making: Perspectives of African-Americans with diabetes. *Social Science and Medicine* 71: 1–9.

Penner, L. A., Harper, F. W. K., Dovidio, J. F., et al. 2017. The impact of black cancer patients' race-related beliefs and attitudes on racially-discordant oncology interactions: A field study. *Social Science and Medicine* 191: 99–108.

Pensola, T. H., Martikainen, P. 2003. Cumulative social class and mortality from various causes of adult men. *Journal of Epidemiology and Community Health* 57: 745–51.

Peterson, E. D., Shaw, L. K., DeLong, E. R., Pryor, D. B., Califf, R. M., and Mark, D. B. 1997. Racial variation in the use of coronary-revascularization procedures. Are the differences real? Do they matter? *New England Journal of Medicine* 336: 480–86.

Peterson, E. D., Wright, S. M., Daley, J., Thibault, G. E. 1994. Racial variation in cardiac procedure use and survival following acute myocardial infarction in the Department of Veterans Affairs. *JAMA* 271: 1175–80.

Phelan, J. C., Link, B. G. 2015. Is racism a fundamental cause of inequalities in health? *Annual Review of Sociology* 41: 311–30.

Phelps, E. A., O'Connor, K. J., Cunningham, W. A., et al. 2000. Performance on indirect measures of race evaluation predicts amygdala activation. *Journal of Cognitive Neuroscience* 12: 729–38.

Philbin, M. M., Flake, M., Hatzenbuehler, M. L., Hirsch, J. S. 2018. State-level immigration and immigrant-focused policies as drivers of Latino health disparities in the United States. *Social Science and Medicine* 199: 29–38.

Piper, A. M. S. 1990. Higher-order discrimination. In Flanagan, O., Rorty, A., eds., *Identity, Character, and Morality: Essays in Moral Psychology*, 285–309. Cambridge, MA: MIT Press.

Polonsky, T. S., McClelland, R. L., Jorgensen, N. W., et al. 2010. Coronary artery calcium score and risk classification for coronary heart disease prediction. *JAMA* 303: 1610–16.

President's Commission on Combating Drug Addiction and the Opioid Crisis. 2017. Final Report Draft 11-15-2017. Available at https://www.whitehouse.gov/sites/whitehouse.gov/files/images/Final_Report_Draft_11-15-2017.pdf, accessed July 25, 2018.

Profit, J., Gould, J. B., Bennett, M., et al. 2017. Racial/ethnic disparity in NICU quality of care delivery. *Pediatrics* 140(3): e20170918.

Project Implicit. Described at https://implicit.harvard.edu/implicit/, accessed August 9, 2018.

Purdie-Vaughns, V., Williams, D. R. 2015. Stand-Your-Ground is losing ground for racial minorities' health. *Social Science and Medicine* 147: 341–43.

Purnell, T. S., Luo, X., Cooper, L. A., et al. 2018. Association of race and ethnicity with live donor kidney transplantation in the United States from 1995 to 2014. *JAMA* 319(1): 49–61.

Puumala, S. E., Burgess, K. M., Kharbanda, A. B., et al. 2016. The role of bias by emergency department providers in care for American Indian children. *Medical Care* 54(6): 562–69.

Rathore, S. S., Lenert, L. A., Weinfurt, K. P., et al. 2000. The effects of patient sex and race on medical students' ratings of quality of life. *American Journal of Medicine* 108: 561–66.

Regenstein, M., Trott, J., Williamson, A., Theiss, J. 2018. Addressing social determinants of health through medical-legal partnerships. *Health Affairs* 37(3): 378–85.

Rehkopf, D. H., Modrek, S., Cantley, L. F., Cullen, M. R. 2017. Social, psychological, and physical aspects of the work environment could contribute to hypertension prevalence. *Health Affairs* 36(2): 258–65.

Reich, D. 2018a. How genetics is changing our understanding of 'race.' *New York Times,* March 23, 2018.

Reich, D. 2018b. How to talk about 'race' and genetics. *New York Times,* March 30, 2018.

Reinhardt, U. E., Relman, A. S. 1986. Debating for-profit health care and the ethics of physicians. *Health Affairs* 5(2): 5–31.

Renaud, M. 1994. The future: Hygeia versus Panakeia. In Evans, R. G., Barer, M. L., Marmor, T. R., eds., *Why Are Some People Healthy and Others Not?*, 317–34. New York: Aldine De Gruyter.

Reschovsky, J. D., O'Malley, A. S. 2008. Do primary care physicians treating minority patients report problems delivering high-quality care? *Health Affairs (Millwood)* 27(3): w222–31.

Reynolds, P. P. 1997. Hospitals and civil rights, 1945–1963: The case of Simkins v. Moses H. Cone Memorial Hospital. *Annals of Internal Medicine* 126: 898–906.

Rinsky, R. A. 2001. A message from the editor. *Public Health Reports* 116: 385–86.

Risch, N., Burchard, E., Ziv, E., Tang, H. 2002. Categorization of humans in biomedical research: Genes, race, and disease. *Genome Biology* 3(7): comment 2007, pp. 1–12.

Robert Wood Johnson Foundation. 2011. Moving toward Racial and Ethnic Equity in Health Care. Available at http://www.rwjf.org/content/dam/web-assets/2011/03/moving -toward-racial-and-ethnic-equity-in-health-care.

Robinette, J. W., Charles, S. T., Gruenewald, T. L. 2018. Neighborhood cohesion, neighborhood disorder, and cardiometabolic risk. *Social Science and Medicine* 198: 70–76.

Roediger, D. R. 1999. *The Wages of Whiteness: Race and the Making of the American Working Class.* New York: Verso.

Rosenberg, N. A., Pritchard, J. K., Weber, J. L., et al. 2002. Genetic structure of human populations. *Science* 298: 2381–85.

Rosenstreich, D. L., Eggleston, P., Kattan, M., et al. 1997. The role of cockroach allergy and exposure to cockroach allergen in causing morbidity among inner-city children with asthma. *New England Journal of Medicine* 336: 1356–63.

Ross, C. E., Mirowsky, J. 2011. The interaction of personal and parental education on health. *Social Science and Medicine* 72: 591–99.

Roth, G. A., Dwyer-Lindgren, L., Bertozzi-Villa, A., et al. 2017. Trends and patterns of geographic variation in cardiovascular mortality among US counties, 1980–2014. *JAMA* 317(19): 1976–92.

Roubideaux, Y., Zuckerman, M., and Zuckerman, E. 2004. A Review of the Quality of Health Care for American Indians and Alaska Natives. Commonwealth Fund. Available at www.cmwf.org/publications/publications_show.htm?doc_id=239464.

Rubinstein, W. S. 2004. Hereditary breast cancer in Jews. *Familial Cancer* 3: 249–57.

Rutter, M. 2012. Achievements and challenges in the biology of environmental effects. *Proceedings of the National Academy of Sciences U S A* 109 (Suppl. 2): 17149–53.

Sabin, J., Nosek, B. A., Greenwald, A., Rivara, F. P. 2009. Physicians' implicit and explicit attitudes about race by MD race, ethnicity, and gender. *Journal of Health Care for the Poor and Underserved* 20: 896–913.

Sade, R. M. 1971. Medical care as a right: A refutation. *New England Journal of Medicine* 285: 1288–92.

Sadler, R. C., LaChance, J., Hanna-Attisha, M. 2017. Social and built environmental correlates of predicted blood lead levels in the Flint water crisis. *American Journal of Public Health* 107(5): 763–69.

Saigal, S., Feeny, D., Rosenbaum, P., Furlong, W., Burrows, E., Stoskopf, B. 1996. Self-perceived health status and health-related quality of life of extremely low-birth-weight infants at adolescence. *JAMA* 276: 453–59.

Saigal, S., Stoskopf, B., Streiner, D., et al. 2006. Transition of extremely low-birth-weight infants from adolescence to young adulthood: Comparison with normal birth-weight controls. *JAMA* 295: 667–75.

Saloner, B., Stoller, K. B., Alexander, G. C. 2018. Moving addiction care to the mainstream—Improving the quality of buprenorphine treatment. *New England Journal of Medicine* 379(1): 4–6.

Sancar, F., Abbasi, J., Bucher, K. 2018. Mortality among American Indians and Alaska Natives. *JAMA* 319(2): 112.

Sanger-Katz, M. 2018. Bleak new estimates in drug epidemic: A record 72,000 overdose deaths in 2017. *New York Times,* August 15, 2018.

Satel, S. 2000. *How Political Correctness Is Corrupting Medicine.* New York: Basic Books.

Satel, S. 2001. Indoctrinologists are coming: Does either color or sex determine the level and frequency of medical care that individuals receive? *Atlantic Monthly* 287(1): 59–64.

Satel, S. 2002. I am a racially profiling doctor. *New York Times,* May 5.

Schmidt, M. S. 2015. F.B.I. director speaks out on race and police bias. *New York Times,* February 12, 2015.

Schneider, E. C., Cleary, P. D., Zaslavsky, A. M., Epstein, A. M. 2001. Racial disparities in influenza vaccination. *JAMA* 286: 1455–60.

Schoendorf, K. C., Hogue, C. J., Kleinman, J. C., and Rowley, D. 1992. Mortality among infants of black as compared with white college-educated parents. *New England Journal of Medicine* 326: 1522–26.

Schpero, W. L., Morden, N. E., Sequist, T. D., et al. 2017. For selected services, blacks and Hispanics more likely to receive low-value care than whites. *Health Affairs* 36(6): 1065–69.

Schulman, K. A., Berlin, J. A., Harless, W., et al. 1999. The effect of race and sex on physicians' recommendations for cardiac catheterization. *New England Journal of Medicine* 340: 618–26.

Schultz, W. M., Kelli, H. M., Lisko, J. C., et al. 2018. Socioeconomic status and cardiovascular outcomes—Challenges and interventions. *Circulation* 137: 2166–78.

Schwartz, L. M., Woloshin, S., Welch, H. G. 1999. Misunderstandings about the effects of race and sex on physicians' referrals for cardiac catheterization. *New England Journal of Medicine* 341: 279–83.

Schwartz, R. S. 2001. Racial profiling in medical research. *New England Journal of Medicine* 344: 1392–93.

Scott, S. B., Munoz, E., Mogle, J. A., et al. 2018. Perceived neighborhood characteristics predict severity and emotional response to daily stressors. *Social Science and Medicine* 200: 262–70.

Seervai, S., Shah, A., Schneider, E. C. 2018. The U.S. Has Two Opioid Epidemics: The Federal Response Should Consider Both. To the Point, The Commonwealth Fund Mar. 22, 2018. Available at https://www.commonwealthfund.org/blog/2018/us-has-two-opioid-epidemics-federal-response-should-consider-both, accessed July 25, 2018.

Segal, S. P., Bola, J. R., Watson, M. A. 1996. Race, quality of care, and antipsychotic prescribing practices in psychiatric emergency services. *Psychiatric Services* 47: 282–86.

Sehgal, A. R. 2004. Overlap between whites and blacks in response to antihypertensive drugs. *Hypertension* 43: 566–72.

Semenza, J. C., Rubin, C. H., Falter, K. H., et al. 1996. Heat-related deaths during the July 1995 heat wave in Chicago. *New England Journal of Medicine* 335: 84–90.

Semyonov, M., Lewin-Epstein, N., Maskileyson, D. 2013. Where wealth matters more for health: The wealth-health gradient in 16 countries. *Social Science and Medicine* 81: 10–17.

Sen, A. 1999. *Development as Freedom.* New York: Alfred A. Knopf.

Sequist, T. D. 2017. Urgent action needed on health inequities among American Indians and Alaska Natives. *Lancet* 389 (Issue 10077): 1378–79.

Seth, P., Rudd, R. A., Noonan, R. K., Haegerich, T. M. 2018. Quantifying the epidemic of prescription opioid overdose deaths. *American Journal of Public Health* 108(4): 500–502.

Shah, A. A., Zogg, C. K., Zafar, S. N., et al. 2015. Analgesic access for acute abdominal pain in the emergency department among racial/ethnic minority patients: A nationwide examination. *Medical Care* 53(12): 1000–1009.

Sharma, R. K., Freedman, V. A., Mor, V., et al. 2017. Association of racial differences with end-of-life care quality in the United States. *JAMA Internal Medicine* 177(12): 1858–60.

Shaw, J. G., Nelson, D. A., Shaw, K. A., et al. 2018. Deployment and preterm birth among US army soldiers. *American Journal of Epidemiology* 187(4): 687–95.

Shoda, Y., Mischel, W., Peake, P. K. 1990. Predicting adolescent cognitive and self-regulatory competencies from preschool delay of gratification: Identifying diagnostic conditions. *Developmental Psychology* 26: 978–86.

Shonkoff, J. P. 2012. Leveraging the biology of adversity to address the roots of disparities in health and development. *PNAS* 109 (Suppl. 2): 17302–7.

Shonkoff, J. P., Boyce, W. T., McEwen, B. S. 2009. Neuroscience, molecular biology, and the childhood roots of health disparities—building a new framework for health promotion and disease prevention. *JAMA* 301: 2252–59.

Shonkoff, J. P., Garner, A. S., et al. 2012. Technical Report—The lifelong effects of early childhood adversity and toxic stress. *Pediatrics* 129(1): e232–e246.

Shonkoff, J. P., Phillips, D. A., eds. 2000. From Neurons to Neighborhoods—The Science of Early Childhood Development. Institute of Medicine, National Academy Press, Washington, D.C.

Shweder, R. 1997. They call it "poor health" for a reason. *New York Times,* March 9.

Siddiqi, A., Shahidi, F. V., Ramraj, C., Williams, D. R. 2017. Associations between race, discrimination and risk for chronic disease in a population-based sample from Canada. *Social Science and Medicine* 194: 135–41.

Sidney, S., Quesenberry, C. P., Jaffe, M. G., et al. 2016. Recent trends in cardiovascular mortality in the United States and public health goals. *JAMA Cardiology* 1(5): 594–99.

Simandan, D. 2018. Rethinking the health consequences of social class and social mobility. *Social Science and Medicine* 200: 258–61.

Sims, C. 2006. An arm in the air for that cab ride home. *New York Times,* October 15.

Singh, G. K., Kogan, M. D., Slifkin, R. T. 2017. Widening disparities in infant mortality and life expectancy between Appalachia and the rest of the United States, 1990–2013. *Health Affairs* 36(8): 1423–32.

Singh, G. K., Kogan, M. D. 2007. Widening socioeconomic disparities in US childhood mortality, 1969–2000. *American Journal of Public Health* 97: 1658–65.

Singh, G. K., Yu, S. M. 1996. Adverse pregnancy outcomes: Differences between US- and foreign–born women in major US racial and ethnic groups. *American Journal of Public Health* 86: 837–43.

Singhal, A., Tien, Y-Y., Hsia, R. Y. 2016. Racial-ethnic disparities in opioid prescriptions at emergency department visits for conditions commonly associated with prescription drug abuse. *PLoS One* 11(8): e0159224.

Sjogren, J., Thulin, L. I. 2004. Quality of life in the very elderly after cardiac surgery: A comparison of SF-36 between long-term survivors and an age-matched population. *Gerontology* 50: 407–10.

Skinner, J., Weinstein, J. N., Sporer, S. M., Wennberg, J. E. 2003. Racial, ethnic, and geographic disparities in rates of knee arthroplasty among Medicare patients. *New England Journal of Medicine* 349: 1350–59.

Sloan, F. A., Ayyagari, P., Salm, M., Grossman, D. 2010. The longevity gap between black and white men in the United States at the beginning and end of the 20th century. *American Journal of Public Health* 100: 357–63.

Slopen, N., Chen, Y., Guida, J. L., et al. 2017. Positive childhood experiences and ideal cardiovascular health in midlife: Associations and mediators. *Preventive Medicine* 97: 72–79.

Small, K. M., Wagoner, L. E., Levin, A. M., Kardia, S. L. R., Liggett, S. B. 2002. Synergistic polymorphisms of $_1$-and $_{2C}$-adrenergic receptors and the risk of congestive heart failure. *New England Journal of Medicine* 347: 1135–42.

Smedley, B. D., Butler, A. S., and Bristow, L. R., eds. 2004. *In the Nation's Compelling Interest: Ensuring Diversity in the Health-Care Workforce.* Washington, D.C.: National Academies Press.

Smedley, B. D., Stith, A. Y., Colburn, L., Evans, C. H. 2001. *The Right Thing to Do, the Smart Thing to Do: Enhancing Diversity in Health Professions.* Washington, D.C.: National Academies Press.

Smedley, B. D., Stith, A. Y., Nelson, A. R., eds. 2003. *Unequal Treatment: Confronting Racial and Ethnic Disparities in Healthcare.* Washington, D.C.: National Academies Press.

Smith, D. B., Feng, Z., Fennell, M. L., Zinn, J. S., Mor, V. 2007. Separate and unequal: Racial segregation and disparities in quality across U.S. nursing homes. *Health Affairs (Millwood)* 26(5): 1448–58.

Sorkin, D. H., Ngo-Metzger, Q., De Alba, I. 2010. Racial/ethnic discrimination in health care: Impact on perceived quality of care. *Journal of General Internal Medicine* 25: 390–96.

Stafford, M., Marmot, M. 2003. Neighbourhood deprivation and health: Does it affect us all equally? *International Journal of Epidemiology* 32: 357–66.

Stangor, C., Sechrist, G. B., Jost, J. T. 2001. Changing racial beliefs by providing consensus information. *Personality and Social Psychology Bulletin* 27: 486–96.

Statistics Canada. 2016. 2016 Census of Population Questions, Long Form (National Household Survey). Available at https://www12.statcan.gc.ca/nhs-enm/2016/ref/questionnaires/questions-eng.cfm, accessed July 30, 2018.

Stefanick, M. 2017. Not just for men. *Scientific American* 317(3): 52–57.

Stein, E. M., Gennuso, K. P., Ugboaja, D. C., Remington, P. L. 2017. The epidemic of despair among white Americans: Trends in the leading causes of premature death, 1999–2015. *American Journal of Public Health* 107(10): 1541–47.

Steinbrook, R. 2004. Disparities in health care: From politics to policy. *New England Journal of Medicine* 350: 1486–88.

Stoll, B. J., Stevenson, D. K., Wise, P. H. 2013. The transformation of child health research—innovation, market failure, and the public good. *JAMA* 309: 1779–80.

Stone, D. M., Simon, T. R., Fowler, K. A., et al. 2018. Vital signs: Trends in state suicide rates—United States, 1999–2016 and circumstances contributing to suicide—27 States, 2015. *Morbidity and Mortality Weekly Report* 67(22): 617–24.

Subramanian, S. V., Chen, J. T., Rehkopf, D. H., Waterman, P. D., and Krieger, N. 2005. Racial disparities in context: A multilevel analysis of neighborhood variations in poverty and excess mortality among black populations in Massachusetts. *American Journal of Public Health* 95: 260–65.

Subramanyam, M. A., Diez-Roux, A. V., Hickson, D. A., et al. 2012. Subjective social status and psychosocial and metabolic risk factors for cardiovascular disease among African Americans in the Jackson Heart Study. *Social Science and Medicine* 74: 1146–54.

Sundquist, K., Lindstrom, M., Malmstrom, M., Johansson, S. E., Sundquist, J. 2004. Social participation and coronary heart disease: A follow-up study of 6900 women and men in Sweden. *Social Science and Medicine* 58: 615–22.

Taksler, G. B., Rothberg, M. B. 2017. Assessing years of life lost versus number of deaths in the United States, 1995–2015. *American Journal of Public Health* 107: 1653–59.

Tamayo-Sarver, J. H., Hinze, S. W., Cydulka, R. K., Baker, D. W. 2003. Racial and ethnic disparities in emergency department analgesic prescription. *American Journal of Public Health* 93: 2067–73.

Taylor, K. 2015. At a success academy charter school, singling out pupils who have "Got to Go." *New York Times,* October 29.

Taylor, A. L., Gostin, L. O., Pagonis, K. A. 2008. Ensuring effective pain treatment: A national and global perspective. *JAMA* 299: 89–91.

Taylor, A. L., Ziesche, S., Yancy, C., et al. 2004. Combination of isosorbide dinitrate and hydralazine in blacks with heart failure. *New England Journal of Medicine* 351: 2049–57.

Thakrar, A. P., Forrest, A. D., Maltenfort, M. G., Forrest, C. B. 2018. Child mortality in the US and 19 OECD comparator nations: A 50-year time-trend analysis. *Health Affairs* 37(1): 140–49.

Thomson, G. E. 1997. Discrimination in health care. *Annals of Internal Medicine* 126: 910–12.

Thurston, R. C., Matthews, K. A. 2009. Racial and socioeconomic disparities in arterial stiffness and intima media thickness among adolescents. *Social Science and Medicine* 68: 807–13.

Tishkoff, S. A., Kidd, K. K. 2004. Implications of biogeography of human populations for "race" and medicine. *Nature Genetics* 36 (Suppl. 11): S21–26.

Todd, K. H., Deaton, C., D'Adamo, A. P., Goe, L. 2000. Ethnicity and analgesic practice. *Annals of Emergency Medicine* 35: 11–16.

Todd, K. H., Samaroo, N., Hoffman, J. R. 1993. Ethnicity as a risk factor for inadequate emergency department analgesia. *JAMA* 269: 1537–39.

Torres, J. M., Lawlor, J., Colvin, J., et al. 2017. ICD social codes: An underutilized resource for tracking social needs. *Medical Care* 55(9): 810–16.

Tucker, C. M., Herman, K. C., Pedersen, T. R., Higley, B., Montrichard, M., Ivery, P. 2003. Cultural sensitivity in physician-patient relationships: Perspectives of an ethnically diverse sample of low-income primary care patients. *Medical Care* 41: 859–70.

Twaddle, A. C. 1979. The concept of health status. In Jaco, E. G., ed., *Patients, Physicians, and Illness*, 145–61. New York: Free Press.

United Nations. 1948. Universal Declaration of Human Rights. Available at www.un.org /Overview/rights.html.

United Network for Organ Sharing. 2018. Who We Are. Described at https://unos.org/about/, accessed August 20, 2018.

University of Wisconsin School of Medicine and Public Health. 2018. Available at https:// www.neighborhoodatlas.medicine.wisc.edu/, accessed July 24, 2018.

US Agency for Healthcare Research and Quality. 2018. 2016 National Healthcare Quality and Disparities Report, Executive Summary. Content last reviewed June 2018. Available at https://www.ahrq.gov/research/findings/nhqrdr/nhqdr16/summary.html#Key, accessed August 22, 2018.

US Agency for Healthcare Research and Quality. Medical Expenditure Panel Survey. Described at https://meps.ahrq.gov/mepsweb/about_meps/survey_back.jsp, accessed July 9, 2018.

US Burden of Disease Collaborators. 2018. The state of US health, 1990–2016—Burden of diseases, injuries, and risk factors Among US states. *JAMA* 319(14): 1444–72.

US Census Bureau. 2013. Income, Poverty, and Health Insurance Coverage in the United States: 2012. Available at http://www.census.gov/prod/2013pubs/p60-245.pdf, accessed September 19, 2013.

US Census Bureau. 2015. Income and Poverty in the United States. Available at https://www .census.gov/library/publications/2016/demo/p60-256.html.

US Census Bureau. 2017. Data for Median Family Income. Available at https://www.census .gov/, accessed October 22, 2018.

US Census Bureau. 2017. Race & Ethnicity. Available at https://www.census.gov/mso/www /training/pdf/race-ethnicity-onepager.pdf, accessed July 30, 2018.

US Census Bureau. 2018. Current Population Survey. Available at https://www.census.gov /programs-surveys/cps.html, accessed September 25, 2018.

US Census Bureau. 2018. Educational Attainment in the United States: 2017. Available at https:// www.census.gov/topics/education/educational-attainment.html, accessed July 30, 2018.

US Census Bureau. 2018. Health Insurance Coverage in the United States: 2017. Available at https://www.census.gov/library/publications/2018/demo/p60-264.html, accessed October 22, 2018.

US Census Bureau. 2018. Income and Poverty in the United States: 2017. Available at https://www.census.gov/library/publications/2018/demo/p60-263.html, accessed October 22, 2018.

US Census Bureau. 2018. Population Quick Facts. Available at https://www.census.gov /quickfacts/fact/table/US/RHI225217, accessed October 22, 2018.

US Census Bureau. 2018. Questions Planned for the 2020 Census and American Community Survey. Available at https://www2.census.gov/library/publications/decennial/2020 /operations/planned-questions-2020-acs.pdf, accessed July 30, 2018.

US Centers for Medicare and Medicaid Services. Data on National Health Care Expenditures. Available at www.cms.hhs.gov/NationalHealthExpendData.

US Centers for Medicare and Medicaid Services. 2017. Accountable Health Communities Model. Described at https://innovation.cms.gov/initiatives/ahcm/, accessed September 3, 2018.

US Centers for Medicare and Medicaid Services. 2018. The Accountable Health Communities Health-Related Social Needs Screening Tool. Described at https://innovation.cms.gov/Files/worksheets/ahcm-screeningtool.pdf, accessed September 3, 2018.

US Congress, House of Representatives, Committee on Government Reform, Minority Staff Special Investigations Division. 2004. A Case Study in Politics and Science: Changes to the National Healthcare Disparities Report. Available at www.house.gov/reform/min/politicsandscience/pdfs/pdf_politics_and_science_disparities_rep.pdf#search=%22Changes%20to%20the%20National%20Healthcare%20Disparities%20Report%22.

US Congressional Budget Office. 2008. Growing Disparities in Life Expectancy. April 17, 2008. Available at http://cbo.gov/publication/41681, accessed June 26, 2013.

US Department of Health and Human Services. 1999. Mental health: A Report of the Surgeon General. Available at http://www.surgeongeneral.gov/library/.

US Department of Health and Human Services. 2001. Mental Health: Culture, Race, and Ethnicity—A Supplement to Mental Health: A Report of the Surgeon General. Available at http://www.surgeongeneral.gov/library/.

US Department of Health and Human Services. 2011. HHS Action Plan to Reduce Racial and Ethnic Disparities: A Nation Free of Disparities in Health and Health Care. Available at http://minorityhealth.hhs.gov/npa/files/Plans/HHS/HHS_Plan_complete.pdf.

US Department of Health and Human Services. 2011. Implementation Guidance on Data Collection Standards for Race, Ethnicity, Sex, Primary Language, and Disability Status. Available at https://aspe.hhs.gov/basic-report/hhs-implementation-guidance-data-collection-standards-race-ethnicity-sex-primary-language-and-disability-status, accessed September 27, 2018.

US Department of Health and Human Services. 2018. What is the U.S. Opioid Epidemic? Available at https://www.hhs.gov/opioids/about-the-epidemic/index.html, accessed July 3, 2018.

US Department of Health and Human Services, Agency for Healthcare Research and Quality. National Healthcare Disparities Report, 2003. Available at www.qualitytools.ahrq.gov/disparitiesreport/2003/download/download_report.aspx.

US Department of Health and Human Services, Agency for Healthcare Research and Quality. National Healthcare Disparities Report, 2005. Available at www.ahrq.gov/qual/nhdr05/nhdr05.htm.

US Department of Health and Human Services, Centers for Disease Control and Prevention. 2006. Mortality associated with Hurricane Katrina—Florida and Alabama, August–October 2005. *Morbidity and Mortality Weekly Report* 55(09): 239–42.

US Department of Health and Human Services, Centers for Disease Control and Prevention. 2006. Public health response to Hurricanes Katrina and Rita, Louisiana, 2005. *Morbidity and Mortality Weekly Report* 55: 29–55, 35–38.

US Department of Health and Human Services, Centers for Disease Control and Prevention. 2011. Children's Food Environment State Indicator Report. Available at http://www.cdc.gov/obesity/downloads/ChildrensFoodEnvironment.pdf.

US Department of Health and Human Services, Centers for Disease Control and Prevention. 2011. Life Expectancy at Age 25. Available at http://www.cdc.gov/nchs/hus/contents2001.htm#fig32.

US Department of Health and Human Services, Centers for Disease Control and Prevention. 2013. About BMI for Children and Teens. Available at http://www.cdc.gov/healthyweight/assessing/bmi/childrens_bmi/about_childrens_bmi.html.

US Department of Health and Human Services, Centers for Disease Control and Prevention. 2013. Deaths associated with Hurricane Sandy—October–November 2012. *Morbidity and Mortality Weekly Report* 62(20): 393–97.

US Department of Health and Human Services, Centers for Disease Control and Prevention. 2013. Developmental Milestones. Available at http://www.cdc.gov/ncbddd/actearly/milestones/index.html.

US Department of Health and Human Services, Centers for Disease Control and Prevention. 2015. Asthma. Adult Asthma Data. Available at https://www.cdc.gov/asthma/most_recent_data_states.htm, accessed August 24, 2018.

US Department of Health and Human Services, Centers for Disease Control and Prevention. 2017. Chronic Kidney Disease Surveillance System—United States. Available at http://www.cdc.gov/ckd, accessed August 22, 2018.

US Department of Health and Human Services, Centers for Disease Control and Prevention. 2017. Life Expectancy at Birth. Available at https://www.cdc.gov/nchs/hus/index/htm.

US Department of Health and Human Services, Centers for Disease Control and Prevention. 2017. National Diabetes Statistics Report, 2017. Available at https://www.cdc.gov/diabetes/pdfs/data/statistics/national-diabetes-statistics-report.pdf, accessed September 26, 2018.

US Department of Health and Human Services, Centers for Disease Control and Prevention. 2018. Adult Obesity Prevalence Maps. Available at https://www.cdc.gov/obesity/data/prevalence-maps.html, accessed October 22, 2018.

US Department of Health and Human Services, Centers for Disease Control and Prevention. 2018. Age-Adjusted Percentage, Adults with Diabetes—Total, 2015, by State. Available at https://gis.cdc.gov/grasp/diabetes/DiabetesAtlas.html, accessed October 22, 2018.

US Department of Health and Human Services, Centers for Disease Control and Prevention. 2018. Breast Cancer Deaths: Age-Adjusted Death Rate—Female Breast, per 100,000 Persons in 2015. Available at https://gis.cdc.gov/Cancer/USCS/DataViz.html, accessed October 22, 2018.

US Department of Health and Human Services, Centers for Disease Control and Prevention. 2018. Data Trends & Maps—Hypertension. Available at https://www.cdc.gov/dhdsp/maps/dtm/index.html, accessed October 22, 2018.

US Department of Health and Human Services, Centers for Disease Control and Prevention. 2018. Definitions. Available at https://www.cdc.gov/nchhstp/socialdeterminants/definitions.html, accessed October 17, 2018.

US Department of Health and Human Services, Centers for Disease Control and Prevention. 2018. Diagnosed Diabetes. Available at https://gis.cdc.gov/grasp/diabetes/DiabetesAtlas.html, accessed August 22, 2018.

US Department of Health and Human Services, Centers for Disease Control and Prevention. 2018. Division for Heart Disease and Stroke Prevention: Data Trends & Maps—Hypertension. Available at https://www.cdc.gov/dhdsp/maps/dtm/index.html, accessed September 17, 2018.

US Department of Health and Human Services, Centers for Disease Control and Prevention. 2018. Health, United States, 2017. Available at https://www.cdc.gov/nchs/data/hus/hus17.pdf, accessed August 10, 2018.

US Department of Health and Human Services, Centers for Disease Control and Prevention. 2018. Healthy People 2020. Described at https://www.cdc.gov/dhdsp/hp2020.htm, accessed August 22, 2018.

US Department of Health and Human Services, Centers for Disease Control and Prevention. 2018. Infant Mortality Rates, by State: United States, 2016. Available at https://www.cdc.gov/nchs/pressroom/sosmap/infant_mortality_rates/infant_mortality.htm, accessed October 22, 2018.

US Department of Health and Human Services, Centers for Disease Control and Prevention. 2018. Interactive Atlas of Heart Disease and Stroke. Available at https://nccd.cdc.gov/DHDSPAtlas/Reports.aspx, accessed October 22, 2018.

US Department of Health and Human Services, Centers for Disease Control and Prevention. 2018. Rate of New Cancers in the United States. Available at https://gis.cdc.gov/Cancer/USCS/DataViz.html, accessed August 21, 2018.

US Department of Health and Human Services, Centers for Disease Control and Prevention. 2018. Most Recent Asthma Data. Available at https://www.cdc.gov/asthma/most_recent_data.htm, accessed August 15, 2018.

US Department of Health and Human Services, Centers for Disease Control and Prevention. 2018. Most Recent Asthma State or Territory Data. Available at https://www.cdc.gov/asthma/most_recent_data_states.htm, accessed October 22, 2018.

US Department of Health and Human Services, Centers for Disease Control and Prevention. 2018. United States Cancer Statistics: Data Visualizations. Available at https://gis.cdc.gov/Cancer/USCS/DataViz.html, accessed August 21, 2018.

US Department of Health and Human Services, Centers for Disease Control and Prevention. 2018. Vital Statistics Rapid Release—Provisional Drug Overdose Death Counts. Available at https://www.cdc.gov/nchs/nvss/vsrr/drug-overdose-data.htm, accessed August 22, 2018.

US Department of Health and Human Services, National Institutes of Health. 2013 BMI Calculator. Available at http://www.nhlbi.nih.gov/guidelines/obesity/BMI/bmicalc.htm.

US Department of Health and Human Services, Office of Civil Rights. 2006. Racial and Ethnic Health Disparities PowerPoint Presentation. Available at www.hhs.gov/ocr/healthdisparities.html.

US Department of Health and Human Services, Office of Civil Rights. 2013. Discrimination on the Basis of Race, Color, or National Origin. Available at http://www.hhs.gov/ocr/civilrights/understanding/race/index.html.

US Department of Health and Human Services, Office of Civil Rights. 2018. Discrimination on the Basis of Race, Color, or National Origin. Available at https://www.hhs.gov/civil-rights/for-individuals/race/index.html, accessed September 27, 2018.

US Department of Labor. Employment Statistics. Available at www.bls.gov.

US National Center for Health Statistics. 2013. Deaths in the United States, 2011. NCHS Data Brief Number 115. Available at http://www.cdc.gov/nchs/data/databriefs/db115.htm#are, accessed May 9, 2013.

US National Center for Health Statistics. 2015. United States Cancer Statistics. Available at https://gis.cdc.gov/Cancer/USCS/DataViz.html, accessed August 27, 2018.

US National Center for Health Statistics. 2017. Health, United States, 2017. Table 5—Low Birthweight Live Births, by Detailed Race and Hispanic Origin. Available at https://www.cdc.gov/nchs/hus/contents2017.htm#Table_005, accessed August 27, 2018.

US National Center for Health Statistics. 2018. Current Cigarette Smoking Among Adults in the United States. Available at https://www.cdc.gov/tobacco/data_statistics/fact_sheets/adult_data/cig_smoking/index.htm, accessed September 25, 2018.

US National Center for Health Statistics. 2018. Deaths: Final Data for 2016. *National Vital Statistics Report* 67(5), July 26, 2018.

US National Center for Health Statistics. 2018. Health United States 2017. Available at https://www.cdc.gov/nchs/hus/index.htm, accessed October 2, 2018.

US National Center for Health Statistics. 2018. Infant Mortality Dashboard. Available at https://www.cdc.gov/nchs/nvss/vsrr/infant-mortality-dashboard.htm, accessed August 9, 2018.

US National Center for Health Statistics. 2018. *National Vital Statistics Report* 67(5), July 26, 2018.

US National Center for Health Statistics. 2018. User Guide to the 2016 Period Linked Birth / Infant Death Public Use File. Available at ftp://ftp.cdc.gov/pub/Health_Statistics/NCHS/Dataset_Documentation/DVS/periodlinked/LinkPE16Guide.pdf, accessed September 24, 2018.

US National Center for Health Statistics. Statistics on Individual Health Topics. Available at www.cdc.gov/nchs/fastats/Default.htm.

US Preventive Services Task Force. 2016. Breast Cancer: Screening. Available at https://www.uspreventiveservicestaskforce.org/Page/Document/UpdateSummaryFinal/breast-cancer-screening1, accessed August 27, 2018.

US Renal Data System. 2017. 2017 Annual Data Report, Chapter 6. Available at https://www.usrds.org/2017/view/v2_06.aspx, accessed August 20, 2018.

US Supreme Court. 1974. *Washington v. Davis,* 426 U.S. 229. Described at https://supreme.justia.com/cases/federal/us/426/229/, accessed January 23, 2019.

US Supreme Court. 1978. *Regents of Univ. of California v. Bakke,* 438 U.S. 265. Described at https://supreme.justia.com/cases/federal/us/438/265/, accessed January 23, 2019.

US Supreme Court. 2003. *Grutter v. Bollinger,* 539 U.S. 306. Described at https://supreme.justia.com/cases/federal/us/539/306/, accessed January 23, 2019.

Vaccarino, V., Rathore, S. S., Wenger, N. K., et al. 2005. Sex and racial differences in the management of acute myocardial infarction, 1994 through 2002. *New England Journal of Medicine* 353: 671–82.

Valtorta, N. K., Kanaan, M., Gilbody, S., et al. 2016. Loneliness and social isolation as risk factors for coronary heart disease and stroke: systematic review and meta-analysis of longitudinal observational studies. *Heart* 102: 1009–16.

van Ryn, M., Burgess, D., Malat, J., Griffin, J. 2006. Physicians' perceptions of patients' social and behavioral characteristics and race disparities in treatment recommendations for men with coronary artery disease. *American Journal of Public Health* 96: 351–57.

van Ryn, M., Burke, J. 2000. The effect of patient race and socio-economic status on physicians' perceptions of patients. *Social Science and Medicine* 50: 813–28.

van Ryn, M., Saha, S. 2011. Exploring unconscious bias in disparities research and medical education. *JAMA* 306: 995–96.

Vega, W. A., Sribney, W. M. 2017. Growing economic inequality sustains health disparities. *American Journal of Public Health* 107(10): 1606–7.

Velasquez-Manoff, M. 2017. What doctors should ignore. *New York Times,* December 8, 2017.

Verhaeghe, P. P., Tampubolon, G. 2012. Individual social capital, neighbourhood deprivation, and self-rated health in England. *Social Science and Medicine* 75: 349–57.

Victor, R. G., Lynch, K., Li, N., et al. 2018. A cluster-randomized trial of blood-pressure reduction in black barbershops. *New England Journal of Medicine* 378(14): 1291–1301.

Voelker, R. 2018. A day in the life: Facing the opioid epidemic in Huntington, West Virginia. *JAMA* 319(14): 1423–24.

Voigt, R., Camp, N. P., Prabhakaran, V., et al. 2017. Language from police body camera footage shows racial disparities in officer respect. *Proceedings of the National Academy of Sciences of the United States of America* 114(25): 6521–26.

Wakeman, S. E., Barnett, M. L. 2018. Primary care and the opioid-overdose crisis—Buprenorphine myths and realities. *New England Journal of Medicine* 379(1): 1–4.

Ware, J. E., Sherbourne, C. D. 1992. The MOS 36-item short-form health survey (SF-36). *Medical Care* 30: 473–83.

Warfield, S., Pollini, R., Stokes, C.M., Bossarte, R. 2019. Opioid-related outcomes in West Virginia, 2008–2016. *American Journal of Public Health* 109(2): 303–5.

Wennberg, J. E. 1993. Future directions for small area variations. *Medical Care* 31: YS75–80.

Wennberg, J. E., Barnes, B. A., Zubkoff, M. 1982. Professional uncertainty and the problem of supplier-induced demand. *Social Science and Medicine* 16: 811–24.

West, P., Sweeting, H., Young, R., Kelly, S. 2010. The relative importance of family socio-economic status and school-based peer hierarchies for morning cortisol in youth: An exploratory study. *Social Science and Medicine* 70: 1246–53.

Whitman, S., Orsi, J., Hurlbert, M. 2012. The racial disparity in breast cancer mortality in the 25 largest cities in the United States. *Cancer Epidemiology* 36: e147–e151.

Wilensky, G. 2016. Addressing social issues affecting health to improve US health outcomes. *JAMA* 315(15): 1552–53.

Wilkinson, R. G. 1999. Health, hierarchy, and social anxiety. *Annals of the New York Academy of Sciences* 896: 48–63.

Williams, D. R. 2017. Why Discrimination Is a Health Issue. Robert Wood Johnson Foundation Culture of Health Blog, Oct 24, 2017. Available at https://www.rwjf.org/en/blog/2017/10/discrimination-is-a-health-issue.html, accessed August 9, 2018.

Williams, D. R. 2012. Miles to go before we sleep: Racial inequities in health. *Journal of Health and Social Behavior* 53: 279–95.

Williams, D. R., Mohammed, S. A., Leavell, J., Collins, C. 2010. Race, socioeconomic status, and health: Complexities, ongoing challenges, and research opportunities. *Annals of The New York Academy of Sciences* 1186: 69–101.

Williams, D. R., Sternthal, M., Wright, R. J. 2009. Social determinants: Taking the social context of asthma seriously. *Pediatrics* 123 (Suppl. 3): S174–S184.

Wilson, I., Cleary, P. 1995. Linking clinical variables with health-related quality of life. *JAMA* 273: 59–65.

Wise, P. 2009. Confronting social disparities in child health: A critical appraisal of life-course science and research. *Pediatrics* 124 (Suppl. 3): S203–S211.

Witzburg, R. A., Sondheimer, H. M. 2013. Holistic review—Shaping the medical profession one applicant at a time. *New England Journal of Medicine* 368: 1565–67.

Wolinsky, F. D. 1988. *The Sociology of Health: Principles, Practitioners, and Issues.* Belmont, CA: Wadsworth Publishing.

Wong, M. S., Grande, D. T., Mitra, N., et al. 2017. Racial differences in geographic access to medical care as measured by patient report and geographic information systems. *Medical Care* 55(9): 817–22.

Wong, M. D., Shapiro, M. F., Boscardin, W. J., and Ettner, S. L. 2002. Contribution of major diseases to disparities in mortality. *New England Journal of Medicine* 347(20): 1585–92.

Wood, A. J. 2001. Racial differences in the response to drugs: Pointers to genetic differences. *New England Journal of Medicine* 344: 1393–96.

World Bank. Global Burden of Disease and Risk Factors. 2006. Available at https://openknowledge.worldbank.org/, accessed October 22, 2018.

World Bank. Open Data. Available at https://data.worldbank.org/, accessed October 22, 2018.

World Bank. World Development Indicators 2017. Available at http://wdi.worldbank.org/tables, accessed October 22, 2018.

World Health Organization. 2018. Social Determinants of Health. Available at https://www.who.int/social_determinants/sdh_definition/en/, accessed October 17, 2018.

World Health Organization. 2018. World Health Statistics 2018. Available at http://www.who.int/gho/publications/world_health_statistics/2018/en/, accessed October 22, 2018.

World Health Organization. 2018. Levels & Trends in Child Mortality. Available at http://www.childmortality.org, accessed October 22, 2018.

World Health Organization. 2018. WHO Methods and Data Sources for Global Burden of Disease Estimates 2000–2016. Available at https://www.who.int/healthinfo/global_burden_disease/GlobalDALY_method_2000_2016.pdf?ua=1, accessed January 18, 2019.

World Health Organization. Definition of Health. Available at www.who.int/about/definition/en/.

Yan, L. L., Liu, K., Daviglus, M. L., et al. 2006. Education, 15-year risk factor progression, and coronary artery calcium in young adulthood and early middle age: The Coronary Artery Risk Development in Young Adults study. *JAMA* 295: 1793–1800.

Yancy, C. W., Fowler, M. B., Colucci, W. S., et al. 2001. Race and the response to adrenergic blockade with Carvedilol in patients with chronic heart failure. *New England Journal of Medicine* 344: 1358–65.

Yang, T. C., Matthews, S. A., Hillemeier, M. M. 2011. Effect of health care system distrust on breast and cervical cancer screening in Philadelphia, Pennsylvania. *American Journal of Public Health* 101: 1297–1305.

Ylitalo, K. R., Lee, H., Mehta, N. K. 2013. Health care provider recommendation, human papillomavirus vaccination, and race/ethnicity in the US National Immunization Survey. *American Journal of Public Health* 103: 164–69.

Young, C. J., Gaston, R. S. 2000. Renal transplantation in black Americans. *New England Journal of Medicine* 343: 545–52.

Yudkin, J. S., Kumari, M., Humphries, S. E., Mohamed-Ali, V. 2000. Inflammation, obesity, stress and coronary heart disease: Is interleukin-6 the link? *Atherosclerosis* 148(2): 209–14.

Zhou, C., Yu, N. N., Losby, J. L. 2018. The association between local economic conditions and opioid prescriptions among disabled Medicare beneficiaries. *Medical Care* 56(1): 62–68.

Zimbardo, P. G., Boyd, J. N. 1999. Putting time in perspective: A valid, reliable individual-differences metric. *Journal of Personality and Social Psychology* 77: 1271–88.

Zuvekas, S. H., Taliaferro, G. S. 2003. Pathways to access: Health insurance, the health care delivery system, and racial/ethnic disparities, 1996–1999. *Health Affairs* 22(2): 139–53.